PRAISE FOR SAGE-F
NATURA.

MW00850231

"...providing access to this information makes a deeper statement about our right to bodily autonomy...understanding how pregnancy and abortion work helps make women full participants in our reproductive health, not passive recipients of aid...
I'm glad Sage-femme! is furthering this discussion."

—Feministe

"Want reproductive freedom? Buy this amazing book; tell your friends about it; and read it carefully together. Do self-examination together; get to know how your cervices look through your menstrual cycles. Keep this book and your speculum in a safe place. Of course, you continue to fight for our rights, including legal abortion or better yet, the repeal of abortion laws. But, come what may, you know that if you ever face an unwanted pregnancy, whatever the political climate, you have the tools you need.
That, my sister, is reproductive freedom."

—Carol Downer

NATURAL LIBERTY
REDISCOVERING SELF-INDUCED
ABORTION METHODS

◊

SAGE-FEMME!
LAS VEGAS, NEVADA

09-2

Copyright © 2008 by Sage-femme Collective.

Published by
Sage-femme!
848 N. Rainbow Blvd. #2599
Las Vegas, NV 89107
www.sagefemmetoday.com

ISBN 978–0–9645920–0–1 (pbk.)
First Revised Edition.

Cover illustration copyright © Sage-femme Collective.
Cover - 'Papaya Fibonacci Spiral.'
Leonardo of Pisa, known as Fibonacci, in his *Liber Abaci* AD 1202, conceptualized the population potential of a pair of rabbits into a visual mathematical representation and created the golden spiral. Colors were selected from a ripe papaya.

iv

Acknowledgements

Many have contributed to the creation of this work.
We wish to acknowledge and express our gratitude to
the many anonymous individuals who helped to
make *Natural Liberty* a reality.

Table of Contents

vii

Introduction

Corinna is lying near death,
She sought to rid the contents of her womb,
        risked her life, and never said a word.
I should feel anger, but I fear so for her,
        conceived within, and by me.
        Life is unsure, but this I know.
Goddess Isis, of Paraetonium, of
        joyous windswept fields of Canopus,
        of Memphis, and regal palms of Pharos,
        and delta Nile whose waters spread
        to the sea through seven sacred mouths,
I pray by your rattles:
        by the sacred image of Anubis,
        may your husband, Osiris, always love your rites.
        May the snake glide unhurried in your sacred temple,
        and the horned Apis honor your procession.
May your gaze be drawn this way,
        to bestow kindness on her,
        and save two by saving one.
        The life you grant to her returns to me my heart.
She always wore the laurel crown and is worthy of your blessing.
        attending all your special days.
Goddess Ilithyia, comforter of laboring women,
        easing the burden when contractions quake and strain,
        please look fondly on her, and hear my prayers.
I, myself, in robes of white, shall burn incense at your altar,
        and at your feet lay gifts, inscribed:
        Ovid, offers these in gratitude for saving Corinna.
And last, my love, may I be bold amidst my fear?
        Corinna, if you live,
        never again such danger, my dear!

                                        -Ovid (43 BC - 17AD)

1

From the beginning of recorded time, women and men have searched for safe effective abortion methods. It took civilization thousands of years to develop the professional clinical abortion services contemporary women utilize. People rarely pause to recall and appreciate these facts when discussing the issues surrounding abortion. During *thousands* of years of terrible agony and gross errors,[1] millions of women were marred permanently and millions more died from trying to end unwanted pregnancies. Even today the estimated number of women who die each year from unsafe abortion ranges from 70,000 to 200,000.[2] In addition, millions of women per year are believed to suffer temporary or permanent disability from unsafe abortion.[3] The modern world has the capacity to provide safe abortion services for our beloved daughters, girlfriends, mothers, sisters, and wives. Women and men should be rejoicing in the marvels of modern science and praising the wonderful modern world where, if desired, pregnancy termination can be nearly 100% safe for all women. Instead, the rights of women are held hostage, as politicians and sectarian zealots debate when abortion should be allowed, if at all.

For thousands of years, nearly every culture recognized abortion as a natural body function and necessity. According to Chinese folklore, 5000 years ago Emperor Shennong, who wrote the earliest Chinese pharmacopoeia and is believed to have been the father of Chinese medicine and acupuncture, recommended the use of mercury, a toxic metal, to induce abortion.[4] In China, between 500 and 515 BC, the number of abortions induced among the royal concubines is documented.[5] The Egyptians documented the use of agents to terminate pregnancy thousands of years ago. The first written

2

documentation of an abortion technique is in the Egyptian Ebers Papyrus, dated to 1550 BC.[6] The Greeks and Romans further documented what abortifacients were deemed effective and which abortifacients were considered too dangerous. Aristotle recommended induced abortion to maintain the population at optimal size.[7]

Hippocrates forbade the use of abortive suppositories, which he deemed too dangerous to the woman; however, he recommended oral abortifacients as well as physical exertion which he believed caused abortion. Soranus, another Greek physician, in his written work, *Gynecology*, recommended a detailed abortifacient regime for the care and health of the woman. It included abortifacient herbs, baths, exercise, fasting, and bloodletting while discouraging the use of sharp instruments which could perforate the uterus. Soranus qualified Hippocrates' categorical disapproval of pessaries and suppositories to cause abortion, warning that, "one should choose those which are not too pungent, that may not cause too great a sympathetic reaction and heat."[8]

The medical knowledge documented in the writings of ancient physicians indicates that the health of the woman was the primary focus of physicians. The woman's need for abortive services was recognized, and the responsibility of the physician to secure the health of the woman during abortion was emphasized. The valuing of the woman's life and health above that of the unborn was constant throughout history. This vital priority remained until the 1600's, when Roman Catholic thought hardened against induced abortion and equated the life of the mother as equal in importance to that of the unborn.

Today, 42,000,000 abortions take place around the world every year. Research indicates that the incidence of abortions is not reduced by restrictive laws. In fact, the opposite is true. According to a study by the Guttmacher Institute and the World Health Organization, abortion rates are highest in countries with the most restrictive abortion laws. The only factor that reduces the abortion rate is increased education combined with unlimited access to family planning services of contraception and abortion.[9]

Benefits of Abortion

All of society benefits when a woman's natural liberty to abort as she deems necessary is recognized and supported. Positive effects of ensuring women's natural liberty to safe and effective abortion services include: increased health of women, fewer unwanted children, reduced population, reduced crime rate, and increased economic prosperity.

Restricting access to safe abortion forces women to seek other options that may be more dangerous. Laws and restrictions on abortion affect the health of women and the rate of maternal mortality. In areas where abortion is restricted, maternal mortality increases.[10] A 1992 study at the Smt Sucheta Kriplani Hospital in Delhi, India found that 20% of maternal deaths were caused by illegally induced abortion.[11] A Bangladesh study correlated an annual 9% reduction in maternal mortality after 1990 as safer abortion methods became available.[12] A U.S. study in North Carolina of maternal mortality rates in the five years before and after Roe v. Wade, showed a 46% decline in maternal mortality in the five years after the

U.S. Supreme Court's landmark decision to legalize abortion.[13] In areas where abortion is unrestricted, abortion related consequences are also reduced. For example, after Roe vs. Wade in 1973, all abortion-related complications dropped significantly.[14] Conversely, in Chile, where abortion is illegal, up to one-quarter of all obstetrical admissions to the hospital are related to illegally induced abortions.[15] Also, areas which experienced restrictive laws against abortion have shown a higher incidence of kidney failure in women, often related to substances taken to attempt to induce abortion.[16]

Not only do many women suffer (and die) when access to abortion is restricted, unwanted children that are born suffer as well. What happens to a child that is not wanted? Sometimes, the child is put up for adoption, or if kept, the child may or may not receive the nurturing and support needed from the parent. Studies have shown that when women are denied an abortion, they have a greater chance of resenting the child, and often do not provide the care and nurturing the child needs.[17] Orphanages, also, are often unable to provide the direct contact and nurturing children need.[18] It has been estimated that 132,000,000 children are orphaned or awaiting adoption worldwide.[19]

Side effects of lack of contact and nurturing are profound and may affect several generations. In a study of rats, researchers found that if a baby rat received too little care and nurturing from the mother, when that young rat matured, it was unable to produce normal levels of the hormone oxytocin. Oxytocin is a hormone that prompts the mother to nurture and care for her young. Conversely when baby rats received adequate nurturing and caretaking, they produced average oxytocin levels that caused them to display natural maternal behaviors as adults. Likewise, studies on mice have shown that mice which receive above average maternal nurturing (measured by the number of licks they receive from their mother) later produce above average amounts of oxytocin, and were able to nurture their own offspring. However, when baby mice receive less than average maternal nurturing, they are unable to produce average amounts of oxytocin as adults, and are unable to nurture their own offspring with the normal amount of licks. Mice that lack the oxytocin gene are unable to remember other mice in social interactions.[20] Studies of non-human primates show that babies of mothers who push them away or abuse them often become depressed and have been found to have a lack of oxytocin receptors, a condition which continues into adulthood. They often grow up to treat their offspring in the same manner.[21]

Oxytocin has a profound role in the functioning of all mammals.[22] Oxytocin bonds people together on a deep level. Oxytocin is the hormone released with breastfeeding, which encourages a deep bond between the mother and her baby. In adults, oxytocin is released during cuddling and after sexual orgasm. Studies have shown that oxytocin is responsible for a feeling of trust and reciprocation in human social relationships.[23] Children who grew up in orphanages have been found to have lower levels of oxytocin, and their levels of oxytocin did not rise when the children were placed in family groups.[24] Studies suggest that some human adults who are unable to trust and cooperate in a normal way have dysfunctional oxytocin receptors and thus are unable to produce normal amounts of oxytocin hormone.[25]

Lack of access to abortion services affects mother, child, and society. The human population is increasing at rates that were unprecedented before the 20th century. The current rate of human population growth cannot continue without negative consequences to all beings inhabiting the earth. The world's population is expected by some to reach nine billion by 2050. The earth's ability to feed the growing population has decreased since 1994.[26] The United Nations Population Fund estimates that one quarter to one third of the 200 million pregnancies per year are unintended or ill-timed.[27] There is much political and religious argument as to whether there is a human population growth problem. Under ideal conditions perhaps food would be available for all people on earth, yet the reality of budget deficits and grain shortages has caused the United Nations World Food Program to state in 2008 that it would not have enough money to stem a coming tide of global malnutrition.[28] Child poverty has been linked to women and families having children before they have the financial means to care for them.[29] The point will be reached someday where for every baby born, a child somewhere will starve. Starvation has wide-ranging consequences, as studies link starvation to psychosis and genetic mutation, which research suggests affects survivors for multiple generations.[30]

The detriment that the State would impose upon the pregnant woman by denying this choice altogether is apparent...Maternity, or additional offspring, may force upon the woman a distressful life and future. Psychological harm may be imminent. Mental and physical health may be taxed by child care. There is also the distress, for all concerned, associated with the unwanted child, and there is the problem of bringing a child into a family already unable, psychologically and otherwise, to care for it...

The states are not free, under the guise of protecting maternal health or potential life, to intimidate women into continuing pregnancies.

-Justice Harry A. Blackmun, Roe v. Wade, January 22, 1973

Studies indicate that when laws restrict access to abortion the crime rate increases.[31] Nicholae Ceaușescu, the Communist dictator of Romania, made abortion, contraception, and sexual education illegal in 1966, stating "The fetus is the property of the entire society...Anyone who avoids having children is a deserter who abandons the laws of national continuity." The birth rate went up initially, but after one year it began to go down again, reaching the 1966 level in 1983.[32] An underground abortion network became established, and women took matters into their own hands, but not without consequences. Maternal mortality went up to levels unprecedented in Europe. The rate of acute renal failure increased in women who ingested substances attempting self-induced abortion.[33] Thousands of unwanted children were placed in institutions.

Researchers have found that in the instances where abortion was forbidden or denied to a woman who wanted one, she often resented her baby and failed to provide it a good home. Children coming from homes, where they were unwanted, were at a great risk

8

of turning to criminal behavior, as they were less likely to achieve an education and to have success in the job market.[34] The ban on abortion in Romania lasted until 1989 when Ceauşescu was violently deposed. The day after Ceauşescu was deposed; contraception and abortion were legalized again.

A similar pattern of anti-abortion laws and increased crime rate was discovered in the United States. From the early 1960's to 1989, the violent crime rate in the United States rose 80% reaching a peak. It was expected that violent crime would continue to increase but suddenly and without explanation, violent crime began to fall rapidly, eventually reaching the levels of 40 years prior. Where did the criminals go? That was the question asked by Steven D. Levitt and Stephen J. Dubner in their book, *Freakonomics*. Levitt and Dubner looked at the question from many angles and arrived at a surprising correlation. They linked the drop in crime rate in the United States to the legalization of abortion by Roe v. Wade in 1973.[35]

A greater percentage of the children born following Roe v. Wade were wanted children, born into situations where mothers were ready and willing to care for them. By 1990, the Roe v. Wade generation had grown up, and the population in the United States contained a much reduced number of adults who, without Roe v. Wade, would have been unwanted as children and at a greater risk of leading a life of crime. Levitt and Dubner found that increased and decreased crime rates could be directly correlated to increased or decreased restrictions on abortions. Their results were reproduced in multiple states in the United States. The effects were also similar across countries and even across continents.[36]   Access to abortion today reduces crime tomorrow.

When women have the rights of life, liberty, and the pursuit of happiness, they are unrestricted in their ability to contribute to the economic well being of their families and communities. When women are restricted to the home and raising children, fewer women participate in the society's economy, and there is often rapid population growth. World Bank advisor Thomas Merrick suggests societies that recognize the economic and social status of women and women's rights of reproductive control are better able to take advantage of the economic forces of an increased workforce and thus enjoy a rise in living standards.[37]   Societies, that support women and women's control of fertility, limit population growth and experience economic prosperity. In contrast, rapid population growth often coincides with a decline in the economic and social status of women, fewer women in the work force, and restrictions on fertility regulation services. The combined effect leads to a cumulative downward spiral that good economic policies cannot overcome.

In the United States, there is a push among anti-abortion forces to reverse the federal law of Roe v. Wade. The effect would turn the legislation of abortion over to the states. The 1989 U.S. Supreme Court decision, Webster v. Reproductive Health Services, upheld various provisions of a Missouri law that restricted abortion, including: allowing states to prohibit abortion in publicly funded spaces or by publicly funded employees, and allowed a state to declare, "the life of each human being begins at conception." Webster opened the door to permit greater states' rights to restrict access to abortion

10

services. Conservative Christian organizations have been preparing for the overturn of Roe v. Wade by promoting fetal homicide bills. These new state laws would increase the rights of the unborn in a majority of states if Roe v. Wade is overturned, and the state laws go into effect. From 1995 to 2008, nationwide, state governments enacted 335 anti-choice legislative measures.[38] If the United States Supreme Court rules that abortion law is a state issue, then the availability of abortion will become much more restricted than it is now.

More restricted than it is now? Even *with* Roe v. Wade, abortion is restricted in the United States. Despite the fact that every year approximately one million women in the United States have abortions, 87% of all counties in the United States have no abortion provider, and 97% of rural counties have no provider.[39] The Hyde Amendment of 1976 restricted federal Medicaid funding for abortion, which makes it all the more difficult for low income women to obtain abortion services.

Just as in the days before Roe v. Wade, in the United States in 2008, women who have adequate financial resources are able to obtain a safe abortion. However, young and poor women face many hurdles if in need of abortion services.

Parental consent or notification laws in many states in the United States force young women who want abortions to choose between informing their parents (who may not consent) and traveling to states with no parental notification laws. Pregnant adolescents are often slow to recognize the pregnancy and access a clinical provider, leading to a greater likelihood of complications with increased gestational age of the pregnancy. The United States has the highest

11

rate of teenage pregnancies in the industrial world, approximately 750,000 teenage pregnancies of which 80% are unintended.[40]

Mandatory waiting periods in some states require women to be in person for counseling and then wait 24 hours for services. This can mean increased costs and problems for a woman who must arrange for leave from work, childcare, and perhaps stay overnight in a distant city. The cost of abortion can prohibit some women from seeking an abortion, and health insurance does not cover abortion services in many states, which presents more difficulties for middle to low income American women.

Challenges to women seeking abortion are great, and doctors and nurses are also challenged. Medical professionals in North America who provide abortion services continue to serve women despite the terrorist tactics of anti-abortion extremists. Since 1993, in the United States, three doctors who provided abortions were assassinated. Five others have lived through assassination attempts in the United States and Canada. Terrorism against abortion service providers has included bombing, arson, vandalism, burglary, and harassment. Anti-abortion extremists have also launched frivolous lawsuits in an attempt to prevent providers from offering services.

The number of licensed medical doctors willing to provide abortion services is dwindling. According to a 2003 study by the Alan Guttmacher Institute, in the four year period from 1996 to 2000 the number of abortion providers decreased by 11%. Another study shows a drop of 37% in abortion providers since 1982.[41]

The number of medical schools in the United States who train medical students in abortion is also declining. A 1998 study found

12

that only 26% of OB/GYN residency programs trained all residents in abortion procedures. Most OB/GYN residency programs trained only residents who expressed interest, and 14% of the programs trained no residents at all in abortion techniques and procedures.[42]

An additional way that abortion may become more restricted in the United States is through censorship of information. Censorship of information has an ancient history. The contents of the Great Library of Alexandria, Egypt were burned as fuel for the baths by the Muslim commander in the Conquest of 642. He was told by the caliph, Umar, that "if what is written in them agrees with the Koran, they are not required; if it disagrees they are not desired. Destroy them therefore."[43] Much later, the witch hunts in Europe during the 14th and 15th centuries eliminated conservatively 60,000 people whose knowledge of the natural world was deemed heresy by the Roman Catholic Church.[44] The witch hunts often focused on female midwives and herbal healers who had information on herbal birth control.[45] It is believed by some scholars[46] that religious powers orchestrated the elimination of birth control and abortion information, as they wanted to encourage growth in the population which had been reduced due to the Black Death, estimated to have taken 30-60% of Europe's population in the 14th century.[47]

We do not need to travel far back in time to visit an example of abortion information censorship. Ireland has some of the most restrictive abortion laws in the world, allowing abortion only if the pregnancy is deemed to threaten a woman's life. In 1983, written information advocating abortion was deemed unconstitutional by the Irish Supreme Court. In Ireland between 1983 an 1992, books about

13

abortion were removed from libraries; British telephone books listing the phone numbers of abortion clinics in England were destroyed. Students who opposed the censorship ruling by printing information about abortion in student handbooks were arrested. British abortion clinics reported an increase in gestational age in women who were forced to travel underground to England from Ireland for abortions[48] and also noted women arrived with less knowledge about abortion options and with more anxiety.[49] In May 1992, Democratic politician T.D. Proinsias De Rossa, utilizing diplomatic immunity to avoid lawsuit, read the phone numbers of English abortion clinics into the official record of the Irish Parliament. Then, the Irish Family Planning Association was able to officially establish an association with the British Pregnancy Advisory Service. And in 1993, the Ireland Supreme Court recognized the constitutional right of women to travel to obtain abortions. Information on abortion has become more widely available in Ireland since 1993, however the 1995 Information Act continues to restrict women service organizations from referring women to abortion services. In June 2008, Ireland refused to sign the European Union's Treaty of Lisbon, largely because of fears that signing this constitution would possibly override Irish anti-abortion laws.

The Comstock Laws of 1873 in the United States banned material considered obscene including contraceptives and prohibited distribution of educational information on contraceptives and abortion. The ban on contraceptives was declared unconstitutional in 1936; however the remaining portions of the 1873 Comstock Laws continue to be enforced today to ban material deemed obscene. For example, the Federal Communications Commission (FCC) regulates

14

the content of broadcast media via the original remaining Comstock Laws.

Amendments in 1996 to the Comstock Laws, led by the late United States Senator Hyde of Illinois, threaten to ban online information on abortion. Senator Hyde introduced Communications Indecency Act language (into the Telecommunications Reform Act) which made it illegal to sell or distribute information or materials on abortion through online activities and communications. In 1996, rather than vetoing anti-pornography legislation, President Clinton signed the act into law commenting only that the Department of Justice under his term would not enforce the abortion-related speech prohibitions because they are unconstitutional.

In federally funded programs, the George W. Bush administration has censored information advocating abortion. In April 2008, the administrators of Popline, world's largest scientific database on reproductive health, received a complaint from the Bush administration about two abortion-advocacy articles. Popline is funded by USAID, and under the Mexico City policy enacted by President Reagan, and reenacted by President Bush, USAID denies federal funding to non-governmental organizations that promote or perform abortions. The administrators of Popline, removed the abortion-advocacy articles and began to block searches on the word 'abortion', concealing nearly 25,000 search results. After the story was released by the media, the administrators restored the search term 'abortion' but did not restore access to the abortion advocacy articles.

The Justice Department, during the administration of President George W. Bush, has not pursued wide-scale prosecution

15

under the Communications Indecency Act abortion-related speech prohibitions; however it remains to be seen whether information regarding abortion will be further restricted in the United States, and if and when the Communications Indecency Act may be deemed unconstitutional. If Roe v. Wade is overturned by the Supreme Court, then the administration at that time may be prompted to order the Justice Department to pursue the wide-scale restriction of abortion information.

Abortion is a political issue, but it is also a philosophical and religious issue. Roe v. Wade is not the final word in ruling to protect abortion services in the United States. In fact, Roe v. Wade may have a serious flaw. Missing in Roe v. Wade is the determination of when life begins, a point that the Supreme Court was unable to officially determine, "When those trained in the respective disciplines of medicine, philosophy and theology are unable to arrive at any consensus," Associate Justice Harry A. Blackmun, speaking for the majority, wrote, "the judiciary, at this point in the development of man's knowledge, is not in a position to speculate as to the answer."[50]

The question remains...When does life begin? This question cannot be answered with scientific certainty to this day and may never be definitively answered. So, for the foreseeable future, the question must be placed in the unknown. Many who think they know when life begins believe their answer in faith, which makes their belief about abortion part of their religion.

In the United States, the separation of church and state is guaranteed by the first amendment to the Constitution. The political debate in the United States about abortion may rest with the Supreme

Court recognizing that "When does life begin?" is a religious issue. Various religions have various positions regarding the moment life begins and when abortion is acceptable. When laws have been enacted giving preference to a particular religious faith's belief, the obligation of the Court is to deem those laws unconstitutional, as they infringe on the rights of others to freely practice their religious beliefs.

Most religions have a stated official view on abortion. Religions vary widely regarding when they consider the fetus to have life, when abortion is acceptable, and when it is not. The Pro-life movement in the United States, with few exceptions, is a Christian religious movement.[51] From this viewpoint, the embryo is recognized as a human being from the moment of conception, and any act that destroys a fertilized egg is considered murder. Individuals and organizations in the Christian Pro-life movement have stated a desire to make their interpretation of God's law in the Bible the law of the United States.[52] Republican nominee for the 2008 presidential election John McCain stated that he believed that the Constitution of the United States established the United States as a Christian nation,[53] and that the reversal of Roe v. Wade, which would allow the abortion question to be ruled on by individual states, would restore balance to the Constitution of the United States.[54] As of 2008, nineteen states had enacted fetal homicide laws, often proposed by pro-life organizations, which recognize the Christian view that life begins at conception.[55]

In Catholicism, the current Pope Benedict XVI holds that "abortion is a grave sin against the natural law."[56] Some popes have not held this view. Pope Innocent III and Pope Gregory XIV held that the life of the fetus does not begin until quickening

17

(approximately 5 months after conception); and Pope John XXI, (before he became Pope) wrote a book, *Treasure of the Poor*, which included emmenagogual and contraceptive recipes.[57]   St. Augustine held that only aborting a fully formed fetus was a sin.   During St. Augustine's time, the moment that a fetus became fully formed was debated as somewhere between 40 - 80 days.

According to Islam, the fetus does not have a soul until 120 days after conception.[58]   After this point, abortion would be considered murder; however Islam provides exceptions for rape and for when the woman's life or health is in danger.

In Buddhism, there are many views concerning abortion. In Japan, Buddhist women who have induced abortion or have had a spontaneous miscarriage sometimes participate in special rituals called Mizuko kuyo to appease the aborted fetus.[59] The 8th-10th century poems written by Buddhist monks comment on the problem of unlimited reproduction: "Domni is giving birth to innumerable children like tadpoles, so she is faced with the problem of feeding them."[60] However, today, Buddhism holds that abortion is a negative. The Dalai Lama holds this view, however he believes there should be exceptions that should be considered on a case by case basis.[61]

Hinduism considers the fetus a living, conscious person deserving of protection, however some contemporary Hindu theologians have stated that the fetus develops personhood sometime between the third and fifth month.[62] Old Hindu scriptures allowed abortion until the fifth month, and the ancient Vedic Atharva Veda Samhita, considered by some orthodox Hindus to be one of the most mystical of scriptures, recognized the value of fertility regulating

18

plants: "Thou art listened to, O herb, as the most best of plants; make thou now this man for me impotent..."[63]

Modern denominations of Judaism often have fairly liberal interpretations of traditional Jewish texts related to abortion issues. However, according to orthodox Jewish law, abortion is prohibited 40 days after conception. Before 40 days, however, there is some leniency. If the life of the woman is threatened by the pregnancy, abortion is always allowed to save the woman's life.

In the United States, the practice of religion is guaranteed by the Constitution. A woman's religious beliefs may affect whether or not she wishes to exercise her right to an abortion. Her right to refuse to abort may be considered part of her practice of religious freedom. Her right to choose not to have an abortion should be protected with as much passion as the right for a woman to choose to exercise her right to have an abortion. No woman should be forced to have an abortion, and no woman should be denied the choice to have a safe abortion.

A free people [claim] their rights aived from
the laws of nature, and not as
the gift of their chief magistrate.

-Thomas Jefferson

The right to abort may be variously defined as a religious practice, but for all women the right to an abortion may be considered a natural liberty. A natural liberty is an absolute freedom, limited only by the laws of nature, exercised on one's private property. What private property is more private than a woman's body? What is more

19

natural than a plant that a woman could simply walk up to and consume? All women have the inherent rights to carry out all acts that preserve their lives and the natural liberty to exercise those rights without any restrictions.

Simple physical biology indicates that the choice regarding a pregnancy lies inherently with the woman, as almost all pregnancies in the animal kingdom are carried by females. Inherently in the woman's biology is a mechanism of spontaneous abortion which is not completely understood, however the mechanism appears to trigger an abortion when the woman feels stress and depression. Factors such as depression and stress are often experienced by women faced with an unwanted pregnancy, and in one study, women who experienced stress or depression in pregnancy and showed signs of high cortisol levels were found to be 90% more likely to have a spontaneous miscarriage in the first three weeks of pregnancy.[64]

Just as a woman's stress and depression can lead to a spontaneous abortion, estrogenic substances can also interfere with the ability of the body to continue a pregnancy.[65] Over 300 plants have been found to contain estrogenic substances, and it has been suggested that all plants that grow have estrogenic substances in them, often concentrated in the sprouts and seeds in plants.[66]

Some plants historically used for fertility regulation have significant amounts of estrogen in the mature growth. Plants with estrogenic substances in the mature growth have been suggested to have co-evolved with humans in a synergistic relationship enabling population control and evolution.[67] Given sufficient dosage of any plant part containing estrogenic substances, an abortion is likely to occur, especially in the early stages of pregnancy. Plants that can potentially cause abortion are everywhere. They are the rule not the exception; dosage and timing are the ruling factors.

...Governments are instituted among Men, deriving their just powers from the consent of the governed, —That whenever any Form of Government becomes destructive of these ends, it is the Right of the People to alter or to abolish it, and to institute new Government, laying its foundation on such principles and organizing its powers in such form, as to them shall seem most likely to effect their Safety and Happiness.
-Declaration of Independence, July, 4, 1776

The deepest and most passionate reason we, as Sage-femme Collective, wrote this book is philosophical. We believe that by placing this information back into the hands of women, to whom the knowledge rightfully belongs, women will rediscover that abortion is an inalienable natural liberty that a just government cannot legislate. We believe the inevitable conclusion to this empowering foundational concept is a renewed focus on reproductive rights to ensure that every woman has access to the best possible abortion experience: one which is safe, effective, legal, and available without restriction in a supportive environment.

The historical and scientific documentation of self-induced abortion is important and fascinating. We have exhaustively compiled this material over many years, searching through thousands of references and talking with many herbalists, healers, and women while

21

participating in the self-help movement. This information on self-induced abortion, now recovered, should never be forgotten, but we hope women will demand that they never have to resort to using any of it!

By far, the modern system for delivering an abortion in a medical clinic setting by trained health professionals is safer and more effective than self-induced abortion. There have been few studies on negative side effects of self-induced abortion methods, and most self-induced abortion methods are dubious regarding effectiveness. The support networks that exist in a clinical setting to counsel and medically serve the women who seek services are not usually available for most women who attempt self-induced abortion.

The object of the book is to provide the most accurate and up to date information on self-induced abortion available, not to promote self-induced abortion. In a world that respects and loves women, safe legal clinical services with the support of counselors and trained doctors would be available without difficulty. However, if these services are unavailable to women, it is better for women to have some knowledge of possible alternatives than to act with desperation on rumor without understanding the possible side effects.

We hope the ancient woman, Corinna, at the beginning of this introduction, dearly loved by Ovid two thousand years ago will be remembered. Corinna is every woman and girl we love. Do not forget her. Secure our future by recognizing her natural liberty to regulate her fertility. Help ensure that the safest and best services our modern society can offer are available to her.

-Sage-femme! Collective, 2008

How to Use This Book

A system of icons is included regarding the most common known side effects for each self-induced abortion method. The four star system of 'reputed effectiveness' is based on anecdotal evidence only. Very few self-induced abortion methods have been scientifically studied.

Icon Key:

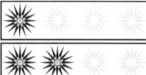 0 – 24% Reputed Effectiveness

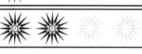 25 – 49% Reputed Effectiveness

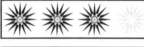 50 – 74% Reputed Effectiveness

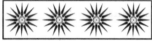 75 – 99% Reputed Effectiveness

 Hormonal Effects

 Liver and/or Kidney Toxic

 Phototoxic

 Contains Thujone

 Deaths Associated

 Heart Effects

 Cathartic Purgative

23

The dating of a pregnancy from the first day of the last menstrual period (LMP) has been used exclusively throughout the book.

The term 'clinical abortion' is used to specify an abortion in a professional medical setting. The term 'medical abortion' is used to indicate an abortion induced via pharmaceutical drugs. Medical abortion with pharmaceutical drugs may be a form of clinical abortion or self-induced abortion.

The term 'menstrual extraction' is used for the self-induced procedure in a self-help group setting while the term 'manual vacuum aspiration' is used for the nearly identical procedure performed by a medical professional in a clinical setting.

An Icon Key and a chart of herbal abortifacients and the most common side effects that have been associated with them is located after the Herbal Introduction in Part III.

The herbal section is organized alphabetically according to common name. The information on each herb follows a precise format: Illustration, AKA (Names), Medicinal Properties, Effects on the Body, Abortifacient Action, Chemical Components, Herbal Lore and Historical Use, Gathering, Preparation, Words to the Wise, and Dosage.

Dosage information has been averaged from several sources. Dosage ranges are suggested for a 150lb. (68 kg) adult. No single dosage recommendation can be appropriate for every individual. Each person has unique sensitivities, constitutions, and physical attributes. Herbs can vary widely in the amount of medicinal components depending on growing conditions, preparation method, storage, etc.

24

The manufacturer's dosage instructions should always be followed for any purchased herbal product. Consumers interested in using the information in this book with regards to their particular case should seek the advice of open-minded physicians, trained acupuncturists, herbalists, homeopathic doctors, and therapists. Self medication or self surgery is dangerous and not recommended.

Part I   Self-Induced Abortion Basics

What is self-induced abortion?

Self-induced abortion is the induced termination of a pregnancy outside of the medical system. Self-induced abortion is sometimes called induced miscarriage. Self-induced abortion methods are sometimes based on traditional clinical abortion methods, like manual vacuum extraction or medical abortion with pharmaceutical drugs. Commonly around the world, self-induced abortion methods are based on methods of folk or alternative medicine, including: herbs, massage, acupuncture, and hyperthermia. In contrast, a spontaneous abortion or miscarriage is an abortion which happens naturally without prompting by external means.

Why would a woman choose self-induced abortion?

A woman may choose to attempt to self induce abortion if restrictions to clinical medical services make receiving professional medical care difficult. Restrictions may be financial, physical, or legal. Abortion may be outlawed or governmental restrictions on abortion services may make receiving clinical abortion services problematic.

Women in middle to low income brackets, in countries where abortions are not covered by national health care, may find the cost to procure a clinical abortion prohibitive. Sometimes the distance necessary to travel to receive clinical abortion services is prohibitive. Parental notification laws in some states in the United States may prohibit some young women from accessing clinical abortion services.

Why would a woman not choose self-induced abortion?

Self-induced abortion is known to be more dangerous and less effective than clinical abortion. Obtaining the necessary supplies, equipment, and support for self-induced abortion may be difficult. Depending on the government of the area, self-induced abortion may be illegal.

Nearly all self-induced abortion substances are suspected or known teratogens. Teratogens cause abnormal growth in the embryo or fetus, and often results in deformities in the child if the abortion attempt is unsuccessful and the pregnancy is brought to term.

Are there certain times in a pregnancy when self-induced abortion is more effective than other times?

Self-induced abortion is easier to accomplish in the earliest stages of pregnancy (the first eight weeks LMP). After the placenta is formed, self-induced abortion becomes more difficult.

What are the contraindications for self-induced abortion?

Answering yes to any of the following questions would indicate a woman is at a greater risk of complications associated with an abortion:

- Am I over 35 years old? Age can be a factor in increased complications. Also, a history of cesarean or previous placental adhesion can cause complications in an abortion.

- Am I overweight, or do I have asthma, allergies, cardiovascular disease, sexually transmitted diseases, glandular disorders, an abnormal uterus, bleeding or clotting disorders? Am I having any other health problems? A history of heavy smoking also increases the risk of complications.

- Do I have an IUD? An IUD must be removed prior to attempting an abortion.

- Do I generally eat in an unbalanced way? Abortion can stress the body, especially a body that is out of balance due to nutritional deficiencies.

- Is my psychological state fragile? The hormones of pregnancy can change suddenly with abortion attempts. Psychological support and counseling is often available in a clinical abortion setting.

- Am I feeling emotionally weak? If a woman has had previous emotional problems, attempting self-induced abortion may not be in her best interest.

- Is my domestic situation problematic? Am I putting myself at emotional or physical risk by attempting an abortion in my current domestic situation? Ideally, a woman attempting a self-induced abortion should have no interference from the people who surround her.

- Am I, due to finances or physical location, unable to access basic telephone, transportation, and backup medical care?

- Am I alone? A woman who is attempting to self abort requires someone close-by who would be able to help her in an emergency.

- Is someone trying to force me into having an abortion? It is not uncommon for women to be manipulated or coerced into an abortion. The counseling system in a clinical abortion service will often screen for women who are being forced into an abortion. Women faced with this issue would benefit from additional support and counseling services. The counseling system in a traditional medical system is set up to support women who are faced with this situation.

- Am I considering self-induced abortion due to financial reasons? Organizations in the United States that may provide financial assistance for clinical abortion are listed in the Resources section.

What methods are used in self-induced abortion?

Medical abortion - A pharmaceutical drug-induced abortion, termed 'medical abortion' is increasingly recognized as an effective and safe self-induced abortion method. Medical abortion is believed to be safest when used with physician oversight, however when physician oversight is unavailable, medical abortion is regarded as the "best and safest way a woman can do an abortion herself."[68] In countries where abortion is restricted or illegal, Womenonwaves.org offers medical abortion prescriptions from foreign doctors and online physician advice. (See Resources).

Menstrual extraction – Menstrual extraction is a modified form of the clinical technique of manual vacuum aspiration. Menstrual extraction groups, sometimes called self-help or friendship groups, form a close community of women who educate each other on proper sterile techniques. They share skills and train by seeing and doing. A simple device called a Del-EM™ is traditionally used. The Del-EM™, consisting of a suction syringe, a check valve, tubing, a glass jar, and a sterile flexible plastic tube called a cannula, is used to extract the menstrual fluids from the uterus. Through the careful use of this method by trained women's self-help groups, many women are finding menstrual extraction to be a safe and effective self-induced abortion option early in a pregnancy.

Herbal abortion – Herbs have been used since ancient times by women to induce abortion.

Homeopathy - Homeopathic remedies (based on herbal abortives) are used in some areas of the world to induce abortion.

Acupuncture – The application of needles inserted and stimulated at specific points on the body has long been used in China for abortive purposes. The development of electronic acupuncture point locators has made this abortion method available to more women.

Massage - The physical manipulation of the body is probably the oldest form of self-induced abortion and still remains popular. The United Nations estimates over 300,000 massage abortions are performed annually in Thailand alone.[69]

Hyperthermia - The application of heat is also an ancient form of abortion. The Greek physician, Soranus, who lived in AD 98-138, prescribed hot baths along with abortive herbs.[70]

Yoga – Yoga, as a menstrual promoting method, is a new discovery. Modern female yoga enthusiasts have learned through experience that some yoga postures and processes have the added benefit of influencing fertility.

Psychic abortion - The use of psychic communication as a fertility regulation method is reported by some women for self-induced abortion.

What steps should a woman take before self-induced abortion?

- Administer a Pregnancy Test

   For a woman who has missed her period and suspects she might be pregnant, the first step in making a decision regarding pregnancy is to find out whether or not she is pregnant. Home pregnancy tests, available at a pharmacy, test the urine for the hormone human chorionic gonadotropin

31

(hCG), a hormone secreted in a pregnant woman's ovary. Some pregnancy tests claim to accurately test on the day of expected menstruation, approximately fourteen days after ovulation. Quantitative hCG blood tests can be accurate 6 – 8 days after ovulation, but are usually only available at a doctor's office.

- Get a Sonogram

A sonogram (ultrasound) at a clinic after the sixth week will help determine if there is an ectopic pregnancy. It is not possible to safely abort an ectopic pregnancy without physician supervision. Ectopic pregnancies are the leading cause of maternal mortality in the first trimester.

In an ectopic pregnancy the embryo implants outside the womb. The most common site for an ectopic pregnancy is the fallopian tube. Ectopic pregnancies can be fatal if the fallopian tube bursts and the woman bleeds to death before emergency attention can be secured. Sometimes the pain of an ectopic pregnancy can seem heavier than normal cramping pains. On average, the symptoms of an ectopic pregnancy appear 7 - 8 weeks LMP. An ectopic pregnancy may feel a lot like a miscarriage, but if the fallopian tube has ruptured the pain will often become so severe that a woman will have trouble standing up. Pain may be on one side of the pelvis or possibly referred to the shoulder. If an ectopic pregnancy is caught early enough, a doctor can administer methotrexate, a drug that inhibits the metabolism of folic acid, to cause an abortion; and surgery can be avoided.

A woman may be at a greater risk for an ectopic pregnancy if she smokes, has had her tubes tied, has an IUD, has had pelvic surgery, endometriosis, pelvic inflammatory disease, a previous ectopic pregnancy, or if her mother took diethylstilbestrol (DES) while she was in the womb. Ectopic pregnancies occur in one of 3,885 pregnancies in the United States.

- Calculate Gestational Age

A woman can have some idea of what she might expect in an abortion if she calculates the gestational age, the time in weeks that the pregnancy has progressed. Since the exact time of conception is unlikely to be known, the first day of the last menstrual period is used to measure how old the fetus is. The fertile time of ovulation is the time when the majority of women conceive. Knowledge of the gestational age of the pregnancy and fetus is a valuable tool when making decisions and knowing what to expect regarding self-induced abortion methods.

To calculate the gestational age: Take the first day of the last normal menstrual period (LMP) and count forward the number of days that the pregnancy has progressed.

- Review Options

    Review available abortion and contraception options (see Resources). Clinical abortion services are usually safer and more effective than self-induced abortion options. Utilize professional clinical abortion services, if possible. Plan to use contraception immediately after abortion, if pregnancy is not desired.

How does a woman care for herself during an abortion?

1. Secure clinical abortion services, if possible.
2. Secure a telephone, be within one hour's drive of emergency medical services, have transportation, antibiotics, and a support person before considering self-induced abortion.
3. Breastfeeding women have special concerns (see Appendix B and Appendix I).
4. Regularly monitor blood loss and body temperature during and after an abortion. A temperature of 101°F (38°C) or above or filling three thick pads in three hours or less requires immediate emergency medical care.
5. Utilize regular uterine massage to help prevent hematometra. Hematometra is when the uterus becomes painfully swollen with blood and clots. The clots can obstruct the release of the uterine contents through the cervical os and prevent the uterus from clamping down to finish the abortion. Hematometra may require uterine aspiration (menstrual extraction). Uterine massage is performed by regularly

34

pressing with force directly above the pubic bone to place pressure on the uterus and help to release clots. Passing clots during uterine massage is normal.

6. Always use clean menstrual pads and change them regularly.

7. Avoid tampons, douching, tub bathing, and sexual intercourse for three weeks after an abortion. The opening to the uterus expands during an abortion. To avoid introducing harmful bacteria to the uterus, nothing should be allowed inside the vagina after the abortion procedure.

8. Receive a RhoGam® shot at a clinic or hospital if she has an Rh- blood type (see Appendix A).

9. Avoid the following herbs and vitamins, which are used historically to *reduce* uterine contractions and halt spontaneous miscarriage: black haw (root bark) *Viburnum prunifolium*, cramp bark (bark) *Viburum opulis*, false unicorn (root) *Chamailirium luteum*, lobelia (leaf and seed) *Lobelia inflate*, queen of the meadow (root) *Eupatorium purpureum*, red raspberry (leaf) *Rubus idaeus*, wild yam (root) *Dioscorea villosa*, and amounts of Vitamin E in excess of 100 I.U. per day.

10. Contact a Traditional Chinese Medicine (TCM) practitioner to assist in the process of healing during and after abortion. One TCM formula, Song Tu Fang, when taken 48 hours prior to abortion, has been shown in one study to decrease both the volume and duration of post abortion blood loss, decrease pelvic pain, and decrease the incidence of post abortion abnormal leucorrhea.[71]

35

How does a woman care for herself after an abortion?

1. Seek medical attention if fever, unusual discharge, or excessive bleeding occurs or if signs of pregnancy do not diminish.

2. Confirm the abortion was complete. Visit a clinic 10 - 15 days after the abortion for confirmation the abortion was completed. A pregnancy test taken three weeks after the abortion will usually show reduced hCG levels.

3. Seek counseling and support when needed (see Resources).

4. Self-induced abortion, whether with herbs or medical abortion pharmaceutical medicines, can be damaging the liver and kidneys. Supplements can help heal and repair the liver and kidneys: lots of pure water, natural juices (cranberry, apple, and beet), and antioxidant supplements Vitamin C and E. Herbal supplements used to help heal the liver and kidneys are: schizandra *Schisandra chinensis*, nettle seed *Urtica dioica*, milk thistle *Silybum marianum*, dandlelion *Taraxacum officinale*, artichoke *Cynara scolymus*, salvia *Salvia officinalis*, and spirulina *Arthrospira platensis* or *Arthrospira maxima*. Seek the advice of a trained herbalist. (For additional supplements, see Post-Abortion Care).

5. Use contraception. A woman should research all options and utilize a birth control method to prevent unwanted pregnancy (see Appendix J).

What signs would indicate something is wrong?

A temperature over 101°F (38°C) may indicate an infection which requires antibiotics. Excessive bleeding, defined as soaking through three or more pads in three hours or less, would indicate hemorrhage. A racing heartbeat or a drop in blood pressure may indicate a systemic infection. Great abdominal pain may indicate an ectopic pregnancy. If any of the above present, immediate emergency medical care must be obtained.

Where can a woman go if something is wrong?

A woman can seek emergency services at a local hospital and say she is having a miscarriage and receive emergency treatment. The symptoms and treatment for miscarriage and self-induced abortion are the same (see Post-Abortion Care).

What are the potential negative health effects of self-induced abortion?

All abortions, including clinical abortions, carry risks to the health of the woman. The risks of self-induced abortion are greater than clinical abortion as training and experience may be lacking. The range of possible negative side effects to self-induced abortifacients varies widely, as there are many abortifacient substances. It is likely there may be unidentified negative side effects, as well. The most serious potential side effects follow:

- Incomplete abortion - Incomplete abortion requires a manual vacuum aspiration procedure (MVA).

- Hemorrhage – Very heavy bleeding soaking through three thick pads in three hours or less requires immediate medical attention. An MVA, medication, surgery, or a blood transfusion may be necessary.

- Teratogenicity - If a woman uses self-abortive means, fails to miscarry, and continues her pregnancy to term, the resulting child may have a wide range of mental and/or physical deformities. Nearly all abortive methods are suspected teratogens. Teratogens are agents which cause the development of abnormal structures in an embryo resulting in a severely deformed fetus. The first 8 weeks of fetal growth is characterized by rapid cell division and is the most crucial period in the development of an individual. All of the embryo's bodily organs and systems are forming and are highly vulnerable to teratogenic agents (medicines, estrogenic substances, viruses, radiation, or infection) during the first eight weeks (LMP) of pregnancy. Estrogenic substances (all estrogenic herbs) are teratogens, and can cause vaginal cancer in female babies in later years. Male embryos exposed to estrogenic substances in the womb and as babies have developed lower sperm count as adults. Progestogens in pregnancy can cause masculinization of females and advanced bone age in later years. Many purgatives and diuretics are also known teratogens. Herbal teratogens can cause low implantation of the placenta, possibly causing complications that can be dangerous to the mother and baby in labor if the pregnancy is brought to term. Fetuses are less vulnerable to

38

teratogens after eight weeks LMP, but these noxious agents may arrest normal functional growth of vital organs, especially the brain, later during a pregnancy, as well.

- Toxicity or Allergy- There is a risk of toxicity or allergic reaction related to self-induced abortifacient substances. The kidney and the liver can be negatively affected by substances ingested in attempt to induce abortion. Toxicity to the kidneys and liver can lead to organ damage or failure. Organ failure can lead to death.

- Infection - Infection is a risk of all abortion methods. The cervical os is more open during abortion, and bacteria can travel from the vagina to the uterus more easily. There is a 5% infection rate in clinical abortion. Self-induced abortion methods involving inner uterine techniques have a greater risk of infection. The risk of infection is relative to the amount of training and experience the practitioner has. If infection occurs and antibiotics are not secured, sepsis (total body infection) may follow. Sepsis can be life threatening.

- Reproductive System Damage - Although rare, damage to the reproductive organs can result from perforation of the reproductive organs or infection which leads to pelvic inflammatory disease (PID).

- Undetected ectopic pregnancy – This is rare, and can be fatal if left untreated.

- Death – It is extremely rare, but death is possible from very serious complications. Death occurs in one out of 100,000

39

clinical abortions. Childbirth is riskier than abortion in the first 20 weeks LMP.

What are the characteristics of a normal abortion?

Wherever the placenta separates from the endometrium, bleeding occurs. The first sign of an abortion is vaginal bleeding, similar or somewhat heavier than an average menstrual period. Clotting and cramping may be similar or somewhat heavier than a woman's normal period. During the first four weeks (LMP) of pregnancy, most women who abort do not notice the little fertilized ovum (egg) encased in its tiny chorionic villi shell amidst the menstrual fluids. By the eighth week LMP, the embryo and sac grow larger and may be noticeable to the naked eye. The placenta passes towards the end of bleeding. Prior to the seventh week, the placenta has not grown large enough to be seen.

From the seventh to the tenth week, the placenta ranges in diameter from ½ - 1¼ in. (15 – 30 mm). The uterus contracts and closes off the blood vessels after the products of conception have passed. The bleeding slows and then gradually stops. Spotting may be present for up to three weeks.

After the abortion, signs of pregnancy begin to disappear. Breasts begin to revert back to their original size. Breasts may be tender and tingly for a few weeks during this transition. The cervix and uterus may be tender for a few weeks as well. An over-the-counter pregnancy test will show negative results around three weeks after the abortion.

40

Understanding Gestational Age and Self-Induced Abortion

Week 1: Menstrual Period

The first day of the last normal menstrual period (LMP) is used to calculate the degree of gestational age. This week a woman is not pregnant and is experiencing a menstrual period.

Week 2: Estrogen Increases

During the second week, a woman is not yet pregnant, her menstrual period has ended, and the ovum in the ovary is beginning to gradually produce estrogen to prepare for ovulation.

Week 3: Ovulation and Conception

The third week begins with ovulation, the monthly time when a follicle in an ovary releases a mature ovum (an egg enclosed in follicle cells) into the abdominal cavity. Ovulation occurs approximately 14 days before the first day of the next expected menstrual cycle (or between 10 - 16 days after the first day of the last menstrual period - LMP). The fallopian tube, moves around the abdominal cavity in search of the released ovum. Fallopian tubes are so agile, that a tube has the capacity to find an ovum released by the *opposite* ovary, if the nearest fallopian tube is damaged or blocked for some reason. When a fallopian tube finds the ovum floating around in the abdominal cavity, wave-like movements of the cilia (tiny finger-like projections inside the fallopian tube) draw the ovum into the flower-like opening and down the funnel of the fallopian tube. The ovum is ripe for fertilization for about 24 hours when the ovum is at the mouth of the fallopian tube. If unprotected intercourse occurs,

41

millions of sperm can swim up the vagina, through the opening of the uterus (called the cervical os), and into the fallopian tube toward egg within its folds. The folds of the fallopian tube that surround the ovum sense the closeness of the sperm and secrete enzymes which loosen the protective follicle cells around the ovum to expose the egg to the sperm for fertilization.

After fertilization, the fallopian tube nourishes and protects the growing and dividing group of cells as the fallopian tube muscles gently contract to make waves that move the fertilized egg along its 4½ in. (11.25 cm) length to the uterus. Meanwhile in the ovary, the follicle that released the ovum develops into the corpus luteum, whose function is to produce the hormone, progesterone. The progesterone secreted by the corpus luteum causes rapid cell division of the endometrium (lining of the uterus) to make a fertile bed for the growing embryo. A woman's basal body temperature, which normally fluctuates a bit higher during ovulation, remains elevated when an ovum is fertilized.

Week 4: Embedding of the Embryo

The rapidly dividing fertilized egg floats around in the uterus at the beginning of the fourth week. With the corpus luteum's secretion of progesterone, the endometrial lining is becoming rich and nutritive. During the first two to three days of the fourth week, the endometrium is prepared, and the fertilized egg implants. The cells of the fertilized egg that touch the endometrium begin to divide rapidly to form a spongy network which reaches an increasing number of maternal blood vessels. Blood begins to flow freely through this thick spongy layer of cells, called the chorionic villi. The chorionic villi begin to absorb nourishment from the blood to support the growing embryo and chorionic shell, which at the end of this week has a 2.5 mm diameter. The progesterone secreted by the corpus luteum also causes growth of the milk ducts in the breasts. Some women may begin to notice a tingling sensation in their breasts at this time. Pregnancy tests cannot detect pregnancy yet, for the chorionic villi have yet to develop and begin to produce human chorionic gonadotropin.

Weeks 2, 3, and 4: Promoting Menstruation

Fertility regulation methods utilized during weeks two through four are emmenagogual. Emmenagogual means to promote menstruation. Methods, if used, are used without definitive knowledge that a woman is pregnant, for technology has yet to create a test that can detect pregnancy at this early stage. Emergency contraception can be used during these weeks to interfere with the hormones required to sustain a pregnancy (see Appendix J). Medical abortion using mifepristone plus prostaglandins can be done as soon as woman knows she may be pregnant. Menstrual extraction is used to extract the menstrual fluids. Self-induced abortion with herbs is believed to be easiest and safest to accomplish during these weeks. Estrogenic herbs taken in week two by women in the ancient world are believed to have worked to provide contraception by increasing estrogen when estrogen is normally at its lowest level. The use of implantation inhibiting herbs (like Queen Anne's lace, cotton root bark, or Vitamin C) in week four blocks, alters, or interferes in the production of progesterone, a hormone on which the pregnancy depends to stimulate the development of the nutritive lining of the uterus. Without progesterone, the lining of the uterus does not grow to be

43

supportive to the fertilized egg, the fertilized egg does not implant, and a woman menstruates as usual. Also, herbs called emmenagogues may be used during weeks three and four to promote menstruation. Most emmenagogues have a direct effect on the uterus. Many emmenagogual herbs are believed to be teratogens, substances that cause the development of abnormal structures in the embryo. Teratogens in the woman's system during the fourth week of pregnancy usually causes the pregnancy to terminate. Hyperthermia, acupuncture, homeopathy, massage, and yoga may also help to bring on menstruation at this early stage of pregnancy. The appearance of the menstrual blood is usually normal to heavy, possibly with more clotting than usual. The very tiny fertilized ovum passes unnoticed amidst the menstrual blood.

Weeks 5 and 6: ``Am I pregnant?''

During the fifth week, the absence of menstruation may be the first indication of the possible pregnancy. The uterine wall is nourishing the fertilized ovum which now measures about 3 mm in length and is covered with the fine root-like threads of the chorionic villi. No human characteristics can be seen on the 2 mm length of the rapidly forming embryo. The chorionic villi begin to produce quantities of a hormone called human chorionic gonadotropin (hCG).

Pregnancy tests taken during the fifth week or later, detect the presence of hCG in the urine. If hCG is present, then the test will indicate that a woman is pregnant.

Physical signs of pregnancy may also become evident. A woman may have morning nausea; her breasts may be feeling tender to the touch; and her vagina and cervix may be turning a bluish to violet

44

color. Pressure on the bladder and increased urination may be noticeable now.

By the end of the sixth week, the uterus will have grown to about the size of a small plum. The fast-growing embryo has a 4 mm length at this time.

Weeks 5 and 6: Abortion

Medical abortion using mifepristone plus prostaglandin is most effective when used at gestations less than seven weeks. Menstrual extraction can be used at this time, however menstrual extraction has been found to be most effective when effective when used at around 7 weeks.

Implantation inhibiting (progesterone blocking) herbs like Queen Anne's lace or cotton root bark may prove effective during the fifth and sixth weeks. Implantation inhibiting herbs block progesterone causing the uterine lining to become a negative environment incapable of nourishing a fetus. When this happens, the chorionic villi separate from the uterine wall causing bleeding like a menstrual period. The os, the opening of the cervix, dilates due to the stimulation of the body's hormonal system, and the uterine contents pass out the body.

In addition to implantation inhibiting herbs, other abortive herbs with uterine contracting (oxytocic) properties, like cotton root bark, papaya, and parsley are used to stimulate uterine contractions, which may help to expel the uterine contents. Hyperthermia, massage, yoga, homeopathy, and acupuncture may also help to abort at this stage of pregnancy.

Abortions during weeks five and six result in a normal to heavy period, usually with more clotting and cramping than usual.

Weeks 7 and 8: Making Decisions

The majority of women who obtain clinical abortions do so during the seventh and eighth weeks. During the seventh week, some physical signs of pregnancy may subside (like nausea), but other signs may become more noticeable to many women. The mucous plug begins to form in the cervical os during the seventh week. Vaginal secretions tend to be thick and acid.

The embryo's arms and legs begin to form during the seventh week. From top of the head to the tail bone, the embryo grows to a 5 – 8 mm length during the seventh week. The facial features of the embryo form, and the heart becomes established and begins to beat in the tiny 8 – 15 mm embryo during the eighth week. The chorionic villi in the endometrium continue to proliferate and begin to form the placenta.

During the eighth week, the woman's breasts become noticeably larger and may feel tighter and tense. The nipples may become more prominent and small bumps, called glands of Montgomery, may begin to develop on the breast in the area around the nipple and the areola.

Weeks 9 and 10: Marked Fetal and Placental Development

During the ninth week, the placenta begins to produce its own estrogen and progesterone. The corpus luteum, having produced estrogen and progesterone up until this time, begins to cease production in most women. The chorionic villi outside the placenta degenerate, and the chorion (the sac membrane) becomes smooth. The head of the fetus grows significantly due to the beginning of intense brain development during the ninth week. The nine week old fetus is now approximately 1.6 - 1.8 cm in length and weighs about four grams.

By the end of the tenth week, the placenta has grown to cover one-third of the uterine wall. The fetus now is 3 cm long and begins to take on a human appearance. The hands and feet are recognizable. Respiratory activity is evident, and weak fetal movements begin. The sac progresses to about the size of a small chicken egg. By the tenth week, the glands of Montgomery around the nipples become pronounced and begin to secrete sebum, which keeps the nipple soft and pliable in preparation for nursing.

Weeks 7 through 10: Abortion

Medical abortion continues to be the safest and most effective form of self-induced abortion during this time period. Menstrual extraction is more successful when used around the seventh week, however the procedure can be used in later weeks, if care is taken to dilate the cervix to accept the appropriate sized cannula. Herbal progesterone blockers may be useful to stimulate the placenta to detach after the seventh week, but the embryo has already implanted and the placenta has begun to embed, so the addition of strong uterine contracting emmenagogues like blue cohosh, papaya, or cotton root bark would probably assist in inducing abortion.

Most abortions and miscarriages before the tenth week are complete, meaning all of the uterine contents are expelled and the uterus clamps down to complete the abortion. The bleeding subsides after the small placenta is passed, and over the next few weeks, the signs of pregnancy disappear. Hyperthermia, massage, yoga, homeopathy, and acupuncture may also help to abort at this stage of pregnancy. However, the effort required to be successful at a self-induced abortion increases as the pregnancy becomes increasingly established. The chances of having negative side effects to herbs increases as cumulative dosage and length of time involved in herbal treatment increases. After the tenth week, the chances of having an incomplete abortion increase.

Weeks 11 to 14: Placental Formation

In the eleventh and twelfth weeks, the placenta and chorionic villi begin to form a compact network of connective tissue which is complete by the end of the fourteenth week. The placenta has a 6 cm diameter and weighs more than the 5 cm long fetus by the twelfth week. By the thirteenth week, the placenta is completely formed, and the circulation between the fetus and placenta is complete; the fetus has a 6 cm length. By the fourteenth week, the fetus grows to 10 cm long. Fingers and toes have more detail; nails form. Fetal muscles contract occasionally. The sex of the fetus may be determined after the fourteenth week. From the eleventh to the fourteenth week, the placenta continues to grow progressively larger and becomes more firmly embedded.

A woman's body is changing, too. A woman pregnant during this time may notice less bladder pressure. Nipples on the breasts darken, and fluid colostrum may be expressed. Cardiac output is greater; blood volume starts to increase.

Weeks 11 – 14: Abortion

Medical abortion using mifepristone plus prostaglandin is officially used up until 63 days LMP. Menstrual extraction may be used up until the eighteenth week, as long as appropriate sized cannulas can be obtained and the woman's cervix allows for adequate dilation. Pharmaceutical cervical dilation is utilized to assist the cervix in opening for the menstrual extraction procedure. Herbal abortion past the tenth week of gestation is usually not effective.

The majority of women who have incomplete abortions have them after the tenth week. The main cause of incomplete abortion is the firm attachment of the placenta. In an incomplete abortion, the thin umbilical cord breaks, and the fetus and enclosing sac expel, but the placenta remains adhered to the uterus. When this happens, bleeding continues, sometimes the bleeding is dangerously profuse. The cervical os remains dilated, and the uterus cannot clamp down to stop the bleeding because of the attached placenta. Incomplete abortion can be an emergency situation, because the woman can hemorrhage and lose a high volume of blood very quickly. It is for this reason that the products of abortion must be carefully examined to be certain that all products of conception have been expelled.

Part II Modern Self-Induced Abortion Methods

Introduction

Modern self-induced abortion methods are methods based on clinical abortion procedures, such as: medical abortion and manual vacuum aspiration (MVA). Modern self-induced abortion methods are believed to be more effective than alternative methods of self-induced abortion, such as: herbal, homeopathy, massage, and acupuncture.

Self-induced medical abortion, the use of pharmaceutical medicines without a prescription, is considered the best method of self-induced abortion, because it is relatively safe and is very effective when used in early pregnancy. Self-induced medical abortion is a popular method of abortion in countries where abortion is illegal. Latin American women who immigrate to the United States sometimes continue to use self-induced medical abortion despite the fact that medical abortion is legally available at clinics in the United States.

Menstrual extraction is based on the clinical abortion method of manual vacuum aspiration. The equipment is slightly different, but the procedure is basically the same. A vacuum and a cannula are used to empty the uterus of its contents. Menstrual extraction is usually used during the first trimester, most effectively around the seventh gestational week, to end a pregnancy.

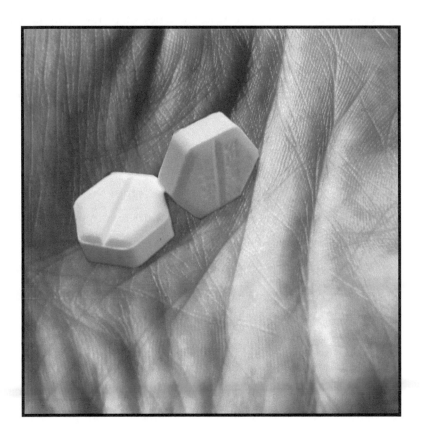

For abortions up to nine weeks, the pills can be provided through primary health care services and women can safely use the method at home or in a clinical setting, according to their own preferences and personal circumstances. Medical abortion after nine weeks and in the second trimester can be carried out in a health centre or hospital.

-International Consortium for Medical Abortion, 2004

51

In medical clinics, medical abortion is an increasingly prevalent abortion technique where a series of pharmaceuticals are taken to terminate a pregnancy. In the majority of medical abortions, a woman is prescribed a pharmaceutical regime. She usually receives two medicines, mifepristone and misoprostol, to block progesterone and cause the uterus to expel the pregnancy, often within eight hours after administration.

The first medicine, mifepristone, (United States brand name Mifeprex™ or Mifegyne™) blocks the progesterone hormone required to sustain pregnancy. Mifepristone has been approved by the FDA for the termination of early pregnancy. Mifepristone is occasionally prescribed for the treatment of endometriosis and glaucoma.

The second medicine prescribed to end a pregnancy, misoprostol, has not been FDA approved to terminate pregnancy, but is FDA approved and prescribed as an ulcer medication. Misoprostol, also known by the brand name Cytotec™, is 85% effective at causing an abortion when used alone. Mifepristone and misoprostol used together are 95% effective at terminating a pregnancy. Misoprostol is more widely used by physicians for off-label application of causing uterine contractions which can induce abortion. Off-label use is the practice of prescribing drugs for a purpose outside the scope of the drug's FDA approved label, an entirely legal practice used in the United States and many other countries, whereby the regulating authority recognizes the physician's medical authority in most cases and allows physicians to practice medicine and use their best judgment.

Research suggests that, with physician oversight, women can safely administer all or part of the mifepristone/misoprostol regime safely at home.[72] When women are allowed to take the misoprostol at home they report more happiness with the medical abortion than women who have to return to the clinic for the misoprostol dose.[73] Studies have indicated that most women are able to ascertain whether or not the abortion was successful at home, by evaluating the tissue passed, any remaining symptoms, and by taking a pregnancy test three weeks after the medical abortion,[74] however how accurately a woman can self-assess the gestational age of her pregnancy has been debated.[75] Also, whether a woman can accurately evaluate her own medical history for conditions contraindicated for medical abortion, such as: evidence of underlying heart disease, respiratory disorders, liver or kidney disorders, or hypertension has also been debated, thus the prevailing thought is that this method of abortion requires physician oversight. However, if abortion is restricted or illegal, self-induced medical abortion with mifepristone and/or misoprostol is recommended as the safest and most effective abortion a woman can do at home.[76]

Financial considerations sometimes influence a woman's choice to pursue a self-induced medical abortion, which may or may not be legal depending on the government of the area and the gestational age of the pregnancy. In 2008, the average cost for a single 200 mcg tablet of misoprostol in the United States was $2.00. In some developing countries, the cost for a single 200 mcg tablet of misoprostol can be as low as $0.50.

Based on the nominal cost of the medication, one would expect that all women could afford an abortion, however that is not the case. In the United States in 2001, the average cost for a clinical medical abortion was $487.00; and approximately 74% of American women paid for abortions with their own money.[77] In the United States, federal funding for abortions is only allowed for rape, incest, and a woman's life being endangered by the pregnancy; and only a handful of states in the United States help poor women access free or reduced price abortion services.

To help women access medical abortion services in countries where abortion is restricted or illegal, WomenOnWeb.org, facilitates physician contact and prescription fulfillment. After a woman fills out an online questionnaire, a physician reviews the woman's medical information and issues a medical abortion prescription, if appropriate. For a donation of 75 Euros (approximately $110.00), the prescription is sent overnight via courier to the woman in need. For women without financial means, a fund fueled by donations can sometimes help. WomenOnWeb.org also provides online support. Most countries allow prescription medicines to be imported, if the medicine is accompanied by a physician's prescription.

WomenOnWeb.org is an offshoot of WomenOnWaves.org, a Dutch ship that provides abortion services in international waters near countries which have restrictive laws on abortion. The presence of the ship brings international media attention to the plight of women in countries where abortion is illegal or restricted.

Medicines Most Commonly Used for Medical Abortion

The medicines most commonly used for medical abortion are mifepristone, misoprostol, methotrexate, and PGE_1 or PGE_2 pessaries:

Mifepristone \miff eh PRIH stone\

Mifepristone (RU486) is synthetic steroid antiprogesterone. Mifepristone blocks progesterone receptors causing the uterine endometrium to be unsupportive to the embryo or fetus, softens and dilates the opening of the uterus, and releases prostaglandins that can cause the uterus to contract. Mifepristone is most effective during the first 9 weeks of gestation before the placenta takes over progesterone production from the corpus luteum. Mifepristone is prescribed by doctors for abortion (FDA approved), emergency contraception, uterine fibroids, endometriosis, depression, glaucoma, cancer, and Cushing's syndrome.

- Mifepristone Brand Names: Mifeprex™ and Mifegyne™.

Misoprostol \mye soe PROST ole\

Misoprostol is a synthetic analogue to prostaglandin E_1. Misoprostol is approved as an ulcer drug in more than 85 countries, but it is commonly prescribed off-label for a variety of obstetrical and gynecological purposes. When used off-label in most countries, it is prescribed without package inserts to inform users of safe dosages, contraindications, and possible side effects. Misoprostol is prescribed off-label for abortion, incomplete abortion, and postpartum hemorrhage. Misoprostol is sometimes combined with the painkiller diclofenac and prescribed for arthritis. This combined medicine is more expensive than the misoprostol alone.

Normal side effects of misoprostol: chills, elevation of body temperature, pain, and cramping. Some women experience headaches, mild dizziness, hot flashes, nausea, vomiting and diarrhea. Usually these side effects go away by themselves. Allergic reactions are rare, but usually present with mild itching and hives.

- Misoprostol brand names: Cytotec™ (United States), Apo-Misoprostol™ (Canada), Novo-Misoprostol ™(Canada), Cityl™ (Colombia), Cyprostol™ (Austria), Cytolog™ (India), Misoprost™ (India), Zitotec™(India), Gastotec™ (Korea), Misel™ (Korea), Gastrul™ (Indonesia), Misotrol™ (Chile), Mibetec™ (Argentina), Isoprolor™ (UK), U-Miso™ (Taiwan), Gymiso™ (France), Prostokos™ (Brazil), Vagiprost™ (Egypt), Arthrotec™ 50 or 75 (United States arthritis medicine with diclofenac), and Oxaprost™ 75 (Central and South America arthritis medicine with diclofenac).

56

Methotrexate \metha TREX ate\

Methotrexate is an antimetabolite drug that interferes in the metabolism of folic acid. Methotrexate inhibits DNA synthesis and affects rapidly dividing cells. In early pregnancy, methotrexate can interfere with implantation and is commonly used to encourage an abortion in the event of an ectopic pregnancy. During the long struggle to get mifepristone (RU486) approved for use in the United States, some physicians began to experiment with low doses of methotrexate in combination with misoprostol for medical abortion. Results were similar to the mifepristone/misoprostol combination. However, side effects and unpredictable bleeding for a few days up to six weeks forced doctors to abandon methotrexate for mifepristone as soon as mifepristone was approved by the FDA for use in the United States.

Methotrexate can cause severe bone marrow and liver damage, so women with alcoholism or liver problems should not take it. Methotrexate can also suppress the immune system; women with immune deficiency should not take it. More mild side effects of methotrexate are: mouth sores, stomach upset, headache, drowsiness, itching, skin rash, dizziness, and hair loss. On rare occasions, methotrexate use has caused lung toxicity which presents with a dry, non-productive cough.

- Methotrexate Brand Name: Rheumatrex™.

Gemeprost™, Prostin E$_2$™, and Cervidil™ Pessaries

Gemeprost™, like misoprostol, is a synthetic analogue to Prostaglandin E$_1$. Gemeprost™ vaginal pessaries are used in the United Kingdom and Sweden for dilation of the cervix prior to a first trimester surgical abortion and for the termination of pregnancy in the second trimester. For first trimester cervical dilation, one Gemeprost™ pessary 1.0 mg is inserted into the vagina up to three hours before the operation. For termination of a second trimester pregnancy, one Gemeprost™ pessary 1.0 mg is inserted every three hours, up to five pessaries total.

Prostin E$_2$™ vaginal pessaries, containing 20 mg of dinoprostone, are used in the United States to terminate pregnancies in the second trimester. Prostin E$_2$™ vaginal pessaries are inserted every four hours, for up to 48 hours, until abortion occurs.

Cervidil™ vaginal pessaries contain 10 mg of dinoprostone are FDA approved to induce labor in full term pregnancies.

Gemeprost™, Prostin E$_2$™, and Cervidil™ pessaries are packed in foil pouches, stored in a freezer, and allowed to come to room temperature before use.

- Gemeprost™ Brand Names: Gemeprost™ and Cervagem™.
- Dinoprostone (PGE$_2$) Brand Names: Prostin E$_2$™ (20 mg) and Cervidil™ (10mg).

Words to the Wise: Contraindications for medical abortion are having an IUD (must be removed prior to medical abortion), long term corticosteroid therapy, chronic heart, liver, respiratory, or kidney disease, severe anemia, uncontrolled high blood pressure, HIV positive status, IV drug use, inflammatory bowel disease, porphyria (a genetic condition), bleeding disorders, active genital herpes infection, known allergy to medical abortion medicines, a scarred uterus (for example, from a caesarean section), and having an infection or sickness.

All successful medical abortions result in bleeding. In medical abortions using mifepristone and misoprostol, most women begin bleeding after taking the misoprostol. Most women abort within five hours of taking the misoprostol. Most medical abortions with mifepristone combined with misoprostol completely evacuate the uterus in seven days, however bleeding and spotting may continue for more than thirty days.

Vitamins containing folic acid should be discontinued while taking methotrexate. Most methotrexate abortions are complete within seven days however up to 20% of women take up to thirty days to complete.

Normal side-effects to medical abortion are bleeding and cramping, usually heavier than a normal period. A woman may feel dizzy, have a fever or chills, diarrhea, nausea, or vomiting. However, a woman should not experience signs of an incomplete abortion, such as heavy or prolonged bleeding, extreme pain, or prolonged fever.

Medical abortion becomes less effective as the pregnancy becomes more established. Most forms of medical abortion have been shown to be effective through the first trimester (12 weeks LMP), and

59

they have also been shown to have some effectiveness into the second trimester.[78] After 9 weeks (LMP), medical abortions have a higher rate of complications. Approximately 8% of medical abortions are unsuccessful. To be absolutely sure that the abortion was successful, an ultrasound can be done ten days after the medical abortion. A pregnancy test taken three weeks after a medical abortion will show reduced gonadotropin hormone, if the medical abortion was successful.

Medical abortion has all the risks of any abortion procedure. Temperature and blood loss should be monitored for signs of infection and hemorrhage. If complications arise, such as prolonged heavy bleeding soaking through three or more thick pads in three hours or less or a fever of 101°F (38°C) indicating infection, a woman should seek immediate emergency medical care. A handful of deaths have resulted when vaginal application of medical abortion pharmaceuticals triggered a rapidly spreading infection which led to sepsis and death.

All abortive agents are potential teratogens which cause abnormal changes in the growing fetus. Many case reports indicate that medical abortion pharmaceuticals are known or suspected teratogens. Mifepristone has been shown to be a teratogen when tested on rabbits, however in tests on rats and monkeys, no teratogenic effect was observed.[79] Very few cases are recorded of ineffective mifepristone medical abortion and the woman choosing to continue the pregnancy; but in these cases the babies born were normal.[80] With misoprostol, several case reports have associated misoprostol use with human limb defects and Mobius syndrome.[81] Multiple case reports show

60

methotrexate acts as a teratogen causing growth retardation in the fetus exposed in the womb to methotrexate.[82] And PGE_1 and PGE_2 pessaries, being similar to misoprostol, are likely teratogens; however scientific studies have yet to show teratogenic effects.[83]

Many scientific studies have been done on medical abortion regimes at different dosages, and their effectiveness has been tested. However, medical abortion is relatively new as an abortion technique, so there is debate regarding the safest and most effective dosage regime to use. Once a dosage regime is chosen, it is most effective to adhere to the regime faithfully.

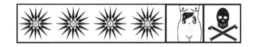

Dosage Regimes and Effectiveness for Medical Abortion

Up to	Effectiveness	Dosage
63 days	85-90%[84]	misoprostol 800 mcg (vaginally inserted then moistened with a few drops of water), repeated after 24 hours.
49 days	92% [85]	mifepristone 200 – 600 mg (sublingually on day 1), and misoprostol 400 mcg (sublingually on day 3). (Scientific studies have shown initial dose of mifepristone can be reduced to 200 mg and still be 92% effective.)
63 days	95% [86]	Same day administration: mifepristone 600 mg (sublingually), and misoprostol 800 mcg (vaginally).
49 days	95% [87]	methotrexate 25 mg (sublingually on day 1), and misoprostol 800 mcg (vaginally on day 7, day 8, and again on day 9 if abortion does not occur)
56 days	90% [88]	mifepristone 200 mg (orally) and misoprostol 800 mcg (vaginally) taken at the same time.
63 days	92% [89]	misoprostol 800 mcg (vaginally on day 1) and misoprostol 800 mcg (vaginally on day 2).
84 days	86% [90]	misoprostol 600 mcg (sublingually every three hours up to maximum of five doses)
84 days	91 - 94.5%[91]	For treatment of incomplete abortion: Single oral dose misoprostol 600 mcg.

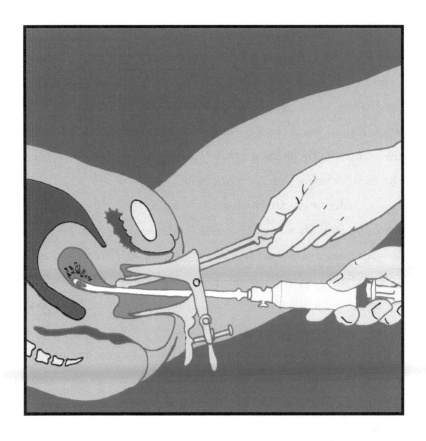

Menstrual extraction is a powerful example of
medical research done by women on and for ourselves.

-Our Bodies, Ourselves for the New Century, 1998

Menstrual extraction is a procedure where the contents of the uterus are removed in a few minutes with a suction device. A procedure similar to menstrual extraction was first developed in the mid-1800s by a physician named Simpson who called the method dry cupping. He states, "I have made frequent use of a tube resembling in length and size a male catheter and having an exhausting syringe adapted to its lower outer extremity been introduced into the cavity of the uterus."[92] The method of 'dry cupping' was not widely taught and this early technique was lost to medicine.

Menstrual extraction was invented in the 1970s in the United States by feminist activists Lorraine Rothman and Carol Downer. A low cost and low-tech device, known as a Del-EM™ was assembled from a flexible plastic cannula (called a Karman cannula), a 50 c.c. syringe, a check valve, some tubing, a rubber stopper, and a mason jar. The procedure was simple, effective, and relatively safe. Rothman and Downer toured the United States educating women's groups on the procedure, and the practice became well known. By 1993, over 20,000 menstrual extractions had been performed in the United States by women in self-help groups.[93]

Today, menstrual extraction, also known as menstrual regulation, is used around the world as a strategy to circumvent anti-abortion laws. Because confirmation of pregnancy is optional, anti-abortion governments (like Bangladesh, Korea, and Cuba) can support 'menstrual regulation' clinics where women are offered menstrual regulation if their period is late, with no pregnancy test required.

Menstrual extraction, when performed in a clinical setting, is called manual vacuum aspiration (MVA). MVA has been in use in the

United States for thirty years. MVA has been found to be 98% effective, only 2% of procedures must be repeated, and those on the second attempt are usually successful. Before twelve weeks LMP, only 1% of MVAs have complications. In the early second trimester, the rate of complications and incomplete procedures for MVA increases.

Menstrual extraction is most effective when used around seven weeks LMP. According to the World Health Organization and the Allan Guttmacher Institute, menstrual extraction can be used up through 12 weeks, and possibly up to 15 weeks, if the necessary sized cannulas can be secured and adequate cervical dilation achieved, and one study indicated that manual vacuum aspiration (MVA) could be used effectively into the first half of the second trimester, for MVA was found to be as effective as electric vacuum aspiration in weeks 14 to 18.[94] Cervical dilation is important in second trimester abortions, and misoprostol has been found to be effective in dilating the cervix in early second trimester abortion.[95]

The procedure of menstrual extraction is valued in the third world especially, because it is inexpensive, portable, quiet, and does not require electricity. Menstrual extraction, with less vacuum pressure than clinical electrical vacuum aspiration units, is also believed by some to cause less disruption of evacuated tissue, making identification of products of conception easier for very early gestations.

Words to the Wise: If the procedure is done too slowly and without sufficient vacuum pressure, clots readily form in the cannula tip and discomfort is increased as the procedure takes longer and can end incomplete. The woman having a menstrual regulation procedure can

65

often experience cramping and possibly nausea, sweating, and lightheadedness as well. To avoid unnecessary duration and discomfort it is essential to establish sufficient vacuum. Most MVA procedures, regardless of gestation are completed in 15 minutes.

Bleeding after menstrual extraction may vary from a few days of spotting to a few weeks of moderate flow, and some women do not bleed at all. It is not unusual to stop bleeding and begin again. Often 48 - 72 hours after the abortion, there is a hormonal shift that may suddenly cause cramping, bleeding, and clots. This is considered normal. (See Post Abortion Care).

Possible Complications Associated with Menstrual Extractions

Although complications are rare because the cannula is very thin and flexible, any use of instruments in the uterus can result in complications.

1. Incomplete evacuation. (1 out of 100 clinical MVAs) 3% of clinical manual vacuum aspirations (before 6 weeks LMP) are incomplete and require a second procedure. The most effective gestational age for menstrual extraction is seven weeks LMP. To ensure complete evacuation, one should watch carefully for the uterus gripping the cannula, the grating sensation, and meticulously examine the collected blood and tissue for signs of conception. A repeat procedure may be needed in an incomplete evacuation.

2. Uterine perforation. (2 out of 1000 clinical MVAs) Uterine perforation occasionally happens during dilation with metal tools in a clinical setting or an instrument goes through the

66

wall of the uterus during the procedure. Uterine perforation is less likely to happen with the flexible plastic cannula used in menstrual extraction. Often, no dilation is necessary for the 6mm cannula used before seven weeks LMP. Surgery or rarely hysterectomy may be needed in the event of uterine perforation.

3. Cut or torn cervix. (1 out of 100 clinical MVAs) Often a tenaculum is used to hold the cervix in a clinical setting. The tenaculum is sharp and can cut the cervix. Using a ring or sponge forceps makes cervical laceration less likely. Rarely stitches are needed to repair a torn cervix.

4. Pelvic infection. Introduction of bacteria into the uterus is the cause of pelvic infection. Infection is a complication that occurs in 5% of clinical abortions. To help prevent infection, follow the no touch technique, monitor for high temperature and low blood pressure, and avoid introducing anything into the vagina for three weeks after the procedure (see Post-Abortion Care). If signs of infection present, seek immediate medical attention and antibiotics. Antibiotics usually clear up the infection. In rare cases, a repeat procedure, hospitalization or surgery is required.

5. Hemorrhage. Hemorrhaging is defined as filling three or more thick pads in three hours or less. This requires immediate emergency medical care. Rarely, an MVA, medication, surgery, or blood transfusion may be required.

6. Hematometra. Uterus becomes distended with blood and clots. When a bimanual exam (see Appendix C) is done the

uterus often feels larger than before the procedure and extremely tender. Hematometra requires that the uterus be re-aspirated. Regular uterine massage after the menstrual extraction procedure can help prevent hematometra.

7. Unrecognized ectopic pregnancy. An ultrasound can diagnose an ectopic pregnancy. After a menstrual extraction, the absence of villi or gestational sac in the expelled contents may indicate a possible ectopic pregnancy. Most ectopic pregnancies present serious symptoms of extreme appendicitis-like pain before 9 weeks LMP.

8. Death. (1 out of 100,000 clinical abortions) Death rarely occurs in abortion; however the risks of self-induced abortion are significantly greater than an abortion in a clinical setting. Childbirth is more risky than clinical abortion up to 20 weeks LMP.

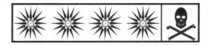

Menstrual Extraction Basics

Menstrual extraction requires careful practice and memorization of the steps of the procedure. Practice of menstrual extraction can be simulated through the use of a ripe papaya to simulate a uterus.[96] The papaya is held still by a partner, and all the steps of menstrual extraction are practiced. A roll of paper may be taped to the papaya to simulate the vagina, and 'no touch technique' can be practiced.

The 'no touch technique' is a technique of menstrual extraction which reduces the risk of infection from cross contamination of the cannula or dilators. With the 'no touch technique' any sterile items that will enter the unsterile vaginal cavity (dilators or cannulas) are not allowed to touch anything except the cervical os. Slowly and carefully with a steady hand the dilators and cannulas are introduced into the vagina (held open with a speculum) without touching anything but the cervical os.

Once comfortable with the procedure with a papaya, practice can be expanded to include women who wish to have their menstruations removed. Only then, after repeated practice, should any group attempt menstrual extraction for the purpose of abortion.

Careful sterilization of all equipment (see Appendix F), washing of hands, wearing sterile gloves, and practice of no touch technique will help prevent infection of the uterus during the menstrual extraction procedure.

Necessary Items for Menstrual Extraction:

1. Del-EM™, MVA syringe, or Mityvac™ hand vacuum pump kit with gauge:

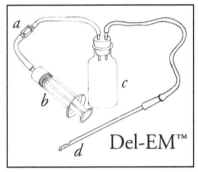

The Del-EM™, invented by Lorraine Rothman in 1971, is a simple construction made from widely available materials:

a – Check valve
b – Syringe
c – Collection jar
d – Karman cannula

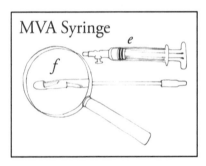

The MVA Syringe is a single use disposable locking plastic syringe attached to a plastic Karman Cannula. MVA syringes are widely used in clinical settings to perform first trimester abortions.

e – Plastic MVA syringe
f – Karman cannula (magnified)

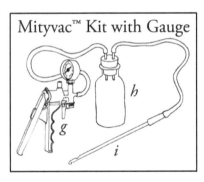

The Mityvac™ hand vacuum pump with gauge, also called a brake bleeder, is available online and at some automotive part stores (see Resources).

g - Mityvac™ hand vacuum pump with gauge.
h – Collection Jar
i – Karman cannula

2. Karman cannula set with sizes ranging from 3 – 14 mm.
3. Ring or sponge forceps.
4. Sterile gloves.
5. A few sterile towels and a cookie sheet or tray.
6. Iodine disinfectant solution and sterile cotton balls.
7. A sterile speculum.
8. Paracetamol, acetaminophen (optional).
9. Antibiotics, preventative regime (see Appendix I).
10. Large pot of boiling water or a pressure cooker to sterilize cannulas and forceps. (See Appendix F).
11. Hydrogen peroxide.
12. Light source: Flashlight, headlamp, or swing arm drafting light.

Note: The Mityvac™ hand vacuum pump, although primarily used to bleed brakes on automobiles, is also sold for a variety of hobby applications. The gauge can be used to establish a specific amount of vacuum; this increases effectiveness and can help indicate if there is a clot blocking the cannula tip or a leak in a connection. An air embolism due to user error of the Del-EM™ is less likely with the Mityvac™, as these hand vacuum pumps are self contained. [97]

Menstrual Extraction Step by Step

1. The group participating in the procedure should be fully familiarized with the equipment and the procedure.

2. Dilate the cervix using pharmaceuticals; if necessary (see Appendix E).

3. Sterilize the cannulas, a tray, several towels, speculum, cotton balls, gloves, and forceps. Also, sterilize some items that can be used to clear a clot in the cannula, such as, a few opened paper clips. All other equipment need not be sterile, as it will

71

not be entering the uterus, however all equipment should be clean. (see Appendix F).

4. Remove tray sterilized from oven; using sterile gloves or forceps place sterile towel on tray. Using sterile forceps, place sterilized cannulas on toweled tray. Place sterile towel over tray holding sterile equipment. Place tray of sterile tools in a safe place near procedure area. Do not allow the tray to be disturbed or to sit for longer than two hours before use.

5. Thirty minutes prior to the procedure, an optional pain relieving medication and/or infection preventative antibiotic can be taken (see Appendix I).

6. Perform bi-manual pelvic exam to assess size and position of uterus; clean single use gloves may be worn to protect the assistant and patient from disease transfer, however gloves need not be sterile (see Appendix C).

7. Wash hands well:
   a. Remove all jewelry.
   b. Scrub all surfaces from fingertip to elbow for 30 seconds with antibacterial soap.
   c. Rinse from fingertip to elbows.
   d. Air dry or dry with a sterile towel, again fingertip to elbow.
   e. Do not allow hands to come in contact with objects that are not disinfected or sterile.
   f. If hands touch a contaminated surface, repeat washing of hands.

8. Carefully put on sterile gloves.

9. Speculum can be inserted. Ideally, the woman having the procedure should have the knowledge and ability to insert her own speculum (see Appendix D).

10. Use a sterile cotton ball or gauze, saturated with iodine solution, held with sterile forceps. Antiseptic iodine solution is applied liberally to entire vagina, speculum surfaces, cervix, and cervical os. Do this three times, each time with a fresh sterile cotton swab, starting at the os and working out to outer vaginal lips and speculum.

11. Slowly and gently grasp cervix (in the 10 or 12 o'clock position) with sterile instrument, either ring forceps or tenaculum.

12. Dilate cervical os with smaller cannulas (4 - 5 mm), as necessary. Use the 'no touch technique' for cannula insertion. Grasp the cannula at the base with sterile gloves and very carefully insert 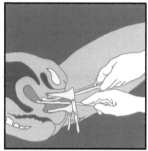 the cannula tip without touching anything else before contact with the cervical os.

13. A 6 mm cannula is usually adequate for pregnancies up to six or seven weeks LMP. The cannula should fit snuggly into the os. Rotate the cannula slightly at the inner os (sometimes known as the cervical canal) to help the cannula pass into the uterus. Note the measurement on the cannula as it passes through the inner os into the uterus.

14. The marks on the cannula indicate centimeters. Move the cannula slowly forward into the uterus until the back of the uterus (the fundus) is touched, but not more than 10 cm. A non-pregnant uterine cavity measures approximately 4 cm.

The cervix itself can have up to a 3 cm length, depending on the number of children a woman has had. A measurement of 8 cm or more (from the back of the uterus to cervical os) usually indicates pregnancy.

15. Establish vacuum. Blood and tissue will begin to flow into the tubing. One source suggests establishing a vacuum of at least 26 in. Hg. (660 mm), for all first trimester vacuum aspirations.[98] Another source[99] calculates the necessary cannula size and amount of vacuum based on the age of the pregnancy:

Weeks LMP	Size of Cannula	In./Hg of Vacuum
4	4 mm	6.3 in. (160 mm)
5	5 mm	7.8 in. (200 mm)
6	6 mm	9.4 in. (240 mm)
7	7 mm	11 in. (280 mm)
8	8 mm	12.6 in.(320 mm)
9	9 mm	14.2 in. (360 mm)
10	10 mm	15.7 in. (400 mm)

16. Gently push the cannula to the fundus. Rotate slightly while pulling back carefully (not past the noted inner os mark). Repeatedly stroke in and out, attempting to reach all parts of the inner uterus while carefully making one rotation of 360 degrees. Repeat if necessary, feeling for areas that feel smooth rather than rough.

17. Pause and empty the collection jar as necessary. Empty contents into a strainer and then a clear baking dish with a small amount of saline/water or vinegar/water solution added.

18. When the evacuation is complete, the person holding the cannula will feel a grating sensation on the uterine lining. The uterus may grip the cannula tightly. Red or pink foam (no tissue) may be seen in the cannula.

19. Release vacuum pressure before removing the cannula.

20. Place the cannula on the sterile tray until the procedure is determined complete.

21. To check for completion:

    a.   Inspect Tissue

          i. Wash the aspired tissue and blood in a fine mesh metal strainer under running water to separate blood and clots.

         ii. Transfer remaining tissue in the strainer into a clear glass dish containing ½ in. (1 cm) of water or saline solution.

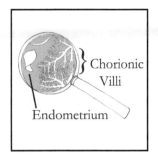

Utilize a light behind the dish to help see the products of conception, which should include chorionic villi and fetal membrane, and after nine weeks LMP, fetal parts. The chorionic villi appear feathery and white, while the endometrium is smooth and transparent.

    b.   Perform a bimanual pelvic exam to check size and firmness of the uterus.

          i. A smaller and firm uterus combined with observation of all expected products of conception in aspirated tissue indicates complete evacuation. (See Post-Abortion Care).

ii. Repeat procedure if uterus is still soft and has not reduced in size or if there is persistent brisk bleeding indicating an incomplete evacuation.

Troubleshooting Menstrual Extraction

Cervix is not visible after speculum insertion.	• Inadequate lighting. • Wrong size speculum. • Cervix above or below speculum, try inserting point of speculum and pointing slightly to the left or right, then straightening out speculum once it is halfway inserted.
Uterus backs away when insertion of cannula is attempted.	• Use ring forceps or tenaculum to hold uterus while cannula is inserted.
Cannula will not pass through cervical inner os.	• Dilate the cervix with smaller sterile cannula. • Use a light rotation at the inner os to ease passage. • Use a sterile lubricant on cannula tip (New unopened small pack of KY Jelly).
No movement or little movement of blood through cannula and tubing.	• Possible vacuum leak – check connections. • Clot clogging cannula tip. Try increasing vacuum a bit, if this does free clotted cannula tip, release vacuum, remove cannula and use a sterile object to clear the tip of cannula, then repeat procedure.

Cannula moves into uterus past the 10 cm mark.	• For most pregnancies prior to 7 weeks LMP, this would indicate uterine perforation Uterine perforation is very rare, but most likely to occur during dilation if metal instruments are used. • Stop procedure, release vacuum, remove cannula from uterus, and seek more information. If uterine perforation is suspected, medical care should be sought immediately. • More advanced pregnancy than expected. Careful pelvic examination will help determine gestational age.
No or only partial products of conception are seen.	• Not pregnant. • Complete abortion already occurred – review medical history. • Possible incomplete abortion, repeat procedure. • Abnormal uterus (possible double uterus). • Possible ectopic pregnancy. If ectopic pregnancy is suspected, medical care should be sought immediately. • Possible molar pregnancy.
Many air bubbles in cannula and tubing, and vacuum decreasing.	• Possible vacuum leak, check connections. • Pulling cannula too far out on pull stroke. • Cannula too small for cervix; increase size of cannula.

Part III   Alternative Self-Induced Abortion Methods

General Introduction

Alternative methods of self-induced abortion are documented in nearly every culture. Some alternative forms of abortion are ancient and some are more contemporary. Ancient methods of self-induced abortion include herbal, acupuncture, and massage. Contemporary alternative forms of abortion include homeopathic, yoga, and psychic. Alternative methods of self-induced abortion are generally believed to be more dangerous and less effective than modern methods of self-induced abortion based on clinical abortion procedures.

Many herbs have been documented as having abortifacient qualities, however much information regarding exact preparations and dosages has been lost. The herbs included in the herbal section that follows are the ones where sufficient information was gleaned from the historical and modern record to piece together the historical significance, the potential effects, and dosage ranges. Some of the information incorporates previously published work by Uni Tiamat,

78

Herbal Abortion: The Fruit of the Tree of Knowledge, published by Sage-femme! in 1994.

Acupuncture is an ancient method of abortion; however information on the techniques of acupuncture is only recently becoming available in western culture. Many significant acupuncture texts have yet to be translated into English.

Massage, as a form of self-induced abortion, is widely practiced in modern-day Asia and Africa, however, massage abortion has an ancient history.

Recent discoveries in self-induced abortion include homeopathy, yoga, and massage. Homeopathic abortive medicines are based on herbs that have a reputation as oxytocic abortifacients. The homeopathic medicines are highly diluted, yet are reputed to have a profound abortive effect with few negative side effects. Female yoga enthusiasts discovered fertility regulating aspects of postures that put significant pressure on the uterus. Psychic methods of self-induced abortion are part of healing modalities that incorporate the mind, body, and spirit.

Herbal Introduction

Knowledge of the abortifacient use of plants has been part of human knowledge for centuries. Sacred images of ancient abortifacient plants have persisted throughout centuries of civilization, even though knowledge about abortifacient use of plants has been largely forgotten.

Herbal abortifacients were considered sacred plants, closely connected to the after-life and the creator. Symbols of the plants became associated with the power of ancient Goddesses, and were worn during rites, used to decorate vessels, and used to decorate textiles. Many iconic images of abortifacient plants persist today, however their ancient symbolism is long forgotten. For example, Aristolochia, highly regarded as an abortifacient medicinal plant since ancient Egypt, was found depicted on a vase from Thebes.[100] Pomegranate, an abortifacient prevalent in many cultures, appears in ancient and contemporary art. Ancient hairpins carved from bone in the shape of a pomegranate have been found in Uzbekistan[101], and pomegranate is still featured on modern pottery vessels from Uzbekistan.[102] In Suzane embroidery from Tajikistan, the bride's wedding cloth is embroidered with the symbolic representation of a blossoming garden, at the center is a pomegranate.[103] Women in ancient Greece wore gold hellebore flower ornaments on their clothing.[104] The ancient decorative use of pineapple as a decorative motif has been dated to AD 200 in Peru on ancient pottery vessels.[105] The paisley decorative design is suggested as evolved from a representation of the dragon arum.[106]

The heart symbol has been suggested as having been derived from the shape of the seed of silphium, an abortifacient plant that grew on the shores of Cyrene, Africa two thousand years ago.[107] The silphium plant was so highly regarded as a fertility regulator that it was traded throughout the Mediterranean. Images of the heart-shaped silphium seeds and Umbelliferae silphium plants were placed on the coinage of Cyrene. Efforts to cultivate silphium failed, and as the supply dwindled, the price increased. The silphium plant became extinct due to over harvesting; however, the heart symbol lived on.

The use of abortifacient herbs has been constant for thousands of years and continues today. However, modern methods of clinical abortion are superior in their effectiveness, safety, and lack of negative side effects. Women seeking abortion should first seek out clinical methods of pregnancy termination if at all possible.

In areas where abortion is restricted or illegal, women will often act on rumor when faced with an unwanted pregnancy. Uninformed women have taken quinine[108] in repeated oral dosages

81

based simply on a whisper, often resulting in continued pregnancy and liver failure. Women have taken a lethal dose of pennyroyal oil for lack of knowledge.[109] Women have sought out back alley abortion providers who may or may not be able to provide a safe abortion, and women have even resorted to shooting themselves in the belly with a gun if other options are unavailable.[110]

Although all self-induced abortion methods are inherently dangerous, some options are less dangerous than others. The goal of this work is to educate women regarding the history, modern use, and possible side effects of many self-induced abortion methods, so that fewer women will mistakenly rely on a hunch when faced with terminating an unwanted pregnancy.

As the knowledge of the risks of certain self-induced abortion methods moves into the collective consciousness through the world-wide web and word of mouth, women become more knowledgeable regarding the most effective and safest methods of self-induced abortion. Uni Tiamat[111] cautioned women about the use of pennyroyal oil to cause abortion. Many women the world over give thanks to Tiamat and others, including: Susan Weed (books and online discussion forums), Sister Zeus (herbal abortion information), Lost Clown at AngryforaReason.blogspot.com (herbal abortion discussion), WomenOnWaves.org (medical abortion information), Rebecca Chalker and Carol Downer's book *Women's Book of Choices* (herbal abortion, medical abortion, and menstrual extraction information), and Hesperian.org (MVA information). Through the dedicated work of these women's rights advocates, better information on self-induced abortion has been made available to women in print and online, and pennyroyal oil poisoning has become very rare.

Abortifacient plants have not been exhaustively studied and are not completely understood in their actions, side effects, or effectiveness. Herbs used medicinally affect the entire body, not just the uterus. Many abortifacient herbs are known to have serious negative side effects. More research should be done.

A glossary of terms is included for the convenience of the reader (see Glossary).

Dosage ranges listed for herbs have been averaged by the author from several sources. The dosages are listed for educational purposes only. Each woman is unique in her body composition, constitution, and sensitivity. No single dosage recommendation is appropriate for every woman, so no woman should act on such information without appropriate professional medical advice after a thorough examination of the facts of her particular situation (See Appendix G).

Of the plants listed, green papaya and fresh cotton root bark stand out for their reputation of having few negative side effects and of being effective to induce abortion beyond the first few weeks of pregnancy. Homeopathic preparations and psychic abortion methods also seem promising. However, further research may bring more light to these abortion inducers. They may have negative side effects that are yet to be discovered, so each woman should do her own research on the latest findings to supplement the data presented in this book.

83

Chart of Herbal Abortifacients/Common Effects Key:

R.E. = Reputed Effectiveness
LMP= Last Menstrual Period

 Hormonal Effects

The following symbols are listed under 'Hormonal Effects':

Symbols	Effects
+BF	Increases Blood Flow to Uterus
+E	Increases Estrogen
-E	Reduces Estrogen
D	Dopamines
-FSH	Reduces Follicle Stimulating Hormone
II	Inhibits Implantation
+LH	Increases Lutienizing Hormone
+O	Increases Oxytocin
+P	Increases Progesterone
-P	Reduces Progesterone
+PG	Increases Prostaglandins
-PG	Reduces Prostaglandins
-PL	Inhibits Prolactin
UC	Contracts Uterus
UR	Relaxes Uterus
+T	Increases Testosterone

 Kidney and/or Liver Toxic

 Phototoxic

 Death associated with use.

 Contains Thujone

 Can Affect the Heart

 Cathartic Purgative

84

Herbal Abortifacient Chart 1 of 2	L M P	R. E.	Hormonal Effects	Liver/ kidney	Photo toxic	Death	Thujone	Heart	Purge
Aloe	6	**	+BF, +E(mild)	•		•			•UC
Angelica	6	**	+ E, +P, +O(UC).	•	•			•	
Arbor vitae	8	**					•UC	•	•UC
Arum	NA	**		•		•		•	
Avocado	8	**	UC, D, +T, -E.			•			
Barrenwort	6	**	D, +T, -E, UR, +BF.						
Birthwort	4	**	Effects pituitary, UC, II.	•		•			•
Black Cohosh	4	**	UR,+BF, +E, -LH.	•					
Black Hellebore	NA	*				•		•	•
Blue Cohosh	6	**	+O, UC, +BF, +E, -LH.	•		•		•	
Castor	6	**	+E, UC.	•		•			•UC
Chamomile	4	**					•UC	•	
Chaste tree	6	**	II, D, -E, +PL,+P, +LH.						
Cotton root bark	12	** *	+O (UC), II, +E, -P.						
Daphne	15	**	-P, +PG (UC).			•			•
Dittany	12	**	UC, II, +PG.		•				
Garlic	6	**	UC, +E, +PG.						
Ginger	4	**	+E,+BF.				•UC	•	
Hibiscus	6	**	-E, -FSH, II.						

Herbal Abortifacient Chart 2 of 2	L M P	R. E.	Hormonal Effects	Liver/ kidney	Photo toxic	Death	Thujone	Heart	Purge
Horseradish	6	**							
Juniper	12	**	UR, II, +BF.			•	•UC	•	
Lupine	15	**	UC.			•			
Male fern	NA	**		•		•		•	•UC
Mistletoe	8	**	UR, UC, +BF.			•		•	
Mugwort	4	**	+BF, +E.				•UC	•	
Nutmeg	NA	*	+O(UC).			•		•	
Onion	6	**	UC, +E, -P, -PG.						
Papaya	12	** *	UC, -P, -E.	•				•	
Parsley	8	**	Effects pituitary, +O(UC).	•	•	•			
Pennyroyal	8	**	+BF, +O(UC).	•		•			
Pineapple	5	**	II, +E.	•	•	•			•UC
Pomegranate	6	**	UC, +E						
Queen Anne's Lace	4	**	II, -P,+E.	•					
Rosemary	4	**	II, +E.	•		•	•UC	•	
Rue	12	**	II, +O(UC).	•	•	•		•	
Saffron	10	**	+BF, +E.			•			
Squirting Cucumber	NA	**				•			•UC
Stoneseed	4	** *	-P, II, -E.	•					
Tansy	6	**	+BF.		•	•	•UC	•	
Wild Ginger	6	**	UC, +E.	•		•			•

Aloe Vera
Aloe socotrina

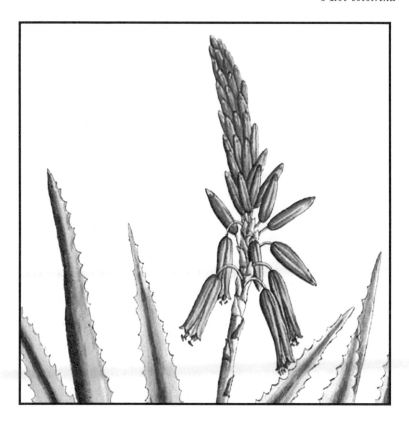

Aloe...is a powerful cathartic, acting particularly on the large intestine, its active principle being termed aloin. Its action is extremely variable, and in large doses it has been known to induce abortion.

- Encyclopedia of Americana, 1918

87

Family Liliaceae

AKA: Aloe vera and burn plant.

Part Used: Fresh leaves, dries leaves, and dried latex.

Medicinal Properties: Anthelmintic, cathartic, demulcent, emmenagogue, estrogenic (mild), oxytocic, purgative, and sedative.

Effects on the Body: Internally: Purges intestines, promotes bile flow, and expels worms. Externally: Antifungal, soothes and heals burns and irritations.

Abortifacient Action: Gastrointestinal Irritation and uterine contraction.

Contains: Phytoestrogen beta-sitosterol and several anthraquinone glycosides: aloin, isobarbaloin, and aloe emodin.

Description: Aloe is a succulent perennial, having grass-green to olive-brown fleshy, long, and narrow leaf blades with spiny teeth running up the sides. New leaves emerge from the center of the aloe plant. Aloe's stem is usually short with strong fibrous roots. Most indoor aloes never bloom, but when growing in their native hot, arid regions, aloes send up 3 ft. (1 m) stalks from which bright yellow to scarlet 1 in. (2.5 cm) tubular flowers bloom in simple or branching clusters from June to September.

Note: *Agave americana* is sometimes called American aloe. Do not confuse American aloe *Agave americana* with true aloe *Aloe socotrina*. They are chemically different.

Aloe Herbal Lore and Historical Use

Many spiritual legends surround the aloe plant. In one legend, aloe is the only plant to come directly from the Garden of Eden.[112] The Mohammedans of Egypt hung the sacred aloe above their doorways to protect the owners against evil. To the Egyptians, aloe was a medicinal plant and a major element in their embalming processes. Nicodemus is said to have purchased a quantity of aloe for the burial of Christ.[113] The ancient Greeks gathered aloe on the island of Socotia as early as the fourth century BC.[114] Aloe was introduced and cultivated in the West Indies and other tropical countries around the 16th century. In Mexico and Columbia, an aloe, called Sabila Sagrada 'the sacred initiate,' is still a magical medicinal plant. The Sabila Sagrada is thought to be home to a goddess who, through offerings and prayers, can be put in a generous mood. Health, wealth, and peace are some of the gifts she is said to give.[115]

Aloe vera, the first-aid plant, is seen on the kitchen windowsills of homes all over the world. Used on a sudden burn to the skin, an aloe leaf's soothing, cell-rejuvenating viscous gel is legendary. Today, farmers commercially cultivate aloe in the Black Sea coastal area and the Caribbean and sell their product around the world to pharmaceutical companies, cosmetic companies, and health food stores. Dried aloe is an ingredient of compound tincture of benzoin, a pharmaceutical product used externally on minor wounds and ulcers as an antiseptic and protective. Many cosmetic companies employ aloe in their skin lotions and hair products. Health food stores stock aloe medicines for their healing use externally and internally. Internally, aloe, in juice and powdered form, is taken for amenorrhea, asthma, colds, convulsions, hemorrhages, to expel pinworms, for ulcers, and most popularly as a purgative for the lower bowels.

In addition, aloe taken internally is often used to promote suppressed or obstructed menstruation. In China[116] and Malaysia,[117] the infusion of the fresh aloe vera leaf is taken orally to encourage menstruation. This same preparation is documented as being used to induce abortion in Samoa.[118] In Nepal[119] and South Korea,[120] the whole aloe plant is used in decoction to induce abortion. In Trinidad[121] and in the West Indies,[122] the gum from aloe is taken orally as an abortifacient. Europeans are known to have historically taken the extract of aloe in wine as an abortifacient.[123] Studies have shown aloe vera stimulates uterine contractions.[124]

Gathering: Aloe's lowest leaves are the most mature and are harvested first. Commercially, the juices of healthy aloes that have had at least two to three years of uninterrupted growth are harvested by cutting the leaves off close to the stem. The yellow juice that exudes is then drained off into containers. The yellow aloe juice becomes more concentrated through evaporation or by boiling. When cold, the honey-like aloe extract solidifies.

Preparation: Aloe's abortifacient action results from gastrointestinal irritation. The medicinal components of aloe (aloin and aloe-emodin) are slow in action, beginning to act approximately 10 - 15 hours after ingestion. To moderate the tendency for aloe to excessively irritate the intestines, dosage of carminatives can be taken with aloe and taken again ten to fifteen hours after ingestion. Angelica, chamomile, ginger, juniper, rosemary, sage, and thyme are carminatives that also have abortifacient properties. Aloe as an abortifacient is reputed to be most effective if used during the first six weeks of pregnancy.

Words to the Wise: Aloe has caused occasional death when a concentrated form of aloe was injected into a tumor or the bloodstream to treat cancer. People suffering from hemorrhoids or degeneration of the liver or gall bladder should not use aloe. Internally, aloe is a cathartic purgative, meaning that aloe irritates the lower bowels. After two weeks, if the desired effect is not produced, one should stop use. Chronic use of aloe may induce hemorrhoids and inflame the kidneys. A large number of inferior aloe products are on the market. It is best to obtain fresh aloe leaves, if possible.

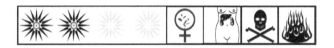

Watch for Signs of Toxicity Specific to Aloe: Severe intestinal pain and red colored urine. As always, reduce dosage at first sign of toxicity. A strong carminative tea, perhaps made from simmering sliced Asian ginger in water, will help to moderate intestinal pain.

Aloe Vera Dosage

Abortifacient Aloe Tea: 3 oz. (85 g) fresh aloe leaves sliced to 1 qt.

> (1 L) water, heat to boiling, strain, and to temper the bitterness add 1 oz. (28 g) sugar. Take early in the morning.

Powdered Extract: 1 - 2 #0 capsules, two to three times a day.

Emmenagogual Aloe Fumigation: Aloe juice is recommended in
steam fumigations, often in combination with a tincture of
myrrh for emmenagogual, contraceptive, and anticancer
purposes. Use one fresh mashed leaf of aloe with twenty
drops of myrrh tincture placed in steaming water. Fumigate
for 20 - 30 minutes, once a day, for two to five days before
expected menses.

Angelica

Angelica atropurpurea (American)
Angelica archangelica (European)
Angelica sinensis (Chinese)

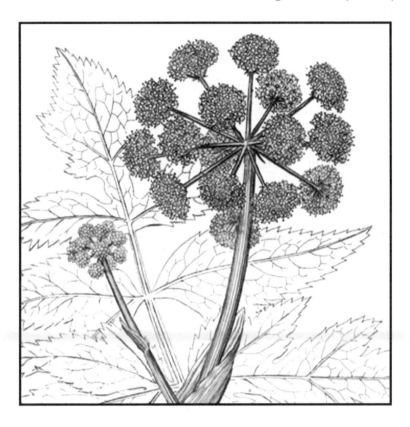

For unmarry'd women [with]
suppression of the courses...take
belly-ache root [angelica] a week before
you expect to be out of order, repeat
the same two days after, the next morning drink
a quarter of a pint of pennyroyal water.

-*Everyman his Own Doctor: The Poor Planter's Physician*, 1763

93

Family Umbelliferae

AKA: Angelica, wild celery, archangel, bellyache root, masterwort, dead nettle, purple angelica, and dong quai.

Parts Used: Root, leaves, flower tops, and seeds.

Medicinal Properties: Leaves and Flower tops: Aromatic, antimutagenic, antiseptic, carminative, diaphoretic, diuretic, and stimulant. Root and seeds: Abortifacient, antimutagenic, anti-spasmodic, carminative, diaphoretic, diuretic, emmenagogue, expectorant, and stomachic.

Effects on the Body: Soothes digestive and respiratory system, stimulates circulation and heart, and regulates menses. Angelica can relax or contract smooth muscle, depending on preparation.

Abortifacient Action: Estrogenic and oxytocic.

Contains: Abortifacient chemicals beta-bisabolene and phytoestrogen beta-sitosterol.

Description: Angelica is tall 4 - 9 ft. (1.3 – 2.7 m) with a 3 ft. (1 m) spread. It is biennial, with white to green sweet-smelling flowers, blooming from June to August in large globe-shaped umbels, 2 – 6 in. (5 – 15 cm) across. Angelica flowers are followed by oblong seedpods each containing two yellow winged seeds that have a licorice-like flavor. Angelica has a smooth, hollow, sometimes-purple stem and pinnate compound leaves with three coarsely toothed oval leaflets that are sometimes further divided into three or five. The root is branched, 3 - 6 in. (7.5 - 15 cm) long and less than an inch (2.5 cm) in diameter. Angelica is seen growing in or near steam banks, marshes, moist fields, and mountain brooks.

Angelica Herbal Lore and Historical Use

Angelica's use by women to treat menstrual irregularities is widespread. A North American variety of angelica, *Angelica atropurpurea,* 'root tonic' was used by Native American Cherokee women for obstructed menses.[125] The early woman colonists from Europe are recorded as having used angelica root decoction's strong emmenagogual properties to promote menstrual flow and produce abortion. *Angelica sinensis,* dong quai, sometimes called 'female ginseng,' has been used since the dawn of history by Chinese wise-women as a tonic for nearly all gynecological problems. Angelica root decoction syrup is used by midwives who give a tablespoon dose after childbirth. The placenta is said to arrive 10 minutes later.[126] European *Angelica archangelica* has been used as a uterine stimulant, as well, to remedy prolonged labor and retention of the placenta.

Spiritually, angelica has been held to be significant in many cultures. *Angelica archangelica* is native to Northern Europe. Its Christianized name, meaning 'angelic herb,' hints at angelica's ancient use in Nordic medicine.[127] Blooming around May 8th, the feast day of St. Michael the Archangel, this angelica came to be known as the root of the Holy Ghost. Its properties are said to have been revealed to a Catholic monk by the Holy Ghost and have the power to protect against evil spirits, witchcraft, poisons and plague. Interestingly, babies conceived as a result of sexual orgies were said to be begotten by the Holy Ghost.[128] Mothers, in the European Dark Ages, made protective necklaces of angelica leaves for their children to wear. Native Americans of the Arkansas tribe mixed the indigenous angelica root with their ceremonial tobacco.

Chinese herbal research scientist, Kee Chang Huang, notes the water soluble component of the dong quai, *Angelica sinensis*, root causes stimulation of the uterus, while the alcohol soluble essential oil exerts an inhibiting or relaxing effect on the uterus. In addition, the alcohol-soluble essential oil has been found to increase DNA synthesis in the uterine tissue and increase the uterine tissue's growth.[129] In alcohol preparations, like tinctures and fluid extracts, dong quai is especially valued in dysmenorrhea (painful menstruation) associated with anemia and in treatments designed to relax the uterus. In decoctions, where the essential oil is allowed to evaporate, dong quai is valued as a uterine contraction stimulant, and is used to regulate menstruation and to release a fully adhered placenta after childbirth.

Angelica has been shown through scientific research to stimulate endometrial secretions, increasing heparin, lysozyme, and capillary blood volume in the uterus.[130] Studies have shown the hot water decoction of angelica to be a uterine stimulant.[131] The water decoction of angelica root, administered intravenously to pregnant dogs and rabbits was abortifacient.[132] Conversely, the dried root of angelica has been suggested through scientific study as a fertility promoter for both women and men.[133] In addition, research on angelica has shown anti-cancer properties and liver protective aspects.[134]

Gathering: Angelica has a two to three year growing cycle. Rarely is the plant mature enough to gather roots in the first year. Roots are best gathered in late autumn, winter, or early spring while the sap is low during the second or third year of growth. Thorough drying of angelica roots eliminates their poisonous qualities that, when fresh, cause irritating reactions in many people. Angelica stems can be eaten fresh or cooked like celery; when gathered in the spring. Angelica leaves are best gathered from summer to autumn in the morning after the dew has dried. Angelica seeds are gathered when ripe. Note: If gathering angelica, always use an accurate field guide. If in doubt, do not collect. Many members of the Umbelliferae family are highly poisonous and all can be easily mistaken for each other.

Preparation: Angelica's uterine contracting root decoction, used throughout time to tone the uterus and stimulate contractions, is probably the most effective abortive angelica preparation. The root must be simmered for several hours to release as much essential oil as possible. Angelica is often used as a simple, meaning used alone, not combined with other herbs. Angelica, as an abortifacient, is most effective if used within the first six weeks of pregnancy.

Words to the Wise: Angelica is estrogenic. Estrogenic herbs contain estrogen-like substances, which act to produce the effects of the female sex hormone estrogen. Estrogenic herbs can cause estrogen-like side effects: abnormal blood clotting, liver problems, and may encourage the growth of estrogen-dependent tumors. Estrogenic herbs should be avoided by anyone taking birth control pills, estrogen medications, or blood pressure medications. Estrogenic herbs may not be as effective for premenopausal women. Estrogenic substances are known teratogens.

Angelica may make the menses heavier. In addition, angelica may raise blood sugar levels. People who have a history of diabetes or heart attacks should not use angelica. Angelica contact can cause dermatitis. Persons with a history of allergic sensitivity to plants should wear long gloves when gathering. All persons taking angelica should stay out of the sun. Phototoxic chemicals in Angelica, called psoralens, produce a rash in people who take them and subsequently expose themselves to sunlight. Some people who take angelica in the evening experience insomnia.

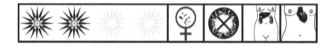

Watch for Signs of Toxicity Specific to Angelica: Stomach pain, nausea, diarrhea, dilated pupils, labored breathing, weak and rapid pulse, and frothing at the mouth and convulsions.

Angelica Dosage

Abortifacient Angelica Decoction (root): Simmer ¼ cup (60 g) cut
        root to 1 qt (1 L) water three hours, drink throughout the day,
        and take no longer than six days.

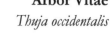

Arbor Vitae
Thuja occidentalis

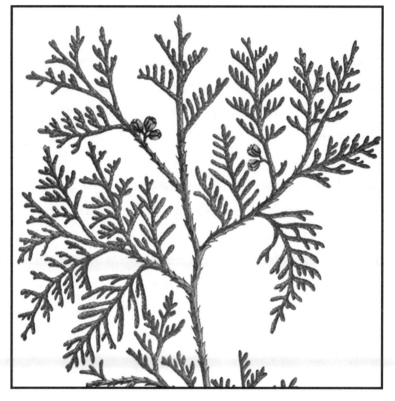

It is asserted that thuja has brought on abortion, acting not so much as
a direct abortivant, but as a gastro-intestinal irritant, producing
violent intestinal disturbances, giving rise, indirectly to miscarriage.

-King's American Dispensatory, 1905

Family Cupressaceae

AKA: Arbor vitae, tree of life, hack-ma-tack, eastern white cedar, swamp cedar, Atlantic red cedar, and feather leaf cedar.

Parts Used: Dried branch tips and leaves.

Medicinal Properties: Anthelmintic, anticancer, anti-inflammatory, antimicrobial, antiviral, astringent, diuretic, emmenagogue, expectorant, irritant, laxative, purgative, and muscle stimulant.

Effects on the Body: Stimulating to circulatory, eliminatory, and reproductive organs.

Abortifacient Action: Contains uterine contracting thujone.

Contains: Camphor-like essential oil (abortifacient), fenchone, thujone, carvone, and Vitamin C.

Description: Arbor vitae, often reaching heights of 60 ft. (18 m) with a 3 – 6 ft. (1 – 2 m) diameter trunk, is a member of the great cypress family. Fragrant scale-like yellow-green leaves cover the flat twigs. Arbor vitae cones are 4 – 6 in. (10 – 15 cm) long, with broad winged seeds. Arbor vitae's bark is deep reddish brown. This attractive cedar, one of the most widely distributed of all conifers, is grown in temperate climates around the world. In North America, arbor vitae is found growing in swampy areas and along stream banks from Eastern Quebec to Manitoba, south to New Jersey, and along the Allegheny mountains to North Carolina and Tennessee, and stretching westward through to Minnesota. In the Adirondack Mountains, arbor vitae can be found as high as 3500 ft. (1067 m).

Arbor-Vitae Herbal Lore and Historical Use

The use of arbor vitae in ceremonial ritual dates back to the beginning of recorded history. Over two thousand years ago, the Sumerians of Mesopotamia believed cedar was the cosmic tree or the tree of life and was held to have magical properties. In ancient Greece, cedar wood was burned at ancient sacrifice altars. The genus name Thuja 'to fumigate' is rooted in the Latin *thuo*, meaning 'to sacrifice'. The ancient surname of the moon-goddess Artemis (protector of women and alleviator of suffering in childbirth) was Artemis Cedreatis, cedar was symbolic of the womb of the Great Mother, and images of Artemis were hung in tall cedars.

In Chinese mythology, cedars were known as 'the trees of faithful loves,' named after a couple who were divided by a king who wished to have the woman for himself. The husband died in grief after being imprisoned, while the woman jumped to her death to escape the hateful attentions of the monarch. The king ordered the two to be buried separately, however a cedar tree sprung from each grave rising to such immense height that the roots and branches of the two trees interlaced at last.

Hippocrates recommended cedar as a vaginal fumigation for uterine prolapse in ancient times. Aristotle, in *Historia Animalium*, mentions oil of cedar used as a contraceptive when combined with olive oil and applied to the vagina. The essential oil of cedar made from the leaves and twigs contains thujone and is known to be a muscular stimulant of the uterus and heart muscle.

Wherever arbor vitae grew the Native Americans used it. The use of arbor vitae in the creation of bows, baskets, canoes, cording,

101

hats, and roofing by Native Americans is documented in *The Original Journal of Lewis and Clark*. Aromatic arbor vitae twigs were ritually placed on hot rocks during a sweat bath as ceremonial incense. Arbor vitae's branches were used by many tribes to make medicinal teas for women's menstrual complaints, male prostate disorders, and to promote perspiration in fevers. Menominee women used an infusion of the dried inner bark of arbor vitae to promote menstruation.[135] To induce abortion, some Native American women used decoctions of arbor vitae branches.[136] The oil, a potent antiviral, was taken both internally and externally for warts. Several Native American tribes used arbor vitae for cancer of the uterus.[137]

Gathering: Leafy young arbor vitae twigs are gathered in the spring. Bark is generally collected off branches that are at least two years old in early spring or late fall when the bark peels easiest. Preparation: Purgative arbor vitae is thought to produce abortion by reflex action on the uterus from gastrointestinal irritation. Carminatives combined with arbor vitae may be helpful in alleviating excessive gastrointestinal pain. Arbor vitae is usually used by itself as a simple up to the eighth week of pregnancy.

Words to the Wise: Do not use arbor vitae's essential oil, commonly called oil of cedar, internally. As with all essential oils, arbor vitae's essential oil is highly concentrated. Sixteen drops of the oil has caused unconsciousness, spasms, and convulsions[138] People with heart conditions or history of heart attack should not use arbor vitae in any

102

form. Arbor vitae contain both fenchone and thujone, which stimulate the heart muscle.

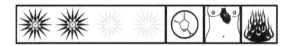

Watch for Signs of Toxicity Specific to *Thuja occidentalis*: Arbor vitae's essential oil has been known to cause heart stimulation, flatulence, and distortion of the stomach, spasms, convulsions, and unconsciousness.

Arbor Vitae Dosage

Abortifacient Arbor Vitae Decoction: 1 oz. (28 g) fresh leaf twigs to
> 2 cups (500 ml) of water. Simmer until the water begins to turn brown. Then, take 1 tsp. - 1 Tbs. (5 - 15 ml), three to six times a day.

Emmenagogual Arbor Vitae Steam Fumigation: Decoction of fresh
> leaves and twigs and/or 2 - 5 drops of the essential oil, use daily for four to five days prior to expected menses.

Arum

Arum dracunculus

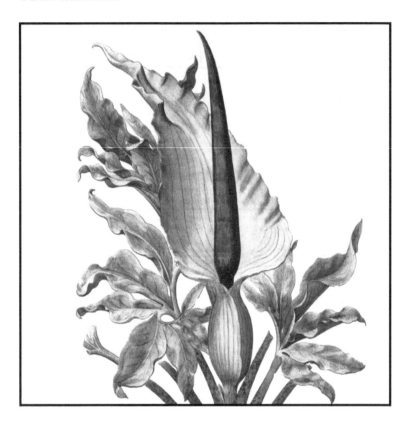

These are all plants that grow, all flowers in God's Land, which were found
by his majesty when he proceeded to Upper Retenu to subdue the country
there according to the command of his father, Amun, who
put them beneath his sandals from the year one to myriads of years.

- Inscription on the botanical room of Tuthmosis III in the
Temple of Amun at Karnak in ancient Thebes, 1500 BC.
(*Arum dracunculus* is depicted there.)

Family Araceae

AKA: Adderwort, dragon flower, snake plant, dragon arum, voodoo lily, viagra lily, stink lily, lords and ladies, and cuckoo pint.

Parts Used: seeds, and fragrance of flower.

Medicinal Properties: Abortifacient.

Effects on the Body: Irritating and acrid.

Abortifacient Action: Possibly embryo toxic.

Contains: Dimethyl oligosulphides.

Description: *Arum dracunculus* attains a height of approximately 2 – 3 ft. (1 m). The leaves are large, and the stalks and the stems are pink with black mottling. The midsummer carrion flowers are composed of a burgundy red spathe with wavy edges and a very dark red spadix.

Great Arum Herbal Lore and Historical Use[a]

Arum was used in ancient times by farmers to gauge a season's fertility. Being one of the first plants to appear in the spring, the size of the arum's spadix was used to estimate the size of the harvest for that year.[139] The ancient Greek physician Dioscorides noted the abortive use of *Arum dracunculus* in 50 BC. Later a myth developed, that when a dragon is slain, wherever the dragon's blood touches the ground, 'dragon arum' sprouts. Ironically, the myth is not far from the truth, as the arum carrion flowers are believed to have evolved to resemble in color, texture, and odor of decaying animals to attract flies as pollinators. The foul smell of arum flower is reputed to

---

[a] The purpose of this book is to recapture information about historical approaches to self-induced abortion. Arum has been included; however the reader must keep in mind that deaths have resulted from ingestion of arum.

abort a newly conceived embryo, which seems hard to believe, but recent studies have shown an increased risk of miscarriage in women who are exposed to inhaled sulphide chemicals.[140] The volatile chemicals emitted by dragon arum flowers to attract pollinating insects are dimethyl oligosulphides.

Sulphur has an ancient reputation as an abortive fumigant. Sulfur has the ability to cause blood to not clot as readily. Dioscorides in his *Materia Medica* prescribed sulphur fumigation to expel a fetus. Onions and garlic contain sulphur and also have a reputation as abortifacients. An 8th century Sanskrit text instructs women wishing to induce abortion to sit over a pot of stewed onions.[141]

Gathering: *Arum dracunculus* grows wild in Crete. The plant parts are gathered in midsummer and the seeds in the fall.

Preparation: Arum would probably be most effective in early pregnancy when teratogenic agents have more influence on the growing fetus.

Words to the wise: *Arum dracunculus* does NOT have a modern medicinal herb record. There are no scientific studies on the possible effects of *Arum dracunculus* internally. Laboratory tests have indicated that inhaled sulfur derivatives can cause serious vascular damage in veins of the brain, the heart, and the kidneys.

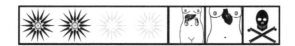

Watch for signs of Toxicity Specific to *Arum dracunculus:* Inhaled sulfides can cause eye irritation, sore throat, coughing, and fluid in the lungs. Inhalation of the fragrance of *Arum dracunculus* flowers has caused dizziness, headache, and vomiting.

Great Arum Dosage

Arum Abortifacient Drink*: 30 *Arum dracunculus* seeds in 4 oz.
(125 ml) of wine. [142]

*Signs of toxicity for internal consumption of the seeds of arum are unknown. Extreme caution!

Avocado

Persea americana

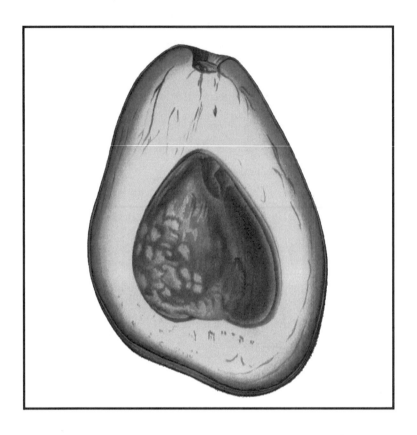

A ha, I only plant them and look!
And LOOK what happens.
They plant more and they plant more.
It is the avocado tree that my father planted, and
I am going to plant it again and again!

-Aztec metaphor[143]

Family Lauraceae

AKA: Aguacate, palta, abacate, ahuacatl, and alligator pear.

Parts Used: Shoots, young leaves, and seeds.

Medicinal Properties: Abortifacient, astringent, carminative, and emmenagogue.

Effects on the Body: Reduces bood sugar and interferes with normal lactation.

Abortifacient Action: Uterine contraction, dopamines may interfere in ovarian hormones, and embryo toxic.

Contains: Volatile oil (methylchavicol, alpha-pinene), tryamine (oxytocic), serotonin (oxytocic), dopamines, flavonoids, and tannins.

Description: The avocado is a vigorous tropical tree, often reaching over 30 ft. (9 m) in height. The avocado tree's dark green leaves are glossy. The pear-shaped avocado fruit is a familiar edible and is commercially grown for distribution around the world. Flesh is pale yellow to yellow green, buttery with a unique, rich, and creamy flavor. The avocado, indigenous to Central and South America, is grown around the world in warm climates. There are many varieties of avocado.

Avocado Herbal Lore and Historical Use[b]

Avocados have an ancient history as a human food, possibly as far back as 5000 BC. Avocado seeds have been found buried with Incan mummies dating to 800 BC. The avocado fruit, although

---

[b] The purpose of this book is to recapture information about historical approaches to self-induced abortion. Avocado has been included; however the reader must keep in mind that deaths have resulted from the ingestion of this herb.

109

poisonous to most birds, was the main diet of the Quetzal, the sacred bird of the Mayans. The Aztecs considered the avocado powerfully sacred, as pairs of avocado fruit were thought to resemble the male anatomy. The word avocado comes from the Aztec word 'ahuacatl,' meaning testicle. The avocado was known to the Aztecs as a fertility vegetable. Young women were forbidden to set foot outside while the avocado fruit was being harvested.

A myth from Guiana about the avocado hints at avocado fertility effects:

> Seriokai often gathered avocados with his wife in the forest of Orinoco. During one of these gathering expeditions, a tapir fell in love with his wife and at last won her heart. When the unsuspecting Serokai climbed down from the avocado tree, the bag on his back filled with heavy fruit, his wife struck him with an axe, cutting off his leg. Gathering up the fruit, she hurried to the tapir's hiding place, and she and the tapir hurried away together. Serokai was nursed back to health by his tribe, and fitted with a wooden peg for a leg. He started after the runaways. Although their path had long been obliterated, Serokai traced them through the forest by the avocado trees that had sprouted from the seeds scattered by his faithless wife. He followed the avocado trees over mountains and forded rivers to find the trees again. The trees grew smaller the nearer he came to the runaways. Eventually, they became sprouts and then only seeds, and then he saw footprints. When he overtook them, he sent an arrow into the body of the tapir, who at that moment bounded off the edge of the world. Seeing her companion so transfixed, the woman leaped also. Hot in his pursuit of vengeance, Serokai followed, and he still hunts the unrepentant ones through space. He is the constellation of Orion, his wife is Pleiades, and the tapir is Hyades, with the bloody eye. [144]

110

Avocados developed a stigma as a sexual stimulant, and individuals who were concerned about appearing chaste did not purchase or consume them in the 19th and early 20th centuries. Growers of avocados pursued a public relations campaign to debunk the stigma, and avocados eventually became popular as a food in North America.

The shoots, young leaves, and seed of the avocado are used as abortifacients in several countries. An infusion of the young leaves occasionally combined with pieces of avocado seed is used in Costa Rica as an emmenagogue and abortifacient.[145] In Cuba, the hot water infusion of avocado shoots is taken orally as an abortifacient.[146] The Kichos Indians of Peru drink the hot water extract of the leaves of avocado as an abortifacient.[147] In Trinidad, the avocado seed is grated into a glass of water, and then the water is taken to induce abortion.[148] In Central and South America, the leaf juice, bark of young stems in decoction, or the avocado seed is cooked and eaten to produce abortion.[149]

In scientific studies, avocado has shown a uterine stimulating effect in the rat uterus.[150] Dopamine has been found in the leaves, and may be the reason that the avocado leaves are used for fertility regulation. Recent scientific studies indicate that dopamine receptors are present in the ovaries.[151] Researchers at the Garvan Institute in Australia have found that avocado contains the fungicidal toxin, persin, which leaches into the flesh of the avocado from the pit. Persin is generally considered safe for human consumption as humans cannot digest it, but persin is very toxic to domestic animals exposed

111

to it. Tests have shown that persin can kill breast cancer cells and enhances the effects of the breast cancer drug tamoxifen.[152]

Gathering: As avocadoes grow year round in tropical climates, leaves and the bark of young branches are harvested as needed.

Preparation: Avocados are widely distributed throughout the world, so they are available in most groceries year round. Avocado seeds may be grown into houseplants or saved for medicinal use by placing them in the freezer for up to six months. Avocado as an abortifacient would probably be most effective during the first trimester. Generally, abortifacients are more effective if used earlier in the pregnancy, and avocado is no exception.

Words to the Wise: Avocado leaves are used to lower blood sugar in diabetics and reduce blood pressure and cholesterol. Dopamine has been found in avocado leaves. Dopamine may interfere with dopamine-receptor antagonist medicines, so individuals who have Parkinson's disease or mental illnesses should not use avocado leaves. Avocado contains a latex substance that can trigger allergic reactions in people allergic to latex or bananas.[153] Avocado leaves and seeds contain an unidentified toxic principle that has caused lung congestion, mastitis, tissue edema, milk reduction, and death (when large quantities of leaves were consumed) in mammals.[154]

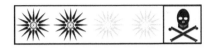

Watch for Signs of Toxicity Specific to Avocado: Gastrointestinal irritation, vomiting, diarrhea, respiratory distress, congestion, fluid accumulation around the tissues of the heart and even death.

Avocado Dosage

Abortifacient Avocado Leaf Drink: Boil three avocado leaves in 28 oz. water for three to four minutes and then steep for two to three minutes. Strain. Drink 3 cups/day, for up to six days.

Abortifacient Avocado Seed Drink: Grate one avocado seed into a glass. Add 1 cup (250 ml) water, allow to steep overnight. Drink 2 – 3 oz. (60 – 90 ml) every three to four hours.

Barrenwort

Epimedium grandiflorinum

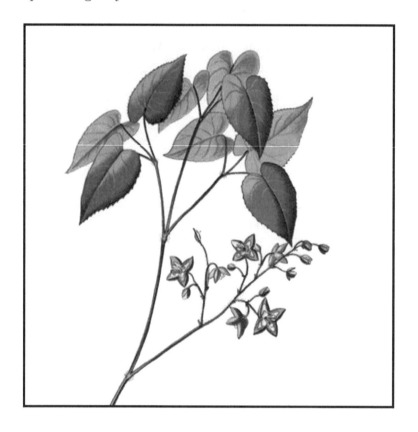

And worts and pansies there which grew

Have secrets others wish they knew.

-Anonymous, from a love poem

Family Berberidaceae

AKA: Horny goat weed, yin yang huo, bhat, and fairy wings.

Parts Used: Root and leaves.

Medicinal Properties: Anti-asthmatic, antitussive, and aphrodisiac.

Effects on the Body: Considered tonic for stimulating hormone secretion to cure impotence, also used for eye ailments. Low doses increase urine output, while high doses decrease urine output.

Abortifacient Action: Increases testosterone, reduces estrogen.

Contains: Ceryl alcohol, hentriacontane, oleic acid, linoleic acid, palmitic acid, stearic acid, phytosterol, and icariin.

Description: Members of the Epimedium genus are hardy perennials native to southern Europe and central, southern, and eastern Asia. Barrenworts are found in the under story of oak forests. Barrenwort's 5 – 15 in. (13 – 38 cm) high stem branches into three sprays of yellow-green, parallel, veined, heart shaped leaves. Barrenwort flowers, which first appear as red buds in spring, can range in color from white and yellow to mauve.

Barrenwort Herbal Lore and Historical Use

Barrenwort's use as medicinal herb dates back to AD 400 to the ancient Chinese medical text *Shen Nong, Canon of Medicinal Herbs*. According to legend, a Chinese goat herder noticed increased sexual activity in his flock after they ate barrenwort. In Asia, barrenwort leaves are eaten as food; its common name means 'friend of the barren.' Chinese research on *Epimedium grandiflorum* leaf extract reports stimulation of sexual activity and sperm production in animals.[155]

Barrenwort stimulates sensory nerves. Barrenwort is believed to stimulate sex drive in women who are androgen deficient.

Dioscorides mentioned the use of barrenwort as a contraceptive; "its leaves [are] beaten and drunk in the amount of 20 g. in wine after the menstrual period for five days preserve in-conception."[156] Barrenwort root was also used historically to cause sterility.[157]

Studies have shown that epimedium raises adrenaline, noradrenaline, serotonin, and dopamine levels in animals. It is the dopamine that may be responsible for the herb's use as a reproductive tonic. Evidence of dopamine receptors in ovaries has been indicated in scientific studies.[158] There is a circular relationship between dopamine, testosterone, and estrogen. Increased dopamine leads to a release of testosterone, and the increased testosterone reduces the number of estrogen receptors. Recent studies have indicated that dopamine receptors are present in the ovaries. Barrenwort's active compound, icariin, inhibits the activity of PDE-5 and increases nitric oxide, which relaxes smooth muscle and dilates blood vessels.

Gathering: Gather leaves during growing season. Flowering sprigs are said to last up to two months in a vase.

Preparation: When purchasing barrenwort leaves, look for a dark green color. Leaves that are yellow or light in color may be bleached from sitting in the sun too long while drying. Barrenwort is used to abort during the first half of the first trimester.

Words to the Wise: Large doses can cause respiratory arrest and muscle spasms. Barrenwort influences dopamine levels. Dopamine may interfere with dopamine-receptor antagonist medicines, so individuals who have Parkinson's disease or mental illnesses should not use barrenwort.

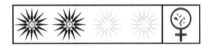

Watch for signs of Toxicity Specific to Barrenwort: Dizziness, vomiting, dry mouth, thirst, and nosebleeds.

Barrenwort Dosage

Barrenwort Abortifacient Infusion: 1 tsp. (4 g) herb to 1 cup (250 ml)
>   water, taken with food, three to four times a day.

Barrenwort Tincture: 1:3, 45% alcohol, then take ½ - 1 tsp.
>   (2.5 – 5 ml), three to four times a day.

Powdered leaves: 1 tsp. (4 g), taken with food, three - four times a day.

Birthwort

Aristolochia serpentaria

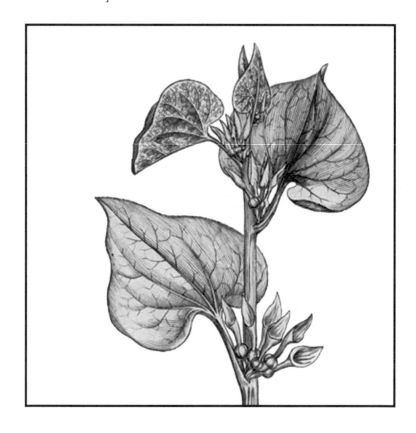

...used among the slaves in Jamaica...
a preparation from the root of this [Aristolochia] is
known to produce abortion, and
is much used for such purposes by Negro females.
-Thomas Strangeways in *Sketch of the Mosquito Shore*, 1822

In some cases... I have found [birthwort] useful...
But,...long-continued use of such medicines is extremely hurtful, and
commonly brings about a general state of disease,
more fatal than the original..
-Dr. Cullen in *Materia Medica*, 1789

118

Family Aristolochia

AKA: Earth apples, snakeroot, mutong (stem), fangji (root), and madouling (fruits).

Part Used: Root.

Medicinal Properties: Alexiteric, antiparalytic, antiperiodic, aphrodisiac, diuretic, diaphoretic, emmenagogue, anti-arthritic, stomachic, purgative, and vermifuge.

Effects on the Body: Said to be useful for snakebite, removing obstructions after childbirth, and preventing infection.

Abortifacient Action: Uterine contraction, embryo toxic, and possibly decreases luteinizing hormone.

Contains: Aristolochic acid, volatile oil, and tannins.

Description: Indigenous to the Mediterranean regions, Asia Minor, and the Caucasus, birthwort is a medium-height perennial that grows in woodland edges and near rivers. The heart-shaped alternate and smooth leaves on erect 3 ft. (1 m) stems spring from an underground web of rhizomes. The yellow flowers have a single flattened lip, are greenish at the swollen base, and are borne in clusters in the axils of the upper leaves through summer. Birthwort is a carrion flower, which has an unpleasant smell to attract insects. The inner parts of the flower have hairs that grab insect pollinators and then release the pollen coated insect.

119

Birthwort Herbal Lore and Historical Use[c]

Birthwort, as suggested by its common name, occupied an important place in the medicine bag of doctors and midwives. Many years ago, birthwort juice was used to promote birth in difficult labor and to help deliver the placenta. An Egyptian vase from Thebes shows a nursing woman with a stylized birthwort plant in the background.[159] Dioscorides recommended birthwort as a vaginal suppository or to be taken orally with pepper and myrrh to expel the menses or embryo/fetus.[160] Ibn Sina's *Canon of Medicine* (AD 1025) recommended birthwort as an emmenagogue and abortifacient.[161] Galen said oral administration of birthwort causes abortion, while a Cairo hospital formulary (ca AD 1200) recommended a vaginal pessary of birthwort to expel a dead fetus.[162] Seeds of birthwort were used historically in Hungary as contraceptive to prevent fertility and to promote menstruation.[163] Birthwort was used as a contraceptive in India and used to induce menstruation in Iran.

Birthwort has been shown in scientific tests to have an antifertility effect. Aristolochic acid stimulates contractions of the uterus. It is 100% effective in blocking pregnancy in mice after a single oral dose (100 mg/per kg) on the 6th or 7th day after sexual intercourse. A dose of 20 - 90 mg/per kg was sufficient to block implantation, and a dose of 30 mg/per kg interrupted midterm pregnancy.[164] Aristolochic acid inhibits phospholipase hydrolysis,

---

[c] The purpose of this book is to recapture information about historical approaches to self-induced abortion. Birthwort has been included; however the reader must keep in mind that many deaths have resulted from the ingestion of herbs in the Aristolochia family.

which checks inflammation and may alter the release of luteinizing and growth hormones from the pituitary.[165]

There are serious negative side effects to birthwort. Modern science has shown a strong correlation between consumption of herbal products containing aristolochic acid and delayed onset renal failure and cancer. Carcinogenic doses of birthwort have been noted at both long-term low doses and short-term high doses, and thus birthwort has been relegated to the back of the shelf because of safety issues.[166]

Gathering: Harvest rhizomes in the fall after the foliage dies down.

Preparation: Chinese medicine requires aristolochia to be diluted in water for oral use.[167] Aristolochia is considered a safe medicine by many traditional Chinese medicinal practitioners, because Aristolochia sp. are used with care and consideration and in relatively small dosages and only for the short term after careful consideration of the individual characteristics of the patient.

It is believed by some traditional Chinese Medicinal (TCM) practitioners and herbalists, that the negative aspects of aristolochic acid are moderated by the plant's use in water based medicinal preparation. However, aristolochic acid has been detected in water-based birthwort decoctions and water based decoctions have recently been blamed for renal failure, too. Acute renal failure has been reported from dosages as low as 60 g. Use extreme caution.

Words to the Wise: There is suggestion that birthwort may be effective as an abortifacient into the second trimester, however the harmful effects of birthwort are well documented. Acute renal failure was reported following a dose of 60 grams. Aristolochic acid is a nephrotoxin and can lead to kidney failure and urothelial cancer. Aristolochic acid stimulates white blood cell activity, is carcinogenic and can damage the kidneys. It should not be used with drugs that influence serotonin or in cases of spleen deficiency, as urothelial cancer is possible.

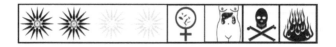

Watch for signs of Toxicity Specific to Birthwort: Vomiting, cramps, and muscle spasms.

Birthwort Dosage*
Fresh Birthwort Tincture: 1:2, 70% alcohol, 5 – 20 drops, two to three times a day, for no more than six days.

*Aristolochia is known to be carcinogenic. Extreme caution!

Black Cohosh
Cimicifuga racemosa

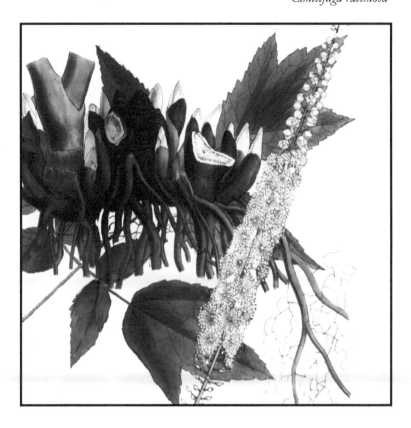

Lydia E. Pinkham's Vegetable Compound
is a positive cure for all the painful complaints and weaknesses so common to
our best female population.

-from an early 20th century American newspaper advertisement

123

Family Ranunculaceae

AKA: Black cohosh, rattle-top, rattlesnake root, fairies candles, squaw root, bugbane, and bugwort.

Part Used: Root.

Medicinal Properties: Alterative, antispasmodic, cardiac stimulant, diaphoretic, diuretic, emmenagogue, estrogenic, expectorant, and sedative.

Effects on the Body: Stimulates liver, kidney and lymphatic system helping to eliminate toxins and purify blood, aids in freeing up mucus, heart stimulant, and relaxing antispasmodic to uterine and intestinal smooth muscle.

Abortifacient Action: Possible estrogenic action and decreases luteinizing hormone.

Contains: Formononetin, a phytoestrogen, known to have abortifacient activity.[168]

Description: Black cohosh is indigenous to North America, but has become naturalized in northern Asia and Europe. Black cohosh found in the United States from northern Maine to Wisconsin and south to Missouri and Georgia. It is an indigenous leafy perennial found growing in upland woods and on hillsides. For example, it ascends to altitudes of 4000 ft. (1219 m) in North Carolina. Black cohosh's stalked leaves are pinnately compound and irregularly shaped. Small multiple white flowers bloom on 3 – 8 ft. (1 - 2.4 m) wand-like racemes from June to September.

Black cohosh's common names describe the herb's physical details. The insect repelling odor given off by the flowers gave rise to the common names bugbane and bugwort. During the winter when

124

the wind passes over the dried-out seed-covered racemes, they rustle like the tail of a rattlesnake, hence the common name 'rattlesnake root.' 'Cohosh' is the term in Native American Algonquin for rough and describes the knotty quality of the medicinal black root.

Black Cohosh Herbal Lore and Historical Use

The common name, squaw root, resulted from the herbal use of black cohosh by Native American women for reproductive organ disorders. The women of the Cherokee tribe considered black cohosh a dependable herb to bring on menstrual flow.[169] Native American women also used black cohosh to relieve pain during labor or during menstruation. Midwives today still widely use black cohosh to stimulate labor.[170]

In 1876, a famous patent medicine (containing several herbs, including black cohosh) was invented by an enterprising woman, Lydia E. Pinkham. Over the years, Lydia E. Pinkham's Vegetable Compound became tremendously popular partly due to its treatment of 'female complaints.' Pinkham's Compound had a reputation for causing abortion if taken in large amounts. Pinkham's Compound can still be purchased, but the black cohosh has been removed from the contemporary recipe.

Black cohosh was thought to have estrogenic properties, acting in the body like the female sex hormone estrogen, however this is being debated. In some scientific tests, black cohosh has been found to lack estrogenic effects in animals.[171] Black cohosh does not contribute to estrogen dependent cancer cells,[172] in fact black cohosh has been shown to inhibit proliferation of breast cancer cells in

125

vitro.[173] In Europe, black cohosh root is widely used in prescription medications for menopausal discomforts. Black cohosh has been shown to affect estrogen receptors in rat uteruses and pituitary glands.[174] Black cohosh has also been shown in scientific tests to suppress luteinizing hormone in ovariectomized rats.[175]

Gathering: The commercial supply of black cohosh grows in the open woodlands and cleared hillsides of the Blue Ridge Mountains. The gathering of wild black cohosh is threatening the species. Conscientious gathering of black cohosh is stressed. Black cohosh root is gathered in the fall (around September in the United States) after the fruit (seed pod) has ripened.

Preparation: Black cohosh, often used in decoction or tincture form, is often combined in equal parts with blue cohosh in labor inducing, emmenagogual, and abortifacient preparations. Black cohosh is sometimes combined with mistletoe or ginger. Black cohosh is most effective if used during the first four weeks of pregnancy.

Words to the Wise: Black cohosh may be estrogenic. Estrogenic herbs contain estrogen-like substances, which act to produce the effects of the female hormone estrogen. Estrogenic herbs can cause estrogen-like side effects: abnormal blood clotting, liver problems, and may encourage the growth of estrogen-dependent tumors. Estrogenic herbs should be avoided by anyone taking birth control pills, estrogen medications, or blood pressure medications. Estrogenic herbs may not

126

be as effective for premenopausal women. Estrogenic substances are known teratogens.

In addition, black cohosh can depress the heart rate; anyone with a history of heart disease should not use black cohosh. Black cohosh may contribute to abnormal blood clotting and liver problems. There have been cases of liver toxicity in women who used black cohosh to regulate menopausal hormones.[176] Large doses of black cohosh may irritate nerve centers causing tremors and convulsions.

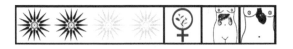

Watch for Signs of Toxicity Specific to Black Cohosh: Nausea, diarrhea, abdominal or joint pain, tremors, headache, visual dimness, depressed heart rate, tremors, and convulsions.

Black Cohosh Menstrual Promotion Dosage

Decoction (root): 3 tsp. (12 g) dried root to 1 cup (250 ml) water.
Simmer 5 - 15 minutes, three to four times a day.
Fresh Root Tincture: 1:3, 60% alcohol, ½ - 1 tsp. (2.5 - 5 ml), two to three times a day.
Powdered (root): 1-4 #0 capsules, three to four times a day.

Black Hellebore

Helleborus niger

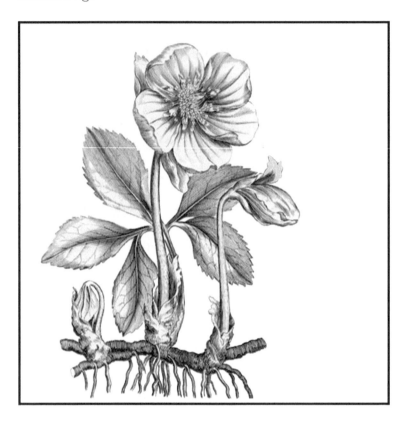

In antiquity, Greek women wore certain gold ornaments called hellebores.
The exact nature of these ornaments was made plain some years ago by
the discovery, in the south of Russia, of four small gold plates of
ancient Greek manufacture. The blossom of the hellebore is represented
on them and there are holes in the plates for fastening them to the dress.

-James George Frazer in *Pausania's Description of Greece*, 1898

Family Ranunculaceae

AKA: Melampode, Christmas rose, Christe herb, melampodium

Part Used: Root

Medicinal Properties: Drastic cathartic purgative, emmenagogue, anthelmintic, violently narcotic.

Effects on the Body: In small doses, black hellebore diminishes the rate of the pulse, increases the force and output of the heart, and causes a rise in blood pressure. In larger doses, hellebore is a narcotic, cardiotoxic, cathartic purgative.

Abortifacient Action: Cathartic purgative and embryo toxic.

Contains: Helleborin (narcotic) and helleborein (cardiac poison and purgative).

Description: Black hellebore is native to the mountainous regions of central and southern Europe, Greece, and Asia Minor. It is a perennial, short plant with dark waxy leaves and flower stalks rising directly from the root with white flowers appear in mid winter.

Black Hellebore Herbal Lore and Historical Use[d]

Hellebore was anciently associated with purging evil spirits and death. Arrows rubbed with hellebore were thought to render animal flesh tenderer. Ancient tradition held that women who became 'soul-sick' with a gloomy temper were sent away on vacation to a city in Greece called Anticyra, where hellebore grew plentifully.[177]

---

[d] The purpose of this book is to recapture information about historical approaches to self-induced abortion. Black hellebore has been included; however the reader must keep in mind that deaths have resulted from the ingestion of this herb.

In Greek mythology, Melampus of Pylos used the milk of goats fed on hellebore to save the daughters of the King of Argos from a hysterical madness, induced by Dionysus. During the siege of Kirka, in 585 BC, the Greeks used hellebore in the water supply to poison the Kirkan troops. The troops were so weakened by diarrhea; they were unable to defend the city from the Greeks.

Hellebore is rarely used in modern medicine, but harking back to Melampus, hellebore homeopathics are used for mental disorders.

Gathering: The black hellebore rhizome is collected from mature plants in autumn and dried. Black hellebore has been known to cause contact dermatitis when touched to the skin; use caution when gathering.

Words to the Wise: Black hellebore root powder can cause violent sneezing. Black hellebore is a narcotic and a cardiac poison no longer used in medicine. Use extreme caution.

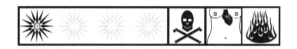

Watch for Signs of Toxicity Specific to Black Hellebore: Gastro-intestinal inflammation, dizziness, inflammation, painful spasms, catharsis, thirst with abdominal heat, dilation of the pupils, cold sweats, convulsions, heart failure.

Black Hellebore Dosage*

Abortifacient Powder: 2 – 3 g powdered root, taken in a single dose.

Abortifacient Decoction: ¼ oz. (7 g) herb to 2 cups (500 ml) of water,
    then 1 fl. oz. (30 ml) every four hours for up to two days.

*Extreme caution! Narcotic and dangerous cardiac poison!

Blue Cohosh

Caulophyllum thalictroides

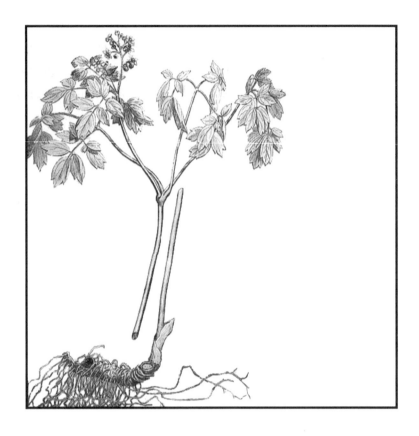

*Blue Cohosh is emmenagogue (excites menstrual flow), and
its use as a parturifacient originated in the custom of the
Indian squaws of employing a decoction of the root for
two or three weeks previous to labor to facilitate childbirth.*

-King's American Dispensatory, 1854

Family Berberidaceae

AKA: Blue cohosh, papoose root, yellow or blue ginseng, squaw root, and blueberry root.

Part Used: Root.

Medicinal Properties: Anthelmintic, antispasmodic, demulcent, diaphoretic, diuretic, estrogenic, expectorant, laxative, oxytocic, parturifacient, sedative, and vermifuge.

Effects on the Body: Uterine stimulant, relieves muscle cramps, complementary to nerves, joints, and blood.

Abortifacient Action: Estrogenic, oxytocic, and decreases luteinizing hormone.

Contains: Caulosaponin (oxytocic), Berberine (abortifacient chemical), methycytosine alkaloid (antispasmodic), and hederagenin (tones uterus).

Description: Blue cohosh is an indigenous perennial herb that grows all over the U.S in rich, moist, deep soils, and in shady areas, often near running streams. A blue cohosh plant is made up of one large triternately compound leaf; the main leaf stem divides into three stems, which again divides into threes, each stem ending in a leaflet. A single stem begins at the light brown knotty root and extends a height of one to three feet (0.3 - 1 m) where it divides into three stems that divide again into three leaflets 2 – 3 in. (5 - 7.5 cm) long, generally oval and 3 - 5 lobed near the apex. From April to May, clusters of yellow-green flowers appear, which are later replaced in August by round deep blue berries. From the thick, crooked root there usually extend 3 semi-straight rhizomes running horizontally a few inches (7 – 10 cm) below the surface from which sprout other plants. Blue Cohosh is a plant

133

that seems to be connected to all others nearby through an underground web of rhizomes.

Blue Cohosh Herbal Lore and Historical Use[e]

Native Americans called blue cohosh 'papoose root' because of its ability to trigger labor and hasten childbirth. Two weeks before the expected date of delivery, women would begin taking the blue cohosh infusion to promote a rapid and painless labor. Present-day Amish women and midwives use blue cohosh infusion effectively in the same manner. Blue cohosh contains a chemical, caulosaponin, which is known to cause strong uterine contractions.

Blue cohosh's tendency to prevent pregnancy is well-known among herbalists and midwives. Native American Chippewa women used a strong decoction of blue cohosh root for contraception. Blue cohosh, like the contraceptive pill, contains estrogenic substances. In scientific tests blue cohosh has been shown to enhance estradiol binding to estrogen receptors and decrease luteinizing hormone.

Although blue cohosh and black cohosh are often combined together and have similar common names, each herb has different individual chemical components and different medicinal properties. Black cohosh has antispasmodic properties causing the uterus to relax, while blue cohosh has stimulant properties, causing the uterus to contract. Blue cohosh and black cohosh have gained a reputation of working better together than alone.

---

[e] The purpose of this book is to recapture information about historical approaches to self-induced abortion. Blue cohosh has been included; however the reader must keep in mind that occasional deaths have resulted from the ingestion of this herb.

Gathering: Blue cohosh rhizomes are collected in the fall when the above-ground parts begin to die back. It is at this time when the sap runs back into the roots for storage in winter.

Preparation: Blue cohosh's uterine-contracting, emmenagogual, and abortifacient properties have been popularly utilized in decoction and tincture form. Blue cohosh is most effective as an abortifacient when utilized to encourage menstruation in the first six weeks of pregnancy. *Mitchella repens* (commonly known as partridgeberry or squaw vine) was combined with blue cohosh by the Native American Rappahannock women and taken five days prior to the expected date of menses to promote menstruation. Blue cohosh has a tendency to stress the kidneys.

Words to the Wise: Caulosaponin, the chemical in blue cohosh that causes uterine contractions, also has the action of narrowing the arteries that supply blood to the heart. People who have a history of high blood pressure, heart disease, or stroke should not use blue cohosh. A constituent of blue cohosh, methycytisine, is similar to nicotine and may lead to symptoms similar to nicotinic toxicity if too much is taken. In fact, nicotinic toxicity has been reported in use of blue cohosh for inducing abortion.[178] Estrogenic blue cohosh may contribute to estrogen-dependent tumors, liver problems, and abnormal blood clotting. Blue cohosh should be avoided by anyone taking birth control pills, estrogen medications, or blood pressure medications. Estrogenic herbs may not be as effective for premenopausal women. Estrogenic substances are known teratogens. Anyone with diabetes, glaucoma, or kidney damage or disease should not use blue cohosh. Powdered blue cohosh root may irritate mucous membranes, so a mask should be worn when processing. Fresh blue cohosh berries are poisonous; children have died from eating them. The berries lose their poisonous qualities when they are toasted, and they have been used as a substitute for coffee.

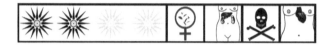

Watch for Signs of Toxicity Specific to Blue Cohosh: Nausea, vomiting, gastritis, headache, sore throat, thirst, elevated blood pressure, dilated pupils, muscle weakness, loss of coordination, cardiovascular collapse, and convulsions. As a rule, always reduce dosage at the first sign of toxicity.

Blue Cohosh Menstrual Promotion Dosage

Decoction (root): 3 tsp. (12 g) herb to 1 cup (250 ml) water. Simmer
20 – 30 min., take three to four times a day for up to six days.

Dried Root Tincture: 1:5, 60% alcohol, 5 - 20 drops, every four to six
hours for up to six days.

Powdered root: 1 - 5 #0 capsules, three to four times a day.

Castor
Ricinus communis

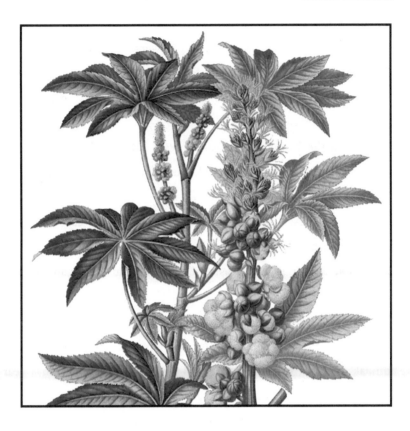

The following is an instance of poisoning by these seeds — the only one with which I have met. The deceased, aged eighteen, was the sister of a gentleman who attended my lectures at Guy's Hospital. The deceased, it appears, ate about twenty castor-oil seeds; one of her sisters ate four or five, and another two…In the night they were all taken ill. About five hours after the seeds were eaten the deceased felt faint and sick; vomiting and purging came on. And continued through the night…She died in five days without rallying; the two other sisters recovered…The effects produced on the sisters who recovered, bear out the statement of Dr. Christison, that two or three of the seeds will operate as a violent cathartic.

-Alfred Swaine Taylor in *On Poisons*, 1848

Family Euphorbiaceae

AKA: Eranda, gana garchak, higuerilla, hintyagi agaci, jarak, pei ma, ricino, tartago, and wonderboom.

Parts Used: seeds, seed oil, and rarely flowers.

Medicinal Properties: Abortifacient, anthelmintic, antitussive, cathartic, contraceptive, emollient, emmenagogue, expectorant, laxative, purgative.

Effects on the Body: Oil increases breast milk, soothes the skin, and is a harmless purgative. Seeds and leaves help to reduce swellings when applied externally.

Abortifacient Action: Seeds: Toxic to embryo, causes uterine contractions, and estrogenic. Oil: Purgative.

Contains: Seeds: Ricin. Castor Oil: Ricinoleic, oleic, and linoleic acids.

Description: Castor is a fast growing perennial shrub which can reach 36 ft. (11 m) in warm climates. In colder areas, castor is grown like an annual, as it can reach a height of 4 – 6 ft. (1.2 – 1.8 m) in a year. Castor's glossy leaves are palmate, 7 – 18 in. (18 – 46 cm) long, with five to twelve deep lobes and toothed margins. Leaf color can range from dark green to dark maroon to bronze. The seed pods, which vary in color, are considered by some to be more attractive than the flowers.

Castor Herbal Lore and Historical Use[f]

Castor seeds have been found in Egyptian tombs dated to 2000 BC. The use of castor in India also dates back 4000 years to the *Susruta Atharvaveda*, and castor is mentioned in the Unani and Ayurvedic medical systems. Castor seed and oil are also documented in ancient Chinese medical texts.

The use of castor to affect fertility is various and widespread. In Africa, the hot water extract of the dried leaf is taken orally to produce sterility and to promote menstruation,[179] and the seed is taken orally as a contraceptive.[180] In Egypt, a hot water extract of the seed is taken orally as a contraceptive.[181] In Spain, castor seed oil is rubbed on the abdomen and genital area to encourage uterine contractions.[182] In Liberia, the hot water extract of the root of castor is taken orally as an emmenagogue.[183] In South Korea, the decoction of the dried seed is utilized as a contraceptive and to induce abortion.[184]

In India, castor is used in many different ways to affect fertility. The hot water extract of leaf, seed oil, or the seed oil alone is taken orally as an emmenagogue.[185] A section of the stem of castor is inserted into and held in the vagina to induce abortion.[186] The dried flowers of castor, hibiscus, and pomegranate along with pomegranate peels are burned and the smoke inhaled to produce abortion.[187] As a contraceptive measure, the castor beans' seed coat is removed and the

---

[f] The purpose of this book is to recapture information about historical approaches to self-induced abortion. Castor has been included; however the reader must keep in mind that many deaths have resulted from the ingestion of castor beans.

cotyledons are dried and taken orally on or about the 5th - 12th day of the menstrual cycle.[188]

Scientific research into the fertility regulating effects of castor has shown abortifacient, estrogenic, uterine contracting, and embryo toxic effects. The seed oil, taken orally by full term pregnant women, was shown to have a labor inducing effect at a dose of 2 ounces (60 ml).[189] The estrogenic effect of castor beans was verified when rats were fed an ethanol extract of the castor bean seed cake combined with papaya enzyme to liberate the estrogenic proteins.[190] Uterine stimulant results were shown with castor bean leaf and stem extract in rats,[191] and the embryo toxic effect of the water extract of castor bean cotyledons was shown in chicken embryos.[192]

Gathering: Sap from the seeds and leaves may cause contact dermatitis. In warmer climates castor seed pods ripen throughout the year and are gathered by hand. Where castor is grown as an annual, the fruiting branches are cut off as soon as the pods begin to pop open, and this harvest is repeated every week until the end of season. The branches are then spread out on a cloth as the pods and seeds dry, and the seeds pop out of the pods.

Preparation: Cold pressed castor oil is odorless and tasteless when pure. Seeds, if purchased for medicinal purposes, should be untreated with germination chemicals and organic.

Castor oil is most effective as an abortifacient when used in early pregnancy. Castor oil is sometimes combined with Asian ginger *Zingiber officinale*. Castor seed is sometimes combined with papaya enzyme, papain.

Words to the Wise: Castor is estrogenic and should be avoided by anyone taking birth control pills, estrogen medications, or blood pressure medications. Estrogenic substances are known teratogens. Castor may not be as effective for premenopausal women. Persons suffering from kidney infections should not take castor oil as a purgative. Castor oil should be avoided by anyone suffering abdominal pain or intestinal infection. The toxicity of castor beans is well documented; however reports of poisoning are rare. In most cases, adults would require in excess of eight beans to achieve a lethal dose; however fatalities have occurred from consuming as few as three seeds. Castor seeds are pretty, and children may think they are candy, so castor seeds should be stored in a locked cabinet.

Ricin is the very deadly poison that is removed in the process of cold pressing and filtering the castor beans to produce castor oil. One gram of ricin has been estimated to be 6000 times more deadly than cyanide and 12,000 times more deadly than rattlesnake venom! The seed pulp left over from castor bean oil extraction contains approximately 5% ricin by weight. A fatal dose for an adult is 0.2 mg of ricin. In the United States, due to fears of bioterrorism, a person caught in possession of ricin can be sentenced to up to 10 years in prison.

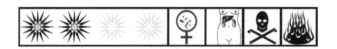

Watch for Signs of Toxicity Specific to Castor Oil: Violent vomiting and diarrhea, dehydration, gastro intestinal bleeding, skin cold and clammy, reduced pulse, and collapse.

Castor Dosage

Castor Oil Menstrual Promoter: 2 oz. (60 ml) castor oil are taken with 8 - 12 oz. (250 -375 ml) lukewarm milk. Asian ginger can be taken to calm the stomach. Purgative effects will be seen in one to two hours.

Castor Bean Contraceptive*: Take ½ -1 castor bean after menstruation to provide contraceptive action for one month. When conception is desired, castor beans are stopped and conception follows after one year.

*One study shows taking a single dose of three castor bean seeds at one time provides contraceptive action for one year.[193] However, this number of castor beans may be fatal, as fatal poisonings of adult humans have occurred with as few as three castor seeds.[194]

Chamomile
Anthemis nobilis

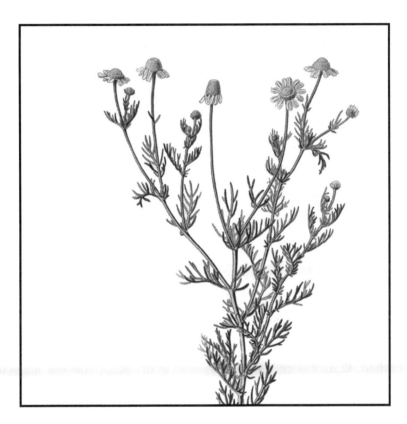

*The...steaming of the parts by sitting over a chamber
filled with hot chamomile tea, is the first step taken by the
nervous wife when the menstrual flow has failed to appear
sharp on time and she still lives in hopes that it is but a cold
which has interfered with the regularity of its return.*

-William Pepper in *A System of Practical Medicine*, 1886

143

Family Compositae

AKA: Chamomile, chamomile, anthemis, matricaria, ground apple, and manzanilla.

Parts Used: Flowers and essential oil distilled from flowers.

Medicinal Properties: Antispasmodic, carminative, diaphoretic, emmenagogue, nervine, stomachic, and tonic.

Effects on the Body: Flowers are soothing to nerves and stomach; essential oil is a tonic stimulant to uterus, kidney, spleen, and liver.

Abortifacient Action: Uterine contracting, prolongs the action of the adrenal hormone adrenaline and decreases capillary permeability in the uterine tissues, and contains beta-bisabolene (abortifacient chemical).

Contains: Essential oil (with azulenes), vitamin P (rutin), thujone, and beta-bisabolene.

Description: Roman chamomile *Anthemis nobilis* is native to the Mediterranean region. Perennial Roman chamomile is more aromatic and robust than annual German chamomile. Roman chamomile is short, 12 in. (30 cm), and grows wild in dry sandy soil and full sun. Hemispherical daisy-like flowers (June-September) with a strong scent appear singly and occasionally in pairs off its many erect branches. Pale green, feather-like leaves line Roman chamomile's downy stems.

Chamomile Herbal Lore and Historical Use

The Egyptians cultivated chamomile and dedicated the plant with its golden cones to the sun. Symbolic religious references to chamomile's holy womanly qualities still exist. In Greek, a variation of chamomile, 'Mater Cara' means 'Beloved Mother.' The Roman Catholic Church dedicated chamomile to St. Anne, mother of the

Virgin Mary. Today, chamomile is valued primarily for its soothing sedative properties and its ability to promote a natural hormone, similar to thyroxin, which has the power to rejuvenate the texture of the hair and skin and is believed to restore the liveliness of youth, both mentally and physically.

Chamomile is a relatively recent herb placed in the emmenagogual class of herbs. Abortifacient and emmenagogual properties are reported from use of Roman chamomile's flower infusion or essential oil. Nicholas Culpepper, an English herbalist of the 17th century, recorded chamomile's ability 'to bring down women's courses.' Culpepper may have been speaking of the hot tea used as a steam fumigation or possibly that of the essential oil, which was in common use during his time. The essential oil, distilled from fresh flowers since medieval times, is known to be a uterine stimulant and a treatment for eczema and asthma. Uterine stimulation by chamomile's essential oil is most likely due to the thujone the essential oil contains. Thujone has been shown to be a uterine stimulant in animals.[195] The hot water extract of dried chamomile flowers is documented as being used as an emmenagogual sitz bath in East Indian Unani medicine.[196] In Germany, the hot water infusion of chamomile flowers is documented in the form of a vaginal douche used to induce abortion.[197]

Gathering: The chamomile flower buds are carefully cut off the mother plant just before they are about to bloom and then dried quickly on stainless steel screen or in a cheesecloth hammock out of

145

direct sunlight. The flowers are turned occasionally as they dry and stored in airtight containers.

Preparation: Chamomile infusion of flowers or essential oil can be used as a sitz bath or fumigation during the first four weeks of pregnancy. Essential oils are extracted by distillation and are very concentrated. Some essential oils can be deadly at a dose of one teaspoon (4 ml)! Essential oils designated for aromatherapy should not be used internally. Chamomile infusion contributes calming qualities when added to a bath. Chamomile infusion with a bit of grated Asian ginger added makes a mildly emmenagogual and carminative tea. Boiling will destroy chamomile's oil; it should not be boiled.

Words to the Wise: People who are allergic to ragweed, aster, or chrysanthemum should be cautious of chamomile, for it is in the same family. Chamomile contains the uterine contracting and possibly toxic thujone, which can stimulate the heart muscle.

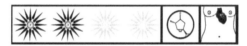

Watch for Signs of Toxicity Specific to Chamomile: Nausea, vomiting, vertigo, convulsions, personality changes, delirium, and hallucinations.

Chamomile Dosage

Emmenagogual Chamomile Fumigation: Chamomile infusion or up to
 five drops of chamomile essential oil may be used in vaginal
 fumigation or sitz bath to encourage menstruation.

Chaste Tree
Vitex agnus castus

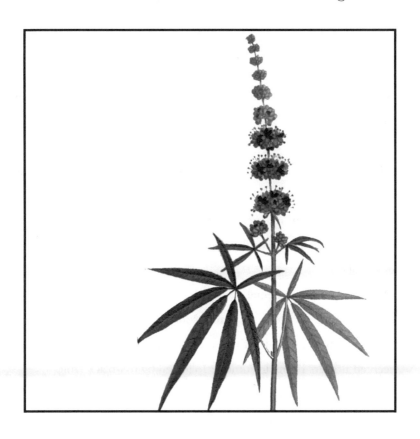

The decoction of the [chaste tree] herbe and seed is good
against pain and inflammations about the matrix, if
women be caused to sit and bathe their privy parts therein;
the seed being drunke with Pennyroiall bringeth downe the menses, as
it doth also both in a fume and in a pessary. . .

-John Gerarde in *General Historie of Plants*, 1597

Family Verbenaceae

AKA: Five-leaved chaste tree, cut leaf chaste tree, Abraham's balm, safe tree, wild pepper, monk's pepper, nirgundi, ching tzu, and huang-jing-zi.

Parts Used: Seeds, roots, twigs, and fruit

Medicinal Properties: Seeds (oral & suppository use): contraceptive, diuretic, emmenagogue, lactogogue. Fruits (in water): vermifuge, emmenagogue. Leaves (decoction): lactogogue, emmenagogue.

Effects on the Body: Regulates hormones, promotes lactation, and relieves pain and spasms.

Abortifacient Action: Increases prolactin.

Contains: Iridoid glycosides, flavones, flavonoids, diterpenoids, and essential oil.

Description: Ornamental deciduous shrub, up to 25 ft. (7.6 m) in height, native to west Asia and southwest Europe, with aromatic palmate leaves divided into five to six pointed leaflets. Small lilac scented flowers borne in summer followed by red-black fruit.

Chaste Tree Herbal Lore and Historical Use

The ancient Greek physician, Dioscorides, noted that chaste tree "destroys generation as well as provokes menstruation."[198] Four hundred years after Dioscorides, Hippocrates mentioned that the chaste tree is used to stem excess menstruation, "If blood flows from the womb, let the woman drink dark wine in which the leaves of the chaste tree have been steeped." Like many herbal abortifacients, chaste tree was intertwined in symbology to the earth mother Goddess – linked intimately with the natural cycle of life and death. According

148

to Greek mythology, the great mother goddess, Hera, was born under a chaste tree. The Greek spring fertility festival, Thesmorphoria, was a three-day women-only reenactment of Persephone returning to Demeter from the underworld. During the Thesmorphoria, chaste tree blossoms were used to adorn hair and costumes, and branches of the chaste tree were placed around Demeter's temple. The branches of chaste tree were made into beds for maidens. In Rome, chaste tree branches were a symbol of chastity carried by the priestesses of Vesta, goddess of the hearth.

Chaste tree has a long history as a hormone regulator, however chaste tree does not contain any plant based hormones. The common names, monk's pepper and Abraham's balm, are believed to stem from chaste tree's use by men as an anti-libido medicine. Modern science has shown that chaste tree reduces the level of male androgens (reducing the male libido) and decreases prolactin levels, which in turn, may increase luteinizing hormone, which triggers increased testosterone levels.[199] Vitex has also been used in Germany for such male complaints as spermatorrhea, prostatitis, orchitis, and sexual neurasthenia.

Chaste tree is known to inhibit implantation if taken in the first week of pregnancy, and it may interfere with ovulation. In 1938, German researcher, Gerhard Madaus found that the leaf, fruit, and bark extract of chaste tree retarded estrus (heat) in female rats; the chaste tree berries were most effective.

Chaste tree has been shown at low doses to have been helpful to women with high prolactin levels and irregular cycles, PMS acne, and

149

corpus luteum insufficiency.[200] Chaste tree berries, in low doses, act on the hypothalamus and pituitary glands by increasing luteinizing hormone (LH) production and mildly inhibiting the release of follicle stimulating hormone (FSH). Low doses of chaste tree reduce estrogen and increase progesterone. In high doses, however, chaste tree berries seem to increase prolactin secretions and seem to have little effect on follicle stimulating hormone (FSH), luteinizing hormone (LH) estrogens, or progestins. Researchers have found that high prolactin levels in early pregnancy (up to 10 weeks LMP) are a cause of recurrent miscarriage.[201]

Gathering: The top four inches (10 cm) of the stem are gathered during summer. Flowers are gathered along with ripening fruit. Berries are collected in autumn by gently rubbing them loose from the stems.

Preparation: Chaste tree was historically combined with dittany. Chaste tree is said to be effective both internally and when used as an emmenagogual fumigant. Chaste tree is most effective if used in early pregnancy (up to 6 weeks). A decoction of chaste tree seeds can be used as a pessary for contraception.

Words to the Wise: Chaste tree may interfere with dopamine-receptor antagonist medicines. Chaste tree berries may have an effect on dopamine levels, so individuals who have Parkinson's disease or who suffer from depression should not take them. Because chaste tree can act like female hormones in the body, chaste tree berries could interfere with oral contraceptives or contribute to estrogen dependent cancerous cells. Breastfeeding women who use chaste tree may find menstruation starts too early after delivery, due to the activation of the pituitary. If chaste tree is taken to reduce PMS symptoms, it may take 6 - 12 weeks before results will be noticeable.

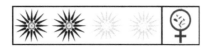

Watch for signs of Toxicity Specific to Chaste Tree: Itching, rash, gastrointestinal disturbances, racing heartbeat, and transitory headaches.

Chaste Tree Dosage

Chaste Tree Menstrual Promoter: 200 mg - 350 mg chaste tree berries, two to three times a day, for up to six days.

Cotton

Gossypium sp.

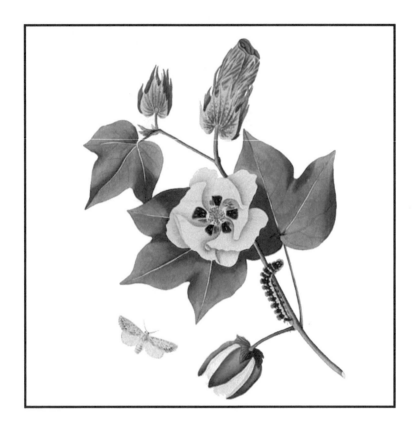

*My attention was called to the bark of cotton root by two or three
planters in Missisippi, during the fall of the year 1857, and
I witnessed its action in one case of abortion. A Negro woman collected
some bark of the fresh root and some green seed (about a pint she told me)
and made a quart of strong tea and drank about half of it. I was sent for
by her master, but the drug had brought about such energetic pains that
it was impossible to check them, and she lost her child.*

-C. C. Ferguson in a letter to J.U. Lloyd,
published in *The Eclectic Medical Journal*, 1860

Family Malvaceae

AKA: Cotton root bark.

Parts Used: Inner bark (cambium) of the root, seed, and fruit.

Medicinal Properties: Emmenagogue, lactogogue, parturient, oxytocic, and vasoconstrictor.

Effects on the Body: Stimulates uterine contractions and stimulates the production of breast milk.

Abortifacient Action: Causes contraction of the uterus and interferes with the corpus luteum and possibly the production of progesterone.

Contains: Gossypol, resinous substance with phenol-carbonic acid, salicylic acid, betaine (abortifacient chemical found in seed), serotonin (abortifacient chemical found in fruit), and phytoestrogen beta-sitosterol.

Description: Cotton grows as an annual herb in cooler climates and as a biennial or perennial shrub 2 – 5 ft. (0.6 - 1.6 m) tall in tropical climates. Branching stems, hairy or occasionally smooth, bear dark green leaves that sometimes have a gray blush. Leaves are usually alternate, three lobed, and around 2 – 6 in. (5 - 15 cm) long. Cotton's beautiful cup-shaped blooms, which open for only one day, have paper-thin cream to yellow petals with a purple to maroon center. After fertilization, three to four segmented seedpods (called bolls) form, each containing multiple seeds covered with grayish lint (cotton fiber). Upon maturity, the boll becomes dry, splitting from the tip and exposing the cotton fiber.

Cotton Herbal Lore and Historical Use

The use of cotton predates recorded history. More than 8000 years ago, the Aztecs grew cotton for textiles. Remains of the cotton plant have been found in Aztec burial mounds, which predate the Egyptian pyramids. Early explorers to North America recorded that the indigenous people were masters at weaving cotton textiles. Native American women of the Alabama and Koasati tribes utilized the medicinal properties of the cotton root. A tea of cotton root bark was used to aid contractions in childbirth, and in high doses cotton root bark was known to induce abortion.[202] Creoles in South America also used cotton root bark as a contraceptive.[203]

African slaves in the American colonies used cotton root bark to induce abortion, a knowledge said to have been passed from mother to daughter in Africa where the cotton plant is believed have originated.[204] Archeological evaluation of plant remains in African American slave cabins in the southwest United States revealed cotton root bark in greater amounts than what would be expected in historical written documentation.[205] Cotton root bark was used by enslaved African women for abortion with no notation of significant negative side effects.[206]

Some slave owners were known to rape slaves. Raping was even considered profitable, for any children that resulted from the offense would increase the number of slaves the rapist owned. Some slave owners found out about the use of cotton root bark for abortive purposes and subsequently forced their female slaves to drink an herbal decoction of the root bark of *Viburnum prunifolium*, which came to be known by the common name black haw. *Viburnum prunifolium* is a

154

strong abortion and miscarriage preventative. Its forced use was intended to insure their slaves would carry pregnancies to term.

During the mid 19th century, women in the United States who sought out cotton root bark tincture at pharmacies were sometimes refused sale and instead ordered the tincture from a company in Canada.[207]

Herbalists today use cotton root bark to produce abortion, stimulate contractions, and encourage the production of breast milk. The cotton seed and root are used in the treatment of nasal polyps, uterine fibroids, and several types of cancer. Chinese tests on rats show that high doses of cotton root bark have an antiprogesterone and corpus luteum effect which can interrupt pregnancy.[208] Interference in the functioning of the corpus luteum interferes in the normal production of progesterone, and the uterine lining becomes unsupportive to the fertilized egg. Cotton is a uterine stimulant. It is believed that cotton root bark has the ability, as an anti-progesterone, to prevent implantation; however other scientific studies have not shown an anti-implantation effect.[209] Cotton root bark is believed to have fewer negative side effects when compared to many other herbal abortifacients.[210]

Gossypol, the dihydroxyphenyl found in cotton seeds and seedlings, is sold in China as a male contraceptive.[211] The toxic effects of gossypol are reduced by combining gossypol with iron salts, which bind to the gossypol, thus inactivating it.[212]

Gathering: Cotton is found growing wild on sand dunes and railroad beds (Caution: toxic chemicals in soil) in southern Florida and the

155

Keys. Cotton is cultivated throughout the southern United States. The bark of the cotton root is gathered before frost sets in, sometimes as late as December in the warmer climates. The inner cambium layer is peeled from the root bark in long strips (1 cm wide). Fresh decoctions or tinctures are created immediately. The dried root is reputed to be worthless medicinally.

Preparation: Cotton root bark has the dual benefit of preventing implantation through an anti-progesterone effect and stimulating uterine contractions. Cotton root bark is usually given by itself as a simple either in the week before an expected menstruation or in the first few weeks after a missed period. Based on historical accounts, cotton root bark may be an effective abortifacient during the first trimester and possibly into the second trimester, as well. However, effectiveness is reduced and the risks to the woman attempting abortion are greater the later the abortion is attempted.

Words to the Wise: Cotton root bark decoction has a reputation as being safe and effective.[213] However, long term use of any medicine can prove to be harmful. Chinese tests with cotton root on animals and humans for periods of eight weeks, showed atrophy of the uterine lining tissue.[214] Abortifacient herbs should never be used as a primary method of birth control. The chemical gossypol in cotton is known to be toxic, but iron salts have shown to inactivate gossypol. Cooking in cast iron pots or multivitamin supplement with iron would help to prevent gossypol toxicity.

Warning! Commercial cotton contains large amounts of toxic chemicals and is not fit for human consumption! According to a 1982 USDA survey, in one season the U.S. cotton crop was sprayed with 7,000,000 pounds of chemical desiccants and defoliants as well as 34,000,000 pounds of herbicides and pesticides! Consumer demand for organic cotton clothing has prompted four U.S. states (Arizona, California, Tennessee, and Texas) to produce small amounts of organic cotton.[215] Organic medicinal cotton root bark tinctures are now available from several reliable distributers (see Resources).

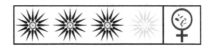

Cotton Dosage

Abortifacient Cotton Root Bark Decoction: Add 4 ounces (113 g) of fresh cotton root bark to 1 quart (1 L) of water. Boil 20 - 30 minutes until the liquid is reduced to 2 cups (500 ml) liquid decoction. Take 4 – 8 Tbs. (60- 120 ml), every thirty minutes to one hour.

Abortifacient Tincture (use only fresh root bark): 1:2, 95% alcohol, 30 – 60 drops, up to three times a day, for no more than six days.

Daphne

Daphne genkwa (Asian)

Daphne mezereum (European)

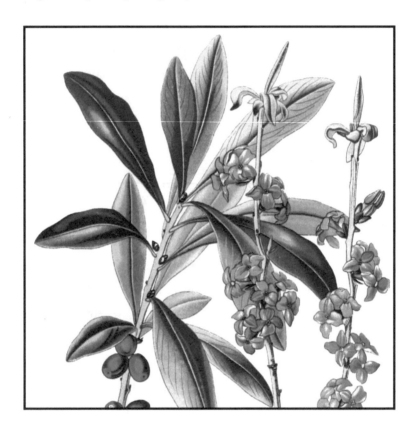

The genkwa flower is good if it has been reserved for as long as several years. Bring it to boil in good vinegar for scores of times of use, remove vinegar, soak it overnight in water, dry it in the sun, and in this way its toxicity will be eliminated. It will give a similar but inferior effect to that of parching the flower with vinegar.

-Shen Nong's Herbal Classic, 2757 BC

158

Family Thymelaeaceae

AKA: Genkwa flower, yuan hua, and nasiniin. Called tu-yǔ or 'fish poison' in China, because when thrown into water it poisons the fish.

Parts Used: Flower buds, leaves, and root bark.

Medicinal Properties: Flower Buds: Abortifacient, anticoagulant, diuretic, antitussive, antiviral, expectorant, pyrogenic, purgative. Leaves: Abortifacient, purgative. Root bark: Abortifacient, anticoagulant, diuretic, purgative, and vesicant.

Effects on the Body: Increases urine, purgative action on the intestines, and reduces blood's clotting ability.

Abortifacient Action: Decreases progesterone, augments uterine contractions, and stimulates production of prostaglandins.

Contains: Isolated methyl esters: yuanhuafine, yuanhuatine, yuanhuacine (used clinically in China intra and extra amniotically at a dose of 70 – 80 mcg to produce abortion with 98% effectiveness), and yuahuadine (used clinically in China intra amniotically at a dose of 60 mcg to produce abortion).[216]

Description: A deciduous 4 ft. (1.3 m) diameter shrub native to Asia. Planted in landscapes for its ornamental scented flowers and bright red berries (poisonous). Daphne flowers appear in early spring on bare stems and do not have petals but are made up of four or five light pink to purple petaloid sepals.

159

Daphne Herbal Lore and Historical Use[g]

Herbal use of *Daphne genkwa* can be traced to 5000 years ago. *Daphne genkwa* is one of the 50 fundamental herbs in traditional Chinese medicine and was first listed in the *Shennong Bencao Jing*, an ancient Chinese text that dates to legendary emperor, Shen Nong, who is considered the founder of Chinese herbal medicine and agriculture.

The ancient Greeks were also aware of the herbal powers of their variety of daphne, *Daphne mezereum*. Greek physician, Dioscorides, advised that *Daphne mezereum* "on a [pessary] pad expels the fetus or embryo."[217] In ancient Greece, the herb daphne shared the name of a Goddess who, struck by Cupid's embittered arrow, refused to allow passion to rule her destiny. The story of Daphne starts with Apollo teasing Eros (Cupid), saying that one so small could not make a difference with his arrows. Angered, Eros dipped one arrow in lead and one in gold. The arrow dipped in lead would cause whoever injured by it, to hate all passion and love, while the one dipped in gold would cause the most insatiable lust for love. Eros turned to Apollo and shot the gold tipped arrow into his chest. Then he turned and shot the lead tipped arrow, hitting Daphne. Apollo chased Daphne desperate for her love, but she ran endlessly away from him. Tiring, Daphne called to her father, the river God Peneus, to help her. Peneus used his power to transform his daughter into a laurel tree. Apollo still enamored of the tree, adorned himself with a

---

[g] The purpose of this book is to recapture information about historical approaches to self-induced abortion. Daphne has been included; however the reader must keep in mind that deaths have occasionally resulted from the ingestion of this herb.

crown of laurel leaves, and from that time on laurel has been viewed as a plant that cleanses the soul.

Modern science has explored the abortifacient powers of daphne. Plant based drugs, yuanhuadine and yuanhuacine, have been isolated from *Daphne genkwa* root and are used in China today to abort with few side effects.[218] Tests with *Daphne genkwa* on rats indicated that daphne stimulates prostaglandins which increase uterine contraction.[219] Extracts of *Daphne genkwa* root injected into the pregnant uterus in monkeys, induced mid-term abortions.[220] Abortion occurred within 69 - 142 hours after the injection of daphne root extract. The fresh root (chewed), or water, oil, and alcohol extracts of the root, have been used to induce labor.[221] The alcohol extract of daphne root was shown to be effective at inducing abortion.[222] The alcohol extract of the root has been used to induce abortion after 12 weeks via intra-amniotic administration.[223]

Gathering: Flower buds should be gathered after morning dew has dried. In China, daphne flowers are thoroughly dried in the sun and stored for several years before use. The root may be gathered at night in late fall. The bark should be peeled from the root and thoroughly dried before storing.

Purchasing: Daphne flower buds (Flos genkwa) can be found in some Asian markets and specialty stores. Some stores also sell genkwa powders, pills and capsules. Daphne root is not generally available, but, as daphne is widely grown worldwide as an ornamental, the root might be obtained fresh.

161

Preparation: Extracts of daphne root bark and flower buds have been shown to be effective as menstrual promoters in early pregnancy and abortive in early and mid-term pregnancy. The flower of daphne is more widely available than the root. In traditional Chinese medicine (TCM), daphne flower buds are fried in a pan with vinegar to reduce toxicity. Use of this vinegar water in a liquid pessary, may be advantageous for abortifacient purposes.[224]

Words to the Wise: Daphne is thought to contain resin compounds that can have an effect on latent malignant cells. Daphne contains cocarcinogenic compounds which do not cause malignant growth, even when applied repeatedly, but they act in a synergistic way with carcinogens, causing rapid malignant cell division when applied after a carcinogen.[225] However, daphne has also been found to contain anti-tumor agents (genkwadaphnin and yuanhuacine) in the root.[226] Licorice *Glycyrrhiza glabra* root interferes in the action of daphne.

Daphne fruits are particularly toxic when eaten, producing a violent irritation of the intestinal mucosa of the digestive tract, resulting in vomiting, sometimes containing blood. Daphne fruits can cause death – especially in children. Symptoms appear 15 minutes to four hours after ingestion. Daphne can cause contact dermatitis.

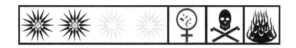

Watch for signs of Toxicity Specific to Daphne: loss of body weight, choking sensation, vomiting, hyper catharsis, and kidney irritation.

Daphne Dosage

Dried Flower Bud Abortifacient Decoction: 1.5 – 3 g flower bud
powder (called flos genkwa in TCM), fry in one cup (250 ml)
vinegar for five minutes, then add 2 cups (500 ml) of water.
Simmer for fifteen minutes. Then take orally, 4 - 8 oz. (125 –
250 ml), two to three times a day. Decoction can be used for
abortifacient vaginal pessary.

Dittany

Origanum dictamnus

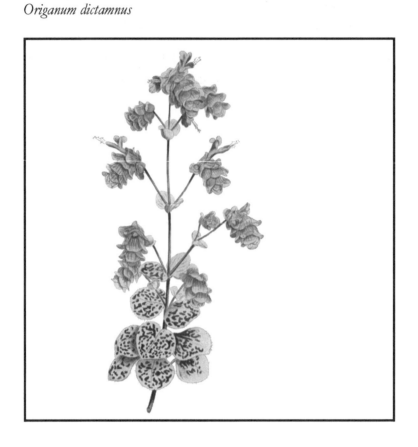

A branch of healing Dittany she brought, which
in the Cretan fields with care she sought.
Rough is the stem, which woolly leaves surround, the
leaves with flowers, the flowers with purple crowned.

- Virgil's *Aeneid*, 25 BC

Family Labiatae

AKA: Dittany of Crete, hop marjoram, dictamnus, winter sweet, and d'ctamo de Creta.

Parts Used: Leaves, flower tops, and seeds.

Medicinal Properties: Antioxidant, antibacterial, antimicrobial, aphrodisiac, oxytocic, stomachic, and vulnerary.

Effects on the Body: Stimulant, relieves gas, increases menstrual flow, and hastens childbirth. Soothes stomach, digestive system, and rheumatism. Helps heal wounds when applied.

Abortifacient Action: Research suggests it stimulates prostaglandins and may inhibit implantation.

Contains: Carvacrol and thymol.

Description: Endemic to Crete, where it grows in the cracks of rocks lining steep ravines in the Cretan Mountains, dittany is a low-growing tender perennial evergreen plant, height 1 ft. (0.3 m). Dittany has procumbent white, woolly stems with small heart-shaped velvety light green to grey leaves and pink or purplish flowers in summer.

Dittany Herbal Lore and Historical Use

Pliny the Elder (AD 23-79) claimed that "of all emmenagogue drugs, dittany had efficacy… so powerful it should not be in the same room as a pregnant woman." Dioscorides commented that dittany "shakes out a dead embryo."[227] Hippocrates in his writings on gynecology recorded that dittany was used to regulate menses. In ancient times, it was believed that a snake (anciently symbolizing phallic power) would allow itself to be burned to death rather than cross the path of dittany of Crete.

Like so many abortifacient herbs, Cretan dittany's herbal powers were woven into the myths and legends of ancient Crete. Cretan dittany is endemic to Crete where locals call it 'eronda,' meaning love, for its aphrodisiac properties. In flower language, dittany symbolizes passion. Dittany's name is derived from Mount Dikte in central Crete. In ancient times, Mount Dikte was presided over by the Mother of Mountains, Cretan Goddess Dictynna, who as the great earth mother was pictured on ancient seals suckling griffons, gripping divine snakes, or holding a double-bladed axe. In ancient times, young Cretan men would climb the very steep rock faces on the sides of the valleys of Crete to gather dittany and offer it as a token of their love and strength to their beloved. Even in the modern day, some Cretan locals believe dittany is magical and can cure anything.

In Europe, Steinmetz's herbal classic *Materia Medica Vegetabilis*, lists dittany as an emmenagogue.[228] A 16th century German pharmacist documented that Cretan dittany was infused in warm water "to expel a dead fetus without any peril to the mother."[229] King's *American Dispensatory* of 1898 said of dittany, "A warm infusion produces diaphoresis, and tends to promote menstruation when recently suppressed from cold." Cretan dittany is featured repeatedly in women's patent medicines of the early 20th century, which were often taken by women to cause abortion. A leaf infusion of dittany is used today by midwives to ease painful labor.

Scientific study has suggested that Cretan dittany inhibits implantation. In 1996, the International Plant Genetic Resources Institute published information indicating that dittany may contain or stimulate the production of prostaglandins.[230] Prostaglandins are

166

hormones that are responsible for cervical ripening and the production of uterine contractions that induce labor.

Gathering: Cretan Dittany is sold in Crete for herbal teas where cultivated plants are the main source of supply. Above ground parts of dittany are best harvested as soon as blooming begins. Cretan dittany is difficult to gather in the wild as it prefers the cracks of tall steep cliffs. Gathering in the wild is not recommended as this plant is considered a vulnerable plant on the International Union for Conservation of Nature (IUCN) red list of threatened plant species 1997.

Preparation: To promote menstruation a warm infusion of the plant is used the week prior to an expected menstruation. For abortive purposes the seeds are used up to the third month of pregnancy. Dittany flowering tops are used in infusion. Sometimes dittany is combined with chaste tree berries to promote menstruation. Dittany seeds are soaked overnight, ground to paste, and added to sweetened water to temper the bitter taste.

Words to the Wise: Stay out of the sun when taking Cretan dittany; phytodermatitis can result from contact or consumption of Cretan dittany and sun exposure. Cretan dittany essential oil has recently become available. Dittany essential oil should not be used internally.

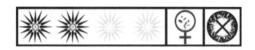

Watch for signs of Toxicity Specific to Dittany: Negative side effects have yet to be documented for Cretan dittany. Reduce dosage or discontinue use if negative side effects appear.

Dittany Dosage

Emmenagogual Infusion: Add ¼ tsp. (1 g) of dittany leaves and flowers to ½ cup (125 ml) of water, and let it simmer covered for seven to ten minutes. Take three to four times a day, for up to seven days.

Emmenagogual Seed: 0.5 g seed/day for no more than five days.

Abortifacient Seed: 3 g seeds/day, for no more than three days.

Garlic
Allium sativa

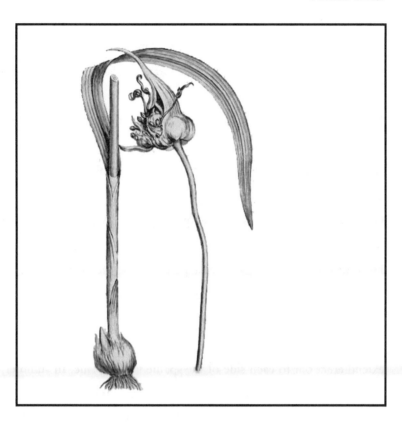

Garlic is good to chew and fumigate.

-8th Century BC Assyrian Health Guide

Family Liliaceae

AKA: Garlic.

Parts Used: Bulb.

Medicinal Properties: Alterative, anthelmintic, antibacterial, antispasmodic, estrogenic, expectorant, diaphoretic, diuretic, hypotensive, and stimulant.

Effects on the Body: Increases sweating and urination and general stimulant.

Abortifacient Action: Contracts uterus, thins blood, and possibly embryotoxic.

Contains: Sulphur, oleanolic-acid, prostaglandin A, and phytoestrogen beta-sitosterol.

Description: Familiar garlic is a perennial or biennial plant with a bulbous corm made up of 10-20 cloves surrounded by white skin. Garlic grows to a height of 2 ft. (0.6 m); the spathe (unbranched stem) having flat, long, pointed leaves, ½ - 1 in. (1.3 - 2.5 cm) wide, that extend erect out to each side of the spathe in one plane. In summer, a long stalk rising from the center of the spathe, forms a bead of one umbel made up of densely compact flowers, of maroon to white hue.

Garlic Herbal Lore and Historical Use

Garlic was originally native to the Kirgiz region of Siberia in Asia. To the ancients, garlic bulbs, along with onion and chive bulbs were recognized as being symbolic of the universe. The layers of skin symbolized the layering of spiritual realms of ancient Egyptian cosmogony.[231] The common peoples' faith in the spirit of garlic was so strong; they would swear their loyalty and trust by garlic when taking

170

an oath.[232]   Garlic was known to drive out sickness, or evil spirits, from the body. Ancient Greek midwives would generously hang garlic throughout the delivery room. The room would be filled with garlic's warm, healing, antibacterial, 'evil spirit' abating vapor. When the baby was born, the women would fasten around the infant's neck a necklace strung with protective garlic clove charms.[233]

The historical evidence of garlic's powers as an emmenagogue and abortifacient is extensive. Dated to 1550 BC, the Egyptian *Ebers Codex* is one of the oldest preserved medical texts. It is in this ancient medical document that the use of garlic to alleviate menstrual disturbances is first mentioned. Garlic was used in a wine solution that was introduced into the vulva to bring about menstruation. In the *Ebers Codex* was another recipe. A plaster made of bread dough, crushed garlic, and the branches and leaves of cedar was placed on the abdomen for the same problem. The ancient Egyptian Kahoun and Carlsberg papyrus medical texts, and the Hippocratic (460 – 377 BC) treatise, *On Sterile Women*, state that if a pealed, clean clove of garlic is inserted into the vulva in the evening, by the next morning, if the woman's breath failed to smell of garlic, one could tell that she would not conceive. In *Diseases of Women*, another work by Hippocrates, a garlic bulb is boiled, cooled, and inserted into the vagina as a suppository to bring about menstruation. In Pliny's (AD 23 - 79) *Natural History*, garlic is crushed with fresh coriander and added to wine, and the wine is taken as both a menstruation promoter and an aphrodisiac. In Dioscorides' (1st or 2nd century AD) *Greek Herbal*, a garlic clove inserted as a suppository was again noted to "bring down the menses." Dioscorides also mentions a species of wild garlic on the

171

island of Cypress called ophioscorodon (serpent's garlic). Boiling the umbel flower of this garlic was good for a sitz bath to help promote menstruation and expulsion of the placenta. For the same purposes it could be used as a smoke fumigation.

Ancient Roman women and men celebrated summer solstice with sexual liberty, and garlic played a part. The summer solstice Cerealia festival was held in honor of Goddess Ceres Legiferer, the lawgiver, who ruled Rome during her matriarchy 600 – 200 BC.[234] The Cerealia was held as a peaceful celebration of the joy of life that Mother Earth Goddess Ceres produced. Ceres, as the earth mother, was the source of all life, all fruit of the land and of the people. Always true, just, and generous with those who kept her rites; her priestesses were known as the foundresses of the Roman legal system.[235] At the time of the Cerealia, the Roman men ate large amounts of the aphrodisiac garlic, which was believed to stimulate the central nerve of the penis, thus contributing to erection.[236] Garlic with coriander seed in wine, as in the emmenagogual recipe by Pliny, was a love potion given by lovers to each other as an aphrodisiac and menstrual promoter.

In ancient Greece, on the night of the full moon, women placed garlic offerings on stone alters at the crossing of three roads in respect to Hecate,[237] Goddess of magic charms and enchantment, who was sometimes called 'most lovely one,' a title for the moon.[238] The full moon harmonized with increased sexual desire of ovulation.[239] Hecate was derived from the Egyptian wise-woman midwife, Heqit, who was in charge of the hekau, meaning mother words of power.[240] The three roads of the crossroads were the feminine trinity of life:

172

heaven, earth, and the underworld. A statue of Hecate with a face pointing in each direction was placed at the crossroads, symbolizing Hecate's three-fold identity: in the heavens in the form of Hecate Selene (the Moon), on the Earth in the form of Artemis (the birth giver and great huntress), and in the underworld in the form of Persephone (the Destroyer).[241]

Later in history, garlic's pagan reputation caused much stress and distain among the clergy and politicians, who enacted law and taboos against garlic's use. A Christian myth says that after Satan left the Garden of Eden, garlic arose in his left footprint, and onion in the right.[242]

Garlic continued to be used for menstrual regulation in many cultures. In India, there is evidence of garlic being used in folk medicine as an abortifacient.[243] The hot water decoction of the garlic bulb is used as an emmenagogue.[244] The seeds of garlic are also recorded as being used for emmenagogual purposes.[245] In Jamaica, the hot water decoction of the garlic bulb is also noted as being used as an emmenagogue.[246] Whereas in Mexico, the same garlic preparation is documented as being used for abortifacient purposes.[247]

Modern science supports the ancient writings indicating garlic is effective as an emmenagogual and abortifacient agent. A strong water extract of garlic bulbs produced contractions in a non-pregnant uterus in one study.[248] Sulphur compounds are released when garlic is chopped, crushed, or chewed. Sulphur has an ancient reputation as an abortive fumigant. Sulfur, as a natural anti-clotting agent, causes the blood to flow more readily. Dioscorides prescribed sulfur fumigation to expel a fetus. Recent studies have shown an increased risk of

173

miscarriage in women who are exposed to inhaled sulfide chemicals.[249] Garlic may have spermicidal contraceptive effects as well. Recent scientific studies have shown garlic's active principle, allitridum, to be highly spermicidal in both animal and human tests.[250]

Gathering: Garlic can be found growing wild in the U.S. from New York to Indiana, and stretching southwest to Missouri. The bulbs of garlic are harvested in late summer before the flowers appear and when the green foliage turns brown. Garlic tops can be braided while green to make an attractive, convenient, strand; or pulled bulbs can be left in the sun for a few days to dry before storing in a cool airy place.

Preparation: Garlic may be used as a suppository in combination with any abortifacient herbal treatment. Parsley combines well with garlic as a suppository. Historically garlic, in clove and umbel flower form, was mentioned boiled.[251] A boiled, cooled clove or small bulb can be inserted like a fresh clove, or the liquid infusion from the boiling of the head or the umbel flowers may be used as a fumigation, vaginal douche, or sitz bath. Garlic is most effective if used very early in pregnancy.

Words to the Wise: Clotting times can double when garlic preparations are used internally. Discontinue if signs of discomfort appear. Do not use garlic as a suppository for longer than two weeks. Garlic may increase blood pressure and the number of leukocytes (white blood cell in the blood). Garlic is estrogenic. Fatalities have been reported when garlic preparations fell into the hands of children. As with all medicines, keep herbs in a safe place that children cannot access. No specific signs of toxicity are reported for garlic as an herbal medicine. Remove garlic pessary if negative side effects are experienced.

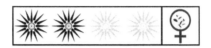

Garlic Dosage

Emmenagogual Garlic Vaginal Pessary: Simmer a garlic bulb in water for ten minutes. Test temperature of water, and when a comfortable warm temperature, douche with the garlic water. When the garlic bulb reaches a comfortable temperature, place in cheese cloth, tie with string and insert into the vagina. Replace every twelve hours for up to six days.

Ginger
Zingiber officinalis

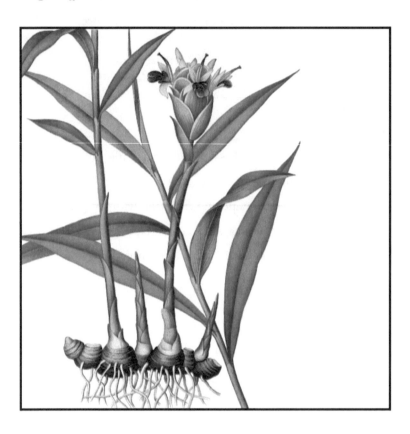

If menstruation has been suddenly suppressed,
it is best to give a hot sitz (hip) bath,
a copious drink of ginger tea, place her in bed…,
and bottles of hot water about her hips and loins.

-R.L Robb in *Robb &Co.'s Family Physician,* 1882

Family Zingiberaceae

AKA: Asian, Jamaican, and Hawaiian Ginger.

Part Used: Root.

Medicinal Properties: Aromatic, carminative, diaphoretic, diuretic, emmenagogue and stimulant.

Effects on the Body: Soothes stomach, stimulates circulatory system, relieves joint and muscle pain, cleans out intestines, and promotes menstruation.

Abortifacient Action: Contains uterine contracting thujone.

Contains: Abortifacient chemical beta-bisabolene (rhizome), phytoestrogen beta-sitosterol, and beta-thujone (rhizome).

Description: Asian ginger, *Zingiber officinalis*, sometimes called Hawaiian or Jamaican Ginger, is cultivated in tropical climates. The knobby root has a smooth shiny tan skin. Inside, the root is cream to yellow with a very strong spicy odor. Grass-like stems emerge from the root nodes.

Ginger Herbal Lore and Historical Use

Asian ginger is the tan shiny root that can be found in nearly every Asian food store and in many mainstream supermarkets. Asian ginger is very effective at promoting menstruation (and possibly abortion) in early pregnancy, and is used for this purpose in China.[252] One prominent herbalist, Susan Weed, notes Asian ginger is quick to act and strong as a menstrual promoter. In experiments on rats, ginger tea caused increased early pregnancy embryo loss.[253]

177

Preparation: Ginger is highly regarded for its power as an emmenagogue and adjuvant, but generally ginger is not considered a strong abortifacient by itself. Ginger's emmenagogual powers are most effective when utilized by taking ginger infusion for five days prior to menses. As an adjuvant, gnger is believed to have the power to enhance the effectiveness of any herbs with which they are combined. Asian ginger also has carminative properties that may combine well with aloe, or other herbs that tend to irritate the digestive organs.

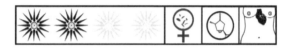

Words to the Wise: Take ginger tea in smaller doses if large doses cause nausea.

Asian Ginger Dosage

Emmenagogual Decoction (root): 1 – 2 oz. (28 - 57 g) sliced fresh root
to 2 cups (500 ml) water. Simmer 20 minutes. Take 1 cup
(250 ml), two to three times a day, on an empty stomach for
up to six days.

Hibiscus

Hibiscus rosa-sinensis
Hibiscus phoenicia
Hibiscus esculentus (okra)

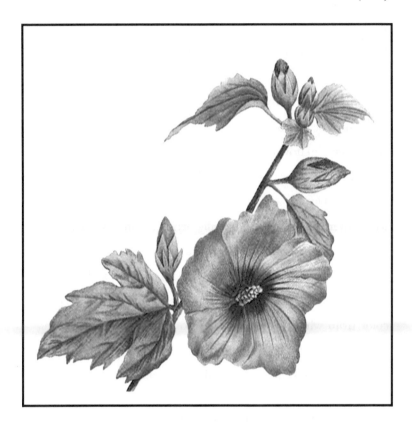

A native of Banda in 1655 (confessed) that
he had caused the abortion of his concubine by
giving her the flowers (Hibiscus rosa-sinensis)
rubbed down with papaya seeds.

-William Dymock in *Pharmacograph Indica*, 1890

Family Malvaceae

AKA: Bunga raya, karkade, kembang sepatu, bebaru, bunga pepulut (Malaysia), pucuk (Indonesia), zhu jin, fu sang, da hong hua (Mandarin), shoe flower, and rose of sharon.

Part Used: Flowers.

Medicinal Properties: Abortifacient, emmenagogue, and contraceptive.

Effects on the Body, Abortifacient Action: Anti-estrogenic and anti-implantation.

Contains: Unknown.

Description: Hibiscus is a small evergreen tropical tree or shrub, growing to a maximum of 30 feet (10 m) high in the wild. Alternate leaves are spirally arranged and often have a toothed or lobed margin. Large trumpet-shaped flowers with five or more petals arise from the upper leaf axils, and grow up to 10 in. (25 cm) in diameter. Flowers, whose petals range in color from white to yellow to red to purple, have a very long style. The fruit of hibiscus forms a dry five lobed calyx (capsule), which splits open to release the seeds at maturity.

Hibiscus Herbal Lore and Historical Use

The origin of hibiscus is unknown. Endemic varieties exist all around the world. According to 'plant lore,' the hibiscus symbolizes beauty and fertility. In Tahitian lore, the hibiscus flower worn over the right ear shows that a person is looking for a mate; and if the flower is worn over the left ear, a mate has been found. Hibiscus flowers also symbolize protection and are reputed to protect from poison and prevent evil spirits and illness.

Around the world, women use hibiscus to affect their fertility. For menstrual promotion and abortion, the fresh flowers are used in a hot water decoction in the following countries: China,[254] Bangladesh,[255] Peru,[256] East Indies,[257] East New Britain,[258] and Rarotonga.[259] In China and Annam, the bark of hibiscus is documented as being used as an emmenagogue. [260] In Jamaica, some tribes use oil from the hibiscus flower to induce abortion.

Hibiscus flowers were said to possess anti-fertility properties by ancient Ayurvedic texts. The flowers of hibiscus are used in Kerala, in southern India, is for their emmenagogue and contraceptive action. In Hindu temples in India, hibiscus flowers are given as offerings to Kali, the goddess known to carry away the dead. The Hindustani name for hibiscus 'pushpa' has multiple meanings: menstruation, vulva, and the honey of flowers. In India, folk-healers of Chhattisgarh, India mix the fresh hibiscus flowers in water and apply the paste externally on the pelvis to produce abortion.[261] The hibiscus flower may have the opposite effect on the uterus if prepared an alternate way; Murray mentions that in Sind (Pakistan) the flowers are fried in clarified butter and are administered for halting excessive menstruation.[262]

Hibiscus rosa-sinensis has a cousin in the okra plant, *Hibiscus esculentus*. Okra is originally from Africa. Three thousand years ago, Egyptians were cultivating okra plants.

African slaves and slave traders brought okra to the Americas. Enslaved women sometimes used okra to achieve abortions via "lubricating the uterine passages by a diet of these pods,"[263] and then inducing abortion with a uterine contracting herb. In West Africa, women today still use okra to induce an abortion.[264]

In Peru, hibiscus flowers were used historically to affect the fertility of both men and women.[265] Recent studies have confirmed that flowers of *Hibiscus rosa-sinensis* have an anti-spermatogenetic effect in male mice.[266]

Scientific studies on animals and humans are confirming the use of hibiscus as an antifertility agent for the female sex. An antiestrogen effect has been shown in mice and rats.[267] The benzene extract of dried hibiscus flowers produced abortion in rats at a dose of 186 mg per kg.[268] The benzene extract of the dried flowers exhibit anti-implantation effects with 80% effectiveness in rats at a dose of 100 mg per kg.[269] An anti-follicle stimulating hormone activity was observed in rats that were given the ethanol extract of flowers at a dose of 150 mg per animal.[270] Antifertility effects have been shown in human females taking ethanol extracts of the dried flowers at a dose of 250 mg, three times a day, on the 7th through the 22nd day of the menstrual cycle.[271]

Gathering: The open flowers of hibiscus are gathered daily in early morning, and dried out of direct sunlight. Leaves may be gathered as needed. Bark and root are best gathered at night.

Preparation: Hibiscus flowers are usually used as a simple, but sometimes combined with papaya seeds, or Asian ginger to induce abortion. Hibiscus flowers are most often used in a hot water decoction during the first eight weeks of pregnancy. When purchasing dried hibiscus flowers, the buyer should be certain that the flowers of hibiscus are purchased, not the calyces (seed pods). The calyces of hibiscus are sold to make herb tea and a drink called Karkady or Agua de Jamaica, pronounced ha-ma-ike-ah in Spanish. Hibiscus calyces are sometimes known as flor de Jamaica, te de Jamaica, hibiscus flores, or even hibiscus flowers, but they are not the flowers; they are the calyx or seed pod. Around the world, *Hibiscus rosa-sinensis* plants are available to purchase as indoor potted plants, and continually flower all year indoors, given enough care, sunlight, and warmth. Purchasing a plant and gathering the blossoms to dry and store for later use may be the best option if the dried flowers are unavailable for purchase.

Words to the Wise: Hibiscus can be a host to whiteflies and aphids that can contribute to allergens and mold spores in and around hibiscus plants. If you are sensitive to allergens, protect yourself when harvesting from hibiscus. No specific signs of toxicity are noted for hibiscus; reduce dosage if negative side effects are experienced.

183

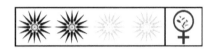

Signs of Toxicity Specific to Hibiscus: Unknown.

Hibiscus Dosage

Emmenagogual Decoction: 1 cup *fresh* flowers to 2 pints (1 L)
hot water, sipped throughout day, for up to ten days.
OR 10 - 16 Tbs. of *dried* flowers to 2 pints (1 L) hot
water, sipped throughout day, for up to ten days.

Horseradish
Cochlearia armoracia

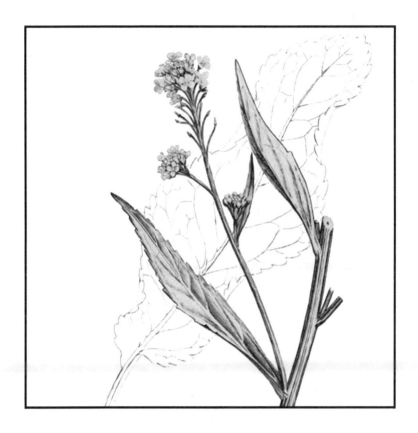

Horseradish was formerly much employed to produce abortion, frequently effecting this object, when other internal agents failed; it was used as follows: A saturated infusion of the recent roots in whiskey was made, of which 4 fluid ounces was the dose, repeating it 3 or 4 times every day, and continuing its use until the desired effect was produced.

-King's American Dispensary, 1898

185

Family Brassicaceae

AKA: Great raifort, mountain radish, rabano rusticana, red cole, wild horseradish.

Part Used: Root.

Medicinal Properties: Antiseptic, antiscorbutic, aperient, digestive, diuretic, expectorant, rubefacient, sialagogue, and stimulant.

Effects on the Body: Stimulates the digestion, promotes sweating thereby lowering fevers, loosens phlegm and moves it out of the system, and stimulates the immune system.

Abortifacient Action: Unknown.

Contains: Vitamin C and peroxidase enzyme.

Description: Horseradish is a long tapering root with brownish beige skin on the outside. Inside, it is very white. Above ground, the leaves can grow up to 3 - 5 feet tall (1 - 1.5 m). Horseradish has small white flowers and sterile seeds, but this is not a problem for horseradish propagates itself well via its root system.

Horseradish Herbal Lore and Historical Use

The ancient Egyptians, as far back as 1500 BC, may have known horseradish, a native to Eastern Europe. The Greeks and Romans may also have known horseradish. They used a wild radish for its medicinal properties, which is believed by some to have been horseradish. Pliny the Elder, in *Natural History* said, "It's called wild radish, esteemed in Arcadia although it originated elsewhere. Besides encouraging urination, it's also very hot. In Italy it's also called armoracia."[272]

186

Horseradish was one of the five bitter herbs (along with coriander, horehound, lettuce, and nettle) historically eaten during the feast of the Passover. In present times, horseradish is still commonly used in the Passover Seder. In the Middle Ages, horseradish's medicinal properties were still valued. Monks brought new herbs to remote areas; horseradish came to Scandinavia with monks around AD 1200. Native Americans of the Cherokee tribe utilized the abortifacient qualities of horseradish.[273]

Gathering: In early spring or fall after the second hard frost, roots that have grown to over one inch in diameter are harvested.

Preparation: Before and during the Jewish Passover holiday in early spring, many markets will stock fresh horseradish, as it is used to make the 'bitter herb' consumed as part of the ritual Seder plate. To select and prepare horseradish, a hard root that feels heavy for its size is chosen. Roots can be frozen for up to six months. To prepare the pungent horseradish into a tincture, gloves and a chemical respirator are worn. Contact lenses are removed. The root is scrubbed and green skin is removed with a peeler. Working outside, the pieces of the horseradish root are ground in a food processor, grated with a cheese grater, or chopped into small pieces with a chef's knife. The fresh horseradish pieces are packed into a wide-mouthed glass jar and covered with alcohol. After preparing horseradish, hands must be washed well. Horseradish tincture is more effective if used during early pregnancy.

187

Words to the Wise: Horseradish can cause contact dermatitis. Horseradish should not be used by individuals with thyroid problems. Large quantities of horseradish can be poisonous due to its content of volatile oils. Horseradish oils can irritate stomach ulcers. Horseradish is considered safe for human consumption, however, cases of livestock poisoning occur when horseradish is used as fodder for animals. Horseradish contains glucosinolates. Glucosinolates contained in kale, cabbage, and broccoli can cause goiters in humans, however the toxicity frequency has dropped dramatically over the past few decades, as researchers have altered the quantity of toxic compounds by creating new cultivars with lower quantities of glucosinolates.

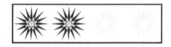

Watch for Signs of Toxicity Specific to Horseradish: Profuse sweating, irritation of the stomach and intestines, loss of strength, and disorientation.

Horseradish Dosage*

Abortifacient Fresh Horseradish Root Tincture: 1:2, 95% alcohol,
>   then 2 - 4 fl. oz. (84 - 112 ml), three to four times a day, for up to three days.

*No deaths are reported, however this dosage may prove toxic.

Juniper

Juniperus communis
Juniperus sabina

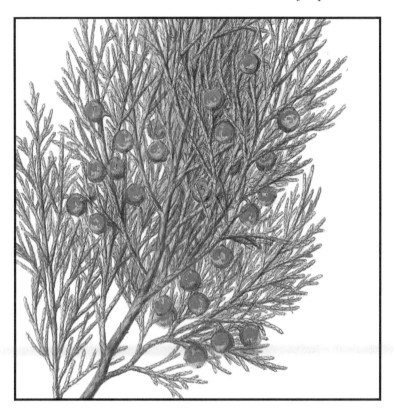

*And when I look, to gather fruit, find nothing but
the savin-tree. Too frequent in nun's orchards, and
there planted, by all conjecture, to destroy fruit rather.*

- Thomas Middleton in *A Game of Chess*, 1624

*She's gane to the garden gay,
To pu' o' the savin-tree;
But for a' that she can say or do,
The babie it would not die.*

- in the 16th century Scottish Ballad, 'Mary Hamilton'

189

Family Cupressaceae

AKA: Juniper, genvier, geneva, bastard killer, horse savin, covershame, hackmatack, kill-bastard, and aiten.

Parts Used: Berries and leaves.

Medicinal Properties: Abortifacient, anodyne, antiseptic, antispasmodic, aromatic, carminative, digestant, diuretic, lithotriptic, rubefacient and stimulant.

Effects on the Body: Uterine stimulant soothes inflammation of the sinuses, regulatory to internal sugar levels, useful in pancreas, kidney, and bladder treatments.

Abortifacient Action: Relaxation effect on the uterus. Contains uterine contracting thujone.

Contains: Abortifacient chemicals: Alpha-thujone, podophyllotoxin, and isocupressic acid.

Description: Juniper varies in form, ranging from a 2 ft. (0.6 m) ground clinging shrub to a 25 ft. (8.3 m) tall tree. Bluish, evergreen, needle-like leaves ¼ - ½ in. (0.5 - 1.3 cm) long, upper surfaces whitish, occur in whorls of three. Small, indistinct greenish-yellow flowers appear on the female plants from late spring to early summer, followed by ½ in. (1.3 cm) diameter fleshy green female cones. Juniper berries are green for two summers and then ripen around October into the characteristic blue-black juniper berries. In the United States, juniper can be found in open woodlands and dry hilltops from Alaska south to Nebraska and east to North Carolina, also found in the northern Rockies south to New Mexico. It is planted as landscaping in other areas.

Juniper Herbal Lore and Historical Use[h]

An origin for any plant that is as widespread as juniper is not easy to pinpoint. Some have suggested that juniper is native to the Mediterranean region, as several medical recipes that list juniper as an ingredient survive in Egyptian papyri dating to 1550 BC. Today there are 13 species of juniper that are believed to be native to North America. In fact, juniper is found in nearly every temperate zone in the northern hemisphere. Throughout history, everywhere juniper grew, the people who lived nearby imbued it with spiritual qualities. The ancient people of the Mediterranean used sacred juniper wood and branches as ceremonial and medicinal incense. Hannibal commanded that the beams of the temple of Diana, Lady of the Grove, be made of the trunks of juniper trees.[274]

Juniper was 'the tree of life' to the ancient Germans, who hung juniper branches on their homes to protect themselves from evil (possibly the origin of the pine wreaths traditionally hung on doors throughout the U.S. during the winter months). The Germans also added the juniper berries to their ritual intoxicating beers. Shamans from Siberia to northwest Pakistan practice an ancient tradition of inhaling juniper smoke to induce a trance, wherein they perform their magical activities.[275] The Native American Cherokee pour a juniper infusion on hot rocks during the ritual sweat lodge.[276] The Native American Peyote church burns the wood chips of *Juniperus oxyderus*

---

[h] The purpose of this book is to recapture information about historical approaches to self-induced abortion. Juniper has been included; however the reader must keep in mind that deaths have resulted from the ingestion of this herb.

during all the peyote ritual activities to protect from evil energies.[277] Like so many herbal abortifacients anciently associated with freedom and sexuality, juniper was reputed to have aphrodisiac powers.[278]

Juniper leaves, berries, and roots have been recorded historically to have contraceptive and abortifacient properties. In *De Materia Medica*, the ancient Greek doctor, Dioscorides (1st or 2nd century AD), recorded the contraceptive use of crushed juniper berries placed on the penis or vulva before intercourse. The Greeks and Romans commonly used the oil of juniper *Juniperus sabina*, also called savin, as an abortifacient. The use of juniper's oil for abortifacient purposes spread from the Mediterranean to Northern Europe, and was mentioned by seventeenth century herbalist Nicholas Culpepper in his *Complete Herbal*.

The effective use of a tea of juniper leaves to relax muscles following delivery by Native American Zuni women is being confirmed by recent scientific testing. Oils from the leaves of juniper have been shown to have a direct effect on the uterus on animals and on isolated human uteri and fallopian tubes[279] causing relaxation of the uterus which if prolonged could lead to an abortion.[280]

Juniper root may have implantation inhibiting properties as well. In a 1986 study using rats, an oral dosage of 200 mg extract of *Juniperus communis* root resulted in blocked implantation in 60% of the rats.[281] One study states that *Juniper communis* extract and *Juniper communis* oil are similar in chemical composition.[282] The needles of juniper can contain isocupressic acid, which is known to reduce blood flow through the placenta, and can cause late term abortion in cows who feed on juniper needles.[283]   Other plants which contain

192

isocupressic acid also have a folkloric tradition as abortifacients. Native American women used water extract of the needles of ponderosa pine *Pinus ponderosa* (which also contains isocupressic acid) to cause abortion.

Gathering: The fleshy blue-black ripe berries are gathered in autumn, around October. Gather leaves in the morning after the dew has dried. Gather the root at night. The berries are dried in open air in the shade and turned frequently. One herbal noted that the highest concentration of the essential oil is in the full grown but unripe berries. As the berries ripen, more and more of the essential oil is converted into resin form.[284]

Preparation: Juniper berries were used anciently in vaginal pessary formulations for abortifacient purposes; however, oral administration of juniper preparations is also recorded. Juniper root may have an implantation inhibiting action. Juniper berries are known to have a uterine stimulating effect. Juniper leaf or berry tincture (which preserves the essential oils in the preparation) has a relaxant action on the uterus and can in large dosages cause an abortion. As an emmenagogue and abortifacient, juniper berries are reputed to be most successful in the first two weeks of pregnancy. Juniper leaves are reputed to be most successful in mid to late term (after 12 weeks) when the placenta is the sole support of the fetus. The Native Americans and the Hunza commonly combine juniper and rue in medicinal preparations. Juniper is sometimes combined with Asian ginger for emmenagogual purposes. Juniper gives gin alcohol its flavor.

Gin is often specified as the menstuum in abortifacient tincture recipes.

Words to the Wise: Anyone with kidney or nerve damage or diseases should not use juniper. Juniper may irritate the kidneys. Juniper berries can cause a drop in blood sugar if food is not consumed within twenty minutes of ingestion. Do not take internally for longer than 6 weeks without a break.[285] Juniper contains uterine contracting and possibly toxic thujone. Juniper, when taken internally, may interfere with the absorption of iron and other essential minerals. Juniper is a diuretic which gives the urine the odor of violet flowers.[286] Late term abortions in cattle due to juniper leaf consumption often have the dangerous complication of a retained placenta.

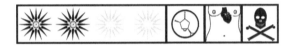

Watch for Signs of Toxicity Specific to Juniper: Diarrhea, purplish urine, blood in the urine, kidney pain, intestinal pain, elevated blood pressure, and a quickened heartbeat.

Juniper Dosage

Juniper Berry Menstrual Promoter: 1 Tbs. berries to 1 cup (250 ml) water. Steep 20 minutes, two to three times a day.

Juniper Implantation Inhibiting Infusion (Needles): One ounce (28 g) needles to 2 cups (500 ml) water. Steep, covered, ½ - 1 hour. Take 1 - 3 Tbs. (15 – 45 ml), two to three times a day for up to six days.

194

Lupine
Lupinus angustifolius

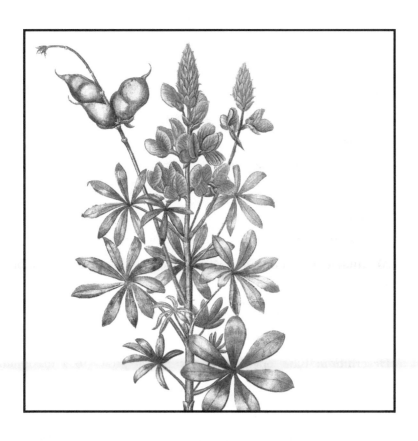

*Many women... "doe use the meale of lupines mingled with
the fall of a goate and some juyce of lemons to make
into a forme of a soft ointment."*

- John Parkinson in *Theatricum Botanicum*, 1640

195

Family Leguminosae

AKA: Blue lupine, narrow-leafed lupine (English), smalbladet lupin (Danish), lupin bleu; lupin à feuilles étroites (French), blaue lupine (German), and Altramuz azul (Spanish).

Other North American lupine varieties that may contain bitter alkaloids: Texas bluebonnet (*Lupinus texensis*), California tree lupin (*Lupinus arboreus*), and wild perennial lupine (*Lupinus perennis*).

Part Used: Seeds.

Medicinal Properties: Diuretic, vermifuge (seeds), anthelmintic, emmenagogue (internal-seeds), and utilized for skin ulcers (external application of seeds)

Effects on the Body: Increases urine output and affects the nerves.

Abortifacient Action: Causes contraction of the uterus and embryo toxic.

Contains: Abortifacient Chemicals: Anagyrine and lupinine.

Concentration of abortifacient alkaloids is highest in mature seed.

Description: Blue lupine is an annual that grows to a maximum height of 1.5 ft. (0.5 m). From velvety stems branch lupine's dark green leaves, which are made up of 5 - 10 narrow oblong 1.5 in. (4 cm) leaflets. Lupine's dark blue flowers form short bunches in summer.

Lupine Herbal Lore and Historical Use[i]

Lupine originated in the Mediterranean area and was cultivated since the days of ancient Egypt. Dioscorides noted lupine's

---

[i] The purpose of this book is to recapture information about historical approaches to self-induced abortion. Lupine has been included, however the reader must keep in mind that many deaths have resulted from the ingestion of this herb.

abortifacient effects "extracts the menses and fetus."[287]   For emmenagogual and abortifacient purposes, Soranus suggested a paste of ground lupine beans combined with wormwood as a poultice on the lower abdomen to cause abortion. He also suggested lupine bean meal with equal parts wallflower and myrtle formed with a little water into a pill the size of a bean to make an abortive vaginal suppository.[288] Although the ancient texts suggest that lupine was used in external applications for abortifacient purposes, in the 'Creation of Man', by Abu al-Hasan al Tabib (AD 1044 - 1101) lupine is listed as an oral abortifacient herb.[289]

Modern science has confirmed that lupine contains compounds that have a direct effect on the uterus. In studies, *Lupinus termis* seeds have increased the motor activity of the uterus at times outside of menstruation, during menstruation, and pregnancy.[290] Lupinine, an alkaloid in bitter lupine seeds, produces contractions of isolated pig uteri.[291]

Bitter lupine seeds are considered a safe food crop, but only when lupine seeds are carefully soaked to remove the poisonous alkaloids is lupine safe for human consumption. Taste is a good indicator of the presence of the bitter alkaloids. Traditionally, lupine seeds of *Lupinus albus* following debittering have been used in the Middle East and Europe to make snack foods. In Europe, lupine seeds are known as lupini beans.

Gathering: There are bitter and sweet forms of *Lupinus augustifolius*. It is the bitter alkaloids that are highly teratogenic and can cause abortion and human death. Modern alkaloid free varieties have white flowers.

197

The bitter lupines usually have blue flowers. Mature blue lupine seeds, gathered in fall, often have a wide range of colors, ranging from uniform grey to speckled brown to nearly black with light spots.

Preparation: Lupine seeds can be purchased online and occasionally can be found in health food stores. A coffee grinder or mortar and pestle can be used to grind dry lupine seeds. Alternately, seeds can be soaked in water overnight, and ground in a mortar and pestle wet. Lupine is used to abort during the first trimester.

Words to the Wise: Lupine seeds are known to cause birth defects in animals. Lupine alkaloids are known to produce birth defects in cattle if eaten during certain early gestational times: cleft palates, crooked legs, distorted spines. It is suspected that human birth defects occasionally are associated with ingestion of milk of sheep or goats that have been grazing on lupine.[292] Teratogenity has been shown in cows if grazing on lupine during 2nd and 3rd month of pregnancy.[293] Lupine alkaloids can affect the nervous system of the person who consumes them, causing a loss in muscle nerve control that is usually reversible.[294] Human deaths have resulted from eating of lupine seeds that were not adequately de-bittered. In lupine seeds, a lethal dose of lupanine has been determined to be about 100 mg/kg. If not properly debittered by repeated soaking and rinsing, 10 g of seeds consumed may lead to death. People with a peanut allergy may also be allergic to lupine flour.[295]

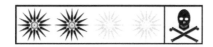

Watch for Signs of Toxicity Specific to Lupine: The alkaloids of lupine target the nervous system: malaise, unpleasant sensations in the head, dimness of vision, cerebral heaviness, dizziness, mental excitation, laryngeal and pharyngeal constriction.

Lupine Dosage*

Abortifacient Lupine Pessary: Grind 1 g bitter lupine seeds to a flour, and mix one part lemon juice and four parts of water to form a thick paste. Place paste into a circle of silk and tie securely with tooth floss to form a small pessary. Insert high into vagina. Replace every twelve hours for up to four days.

Abortifacient Lupine Abdomen Pack: Mix 3 - 5 g bitter lupine seed flour with castor oil to form a thick paste. Apply to lower abdomen. Cover with a piece of plastic, and wrap abdomen with long strip of fabric or wide elastic bandages to hold in place. Sleep on a towel, and place a hot water bottle on top of the lower abdomen. Wear abdomen pack overnight.

* Extreme Caution! Do not take internally! External applications may have toxic effects.

Male Fern

Dryopteris felix-mas

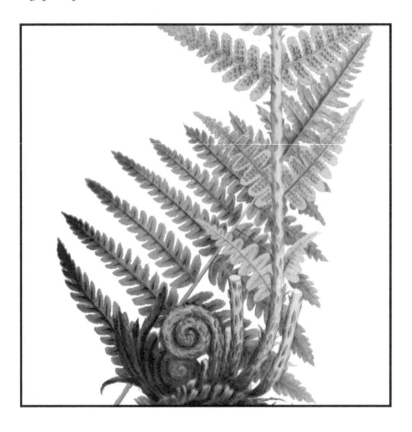

This drug was found to be absolutely without value. An ethereal extract of male fern from one of the most reputable German pharmaceutical laboratories was purchased... but absolutely no results were obtained from its use. The Commission then obtained a fresh solid extract, which gave no better results, although such effects as dizziness, etc., followed its administration.

-H.A. Hare, M.D. in *Therapeutic Gazette*, 1908

200

Family Polypodiaceae

AKA: Shield fern or root, sweet or knotty brake, basket fern, and bear paw's root.

Part Used: Recently dried root.

Medicinal Properties: Anthelmintic and emmenagogue.

Effects on the Body: Cathartic purgative used to expel worms and reflexively promotes menstruation.

Abortifacient Action: Gastrointestinal irritation.

Contains: Oleoresin, filicin, desaspidin, albaspidin, flavaspidic acid and essential oil.

Description: Perennial male fern has stemless oblong-lanceolate erect fronds 2 - 4 ft. (1 m) in height. Leaflets, which hold their yellow-green color through most of the year, are alternate and variously divided and notched. The spore holding sori found on the backs of the leaflets are closer to the mid vein than the margin. Male Fern's numerous kidney-shaped sori appear from summer to autumn, the young color being light green maturing to brown. Male fern has a strong, woody, chaffy rhizome, 8 - 20 in. (20 – 51 cm) long, with a 4 in. (10 cm) diameter. The outer color of the rhizome is dark brown, and the medicinal inside is pale green. Male fern grows in rocky woodlands from Alaska south to Arizona eastward to South Dakota, north to Michigan and Vermont.

Male Fern Herbal Lore and Historical Use[j]

Male fern was traditionally gathered as part of the summer solstice celebration of Midsummer's Eve. The ritual gathering of herbs before sunrise on Midsummer's Eve goes back to ancient Babylonia, 700 BC. The Midsummer's Eve celebration evolved to a Roman summer solstice celebration in honor of the Great Mother Earth Goddess, Ceres, (later known as Diana) who protected and nurtured the grains of the fields. Ecstatic dancing and merrymaking around the fires went on all though the night. Leaping over the fire was believed to protect the individual from harm and protect the vigor of the crops as well. A midsummer tree or maypole (a phallic symbol honoring the union of the sun and moon on the solstice) was erected to bring good luck and fertility. Male fern was associated with fire and lightning, and was gathered by moonlight on the summer solstice. Traditionally, a root of male fern was dug and all but five fronds were cut away. The five-fingered fern was known as 'Lucky Hand' or 'St. John's Hand.' The Male Fern 'Lucky Hand' was dried and hardened by smoking it in a Midsummer's Eve fire. Afterwards the 'Lucky Hand' was said to protect the owner and family from illness or evil spirits in the coming year.[296] Glass made from the ash of male fern was thought to possess magical qualities. His followers believed the ring worn by Genghis Khan contained male fern glass, and that it granted him the power to understand the ways of plants and the speech of birds.[297]

---

[j] The purpose of this book is to recapture information about historical approaches to self-induced abortion. Male fern has been included; however the reader must keep in mind that many deaths have resulted from the ingestion of this herb.

Syrian women about to be married bound the male fern (known to them as bride's gloves) to the bride's hands and dyed the hands with henna. The form of the fern remained on the hands as long as the henna dye lasted protecting the bride from magic. Another belief was that any pregnant women who happened to step on a male fern would miscarry.[298] Tartarean women used male fern root infusion as a contraceptive.[299]

Male fern is known to have an abortifacient effect related to its purgative powers. The abortifacient action of strong purgatives is believed to result from severe gastrointestinal irritation, which stimulates the pituitary gland to produce oxytocin, which causes uterine contractions. Male fern has been known since ancient times as a very strong vermifuge, driving out flatworm. To drive out worms, the person consumes only a fat-free diet for 2 - 3 days. Then, a dosage of male fern root tea is given. The oleoresin in male fern causes paralysis in the worm, and it loosens its grip on the intestine. Around two hours after taking the male fern tea, the person is given a saline laxative, such as epsom salts, which assists in expelling the worm from the body. Male fern is so potent and potentially toxic, its use is thought of as a last resort, only used after other vermifuges, easier to use and having no side effects, have failed to expel the worms.

Gathering: Male fern root should be gathered before sunrise (July-September) on a sunny and warm day that is fore. Dry root in the shade as quickly as possible. Carefully brush dirt off from root with a dry toothbrush as it dries. Male fern's medicinal activity is impaired by storage; collect fresh male fern root for use immediately if at all possible. If the root is dried, only inner portions of the male fern root that have retained their original pale green color are used.

Preparation: Internal use of purgative male fern root decoction causes abortion due to severe gastrointestinal irritation. The use of male fern internally should be avoided due to serious side effects. Words to the Wise: Male fern can cause serious side effects even at therapeutic dosages. Fatal poisoning has resulted from male fern's use as an abortifacient.

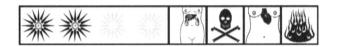

Watch for Signs of Toxicity Specific to Male Fern: Nausea, vomiting, cramping, headache, shortness of breath, albuminuria. and bilirubinuria. Toxic overdoses result in: loss of reflexes, optic neuritis, impairment of vision, temporary blindness, coma, convulsions, and death due to cardiac and respiratory failure.[300]

Male Fern Bath for Muscle Pains
The following recipe is for external use only! Do not use internally!
Simmer 3 – 6 oz. (100 - 150 g) of male fern root in 1 quart (1 L) of water, simmer five to ten minutes, then move pan away from heat and leave to infuse for another ten to fifteen minutes. As a footbath, this decoction may be helpful for menstrual cramps. Traditionally, this male fern decoction was used added to bath water for arthritis and on warm compresses to relieve pain associated with neuritis and rheumatism.

Mistletoe
Phoradendron flavescens (American)
Viscum album (European)

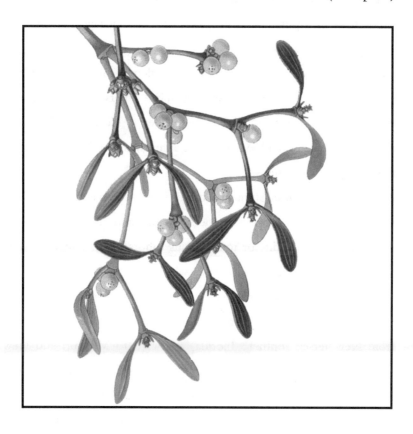

In the palmy days of 'Cranborne Chase,' the season for killing 'dry' does began at Martinstide (Nov.11) and ended at Candlemas (Feb.2). Now it was customary with the keepers to produce the effect of natural sterility by inducing abortion in the female deer, and this they did by laying branches of mistletoe in their feeding grounds some two or three months before the season commenced. The plan succeeded, but it was said that the venison in such cases was deficient in flavor.

-Martin de Albuquerque in *Notes and Queries*, 1865

Family Lorathaceae

AKA: The golden bough and birdlime.

Parts Used: Leaves, flowers, and young twigs.

Medicinal Properties: Antispasmodic, emmenagogue, emetic, diuretic, nervine, oxytocic, and tonic.

Effects on the Body: American mistletoe: Stimulates uterine contractions, raises blood pressure, relaxes nerves, and contains tumor-inhibiting proteins. European mistletoe: Heart stimulant, will first raise then lower blood pressure; stimulates glands, and contains tumor-inhibiting proteins.

Abortifacient Action: Stimulates uterus to relaxation and contraction.

Contains: Amines, beta-phenylethylamine and tyramine protein substances called lectins or toxalbumins (phoratoxin); viscin, choline, sugar, a fixed oil, tannin, and various salts.

Description: American mistletoe, *Phoradendron flavescens*, is a native North American parasitic shrub that can grow on all deciduous trees, from New Jersey south to Florida, westward to Missouri and New Mexico. It is also found in northern California to coastal British Columbia. American mistletoe has strong smooth branches that tend to be brittle at the base. Occurring in opposite pairs, leaves are leathery, dark green, and obovate, up to 3 in. (7.6 cm) long. From May to July, small white flowers appear which mature into white sticky round, ¾ in. (2 cm) diameter berries, each containing 1 seed.

European mistletoe, *Viscum album*, is a native from northwest Europe to China and south to Iran. European mistletoe is a parasitic shrub that can grow on all deciduous trees. European mistletoe has regularly branching stems, up 3 ft. (1 m) long. The 2 in. (5 cm) long leaves are

206

light green, leathery, and blunt and occur in opposite pairs. Flowers mature into small, ½ in. (1.25 cm) diameter, white sticky berries.

American Mistletoe Herbal Lore and Historical Use

Native American women of northern California used mistletoe leaf infusion during labor to regulate contractions, quiet the nerves, expel the placenta, and arrest hemorrhage. The Pomo Native American women used a decoction of leaves and an infusion of roots of the American mistletoe to promote menstruation. The Kawaiisu Native American women used an infusion of American mistletoe plant growing on the Douglas oak tree during the first two months of pregnancy to cause an abortion.[301] Native American women living in northern California were documented as having said that mistletoe leaf abortifacient infusion from mistletoe growing on a buckeye tree was better than that found growing on other trees.[302]

Members of the North American voodoo religion carry mistletoe as a love charm and amulet. In the voodoo religion, mistletoe is sacred to the sensual and the pleasure-loving voodoo Loa Erzulie, a goddess of love.[303] Erzulie is, protector of women, representative of seduction and fertility and is often compared to the Greek goddess Aphrodite.[304]

American mistletoe is known to cause an increase in uterine and intestinal contractions and also an increase in blood pressure. Mistletoe has been shown to increase uterine contractions in non-pregnant cats.[305] The abortifacient effects of mistletoe are attributed to ribosome inhibiting proteins (RIPs). RIPs halt cellular metabolism by inhibiting the final stage of protein production in the cell.[306]

207

European Mistletoe Herbal Lore and Historical Use[k]

European mistletoe was a sacred plant to the Celtic druids, being the golden key (phallus) that gave access to the magical powers of the underworld (womb of the mother earth). Growing on a branch of the oak tree, raised high above the earth, the evergreen (immortal) Mistletoe, with its white, sticky, semen-like berries, was symbolic of the genitals of the oak god to the druids.

The sacred oak god was a lover of the three-fold moon goddess. At the full moon after the winter solstice, the druids would sacrificially castrate the oak god by cutting off his mistletoe with a golden moon sickle, and catching the falling mistletoe in a white cloth, before it touched the ground. The gathering of the abortive mistletoe was symbolic of the woman's moon energy keyed into the magical powers of the underworld (earth mother) energy sufficient to cut off (castrate) the life power of the sexual act and hold the life spirit suspended in the spirit world, between heaven and earth. A sexual celebration ensued after the gathering of the mistletoe. Each worshiper took some of the cut mistletoe home to use to keep away 'evil spirits.' Some of the protective mistletoe was hung in the home by the druids and more was made into magical drinks that were known to heal all illness, give strength and courage, render all poisons ineffective, and make both humans and animals fertile.[307]

Like so many abortifacients anciently associated with orgiastic ceremonies, mistletoe gained an aphrodisiacal reputation. In England

---

[k] The purpose of this book is to recapture information about historical approaches to self-induced abortion. Mistletoe has been included; however the reader must keep in mind that deaths have resulted from the ingestion of this herb.

208

and Ireland, mistletoe was held to have the power to revitalize the sexual organs.

With the advent of Christianity, women and the symbols of powerful women were propagandized to be evil. Christianized Saxons, who had previously associated mistletoe in a manner similar to the Celtic druids, are recorded as claiming that mistletoe was the "forbidden tree in the middle of the trees of Eden."[308] Until the mid 20th century, mistletoe was banned in England's churches, as it was considered to be a symbol of pagan worship.[309]

Gathering: The leafy young branches are gathered from late autumn to December. They may be processed into tinctures immediately or dried in the shade and stored in an airtight container.

Preparation: American mistletoe's abortive action is believed to result from the stimulation of the uterus and intestines causing intense contractions. Conversely, European mistletoe's abortive action is believed to result from its antispasmodic action on smooth muscles (like the uterus and intestines). American and European mistletoe are often used singly as a simple, but they have been combined with other herbs to produce various results. American and European mistletoe's dosage is the same. Mistletoe is most effective if used in early pregnancy.

Words to the Wise: Mistletoe's abortion producing dose is precariously close to its fatal dose. Some women have died attempting to produce an abortion using high dosages of mistletoe. Anyone taking antidepressant MAO inhibitors (such as Marplan, Nardil, and Parnate) should not use mistletoe. The combination of these drugs and mistletoe may result in serious elevation of blood pressure and possibly unconsciousness.[310] Anyone with a history of stroke or heart disease should not use mistletoe due to its tendency to increase blood pressure. Mistletoe berries may cause contact dermatitis in sensitive individuals. Do not eat mistletoe berries. Mistletoe berries, in large amounts, may cause gastroenteritis in adults, and there are cases where children have died due to ingestion of mistletoe berries.

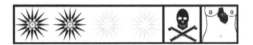

Watch for Signs of Toxicity Specific to Mistletoe: Headache, hallucinations, nausea, acute cramping, gastroenteritis, vomiting, diarrhea, weak pulse, decreased heart rate, muscle spasms and convulsions. At high doses, death typically occurs from cardiovascular collapse within ten hours of ingestion.

Mistletoe Dosage*

Abortifacient Mistletoe Infusion (leaves): One ounce herb (28 g) to 2
cups water (250 ml). Steep overnight. Then, take ¼ cup
(63 ml) doses, three to four times a day for up to six days.
Abortifacient Tincture (fresh leaves): 1:5, 50% alcohol, 15 – 20 drops,
two to three times a day, for up to six days.
*Extreme caution! Fatal dose very close to abortifacient dose!

Mugwort
Artemisia vulgaris

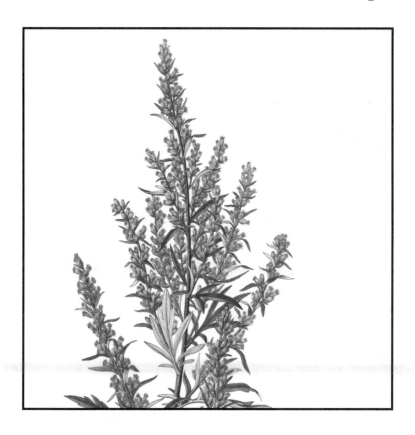

If they would eat nettles in March,
and eat muggins [mugwort] in May,
Sae mony braw maidens
wad not go to clay. [311]

- a song by a mermaid, in an old Scottish legend, who
arose from the Clyde River near Glascow and
admonished those attending a young woman's funeral.

Family Compositae

AKA: Muggins, St. John's girdle, felonherb, cingulum santa, sailor's tobacco, wormwood, bulwand, and green ginger.

Parts Used: Leaves and root.

Medicinal Properties: Anti-inflammatory, anti-spasmodic, bitter digestive tonic, diuretic, diaphoretic, emmenagogue, estrogenic, nervine, stimulant, stomachic, tonic, and vermifuge.

Abortifacient Action: Estrogenic and uterine contracting.

Contains: Alpha-thujone, an abortifacient chemical, and beta-sitosterol, a phytoestrogen.

Description: Mugwort is an aromatic perennial 1 – 5 ft. (0.3 - 1.6 m) in height, having many branched stems that are angular and purplish. Leaves are toothed and deeply lobed 1 – 4 in. (2.5 – 10 cm) long, smooth dark green on top and soft cottony white to light green underneath. Mugwort's numerous yellow to reddish flowers appear in late summer in long clusters. Seeds are long and thin. Mugwort, brought to America by European settlers, is indigenous to Asia. Mugwort has now spread to nearly every temperate zone in the world. In North America, this plant grows wild in waste places and near streams. It is found from Nova Scotia to Ontario, and from the northeast United States south to Georgia, and west to Michigan.

Mugwort Herbal Lore and Historical Use

Ancient myth indicates that women beyond recorded history have used mugwort as a medicinal plant. Mugwort's scientific name (*Artemisia vulgaris*) was derived from the ancient name for Artemis, the moon goddess and mother of all creatures of the Amazons. In

212

Ephesus, Artemis's name was Diana, and statues have been found that show her entire torso covered with breasts, symbolic of how she nurtured and fed all living things. She was the fate goddess, the moon mother who, with her sacred dogs, guarded the gate of the afterworld. Artemis was equally the huntress, death bringer to the very creatures she brought forth.[312] Artemis led the nocturnal hunt, her priestesses wearing the masks of hunting dogs.[313] Her huntress aspect was a form of the destroying crone or waning moon, the moon time when medicinal herbs were gathered for the use of the people. At the new moon, the people of Greece would offer Artemis sacrifices and lavish orgiastic entertainment. A mugwort garland was traditionally worn around the waist or head while dancing round the fire on the European midsummer solstice celebration, which evolved from the Roman Cerealia celebration, held in honor of the Mother Earth Goddess Ceres. The midsummer mugwort garland would be thrown into the flames at the end of the evening to protect the wearer against sickness in the coming year.[314]

Mugwort was said to be one of the nine sacred herbs that were given to the world by the Saxon and Frankish god, Woden.[315] Woden, like Artemis, was the conductor of souls, riding with ghosts through the night on Halloween.[316] The number nine, for the nine sacred herbs given to the world, was an ancient number sacred to women in childbirth. Nine, as three times three, was the triple triad, symbolic of the infinite female Trinity. The word nine was originally derived from the Ennead, the nine-fold goddess of ancient Egypt.[317] The ancient sacred nature of the number nine is still evident in its meaning to the ninth degree, or as in 'dressed to the nines.'

Mugwort was the herb used to flavor beer before the introduction of hops. Beer, originally considered a magical drink used to alter the consciousness, was ritually offered to the goddesses and gods. The distinguishing ingredients in old ritual beers were the herbs added to them, called 'beer worts.' These beers, containing between 5 - 27% herbs and 3 - 10% alcohol were used to alter the mind.[318] Many of these beers were similar to medicinal tinctures used today.

Sometimes called *mater herbarium,* meaning 'mother of all herbs,' mugwort is still deeply respected by many in Europe, Asia, China, and the United States. Mugwort is hung near the bed or burned as incense before retiring to bed to encourage vivid dreaming. The white downy substance on the underside of mugwort's leaves is used in China as 'moxa'. Rolled into little balls and burned above or on the skin at acupuncture points, moxa is used along with acupuncture needles in some acupuncture treatments.

Mugwort, with its menstrual promoting properties, has been used by many around the world. Europeans are known to use mugwort to bring on menstruation. The people of the Philippines use a mugwort native to their area for the same purpose, and Native Americans as well as Russians use a decoction of the leaves of mugwort to stimulate menstruation.[319] Mugwort was used as ceremonial medicine in purification rites by Native American Dakota women after menstruation.[320] Alma Hutchens, in *Indian Herbology of North America*, says mugwort is "safe for suppressed menstruation of mother and daughter."[321] Mugwort is estrogenic; it stimulates uterine contractions.

Gathering: Mugwort may be gathered in late summer when it is in full flower, on a warm morning after the sun has dried off the dew. Mugwort's upper green portion is gathered and processed into tinctures or dried in the shade. The roots of mugwort can be collected in the fall when the above-ground parts have begun to die back. The root is rinsed in pure water and dried in the shade. It should be stored in airtight containers when completely dry.

Preparation: Mugwort is well known and respected as a menstrual promoting emmenagogue, but mugwort does not have much specific documentation detailing its use as an abortifacient. To utilize mugwort's menstrual promoting powers, mugwort is best used in the days prior to the onset of menstruation. Mugwort is sometimes combined with onion in a vaginal pessary (see Onion).

Words to the Wise: Mugwort contains the uterine contracting toxic chemical thujone. Thujone can stimulate the heart. Mugwort is estrogenic and should be avoided by any woman on blood pressure medications. Mugwort may not be as effective in premenopausal women. Estrogenic substances are known teratogens. Mugwort contains the uterine contracting and possibly toxic thujone. Do not use mugwort for longer than seven days, because prolonged use can injure the nervous system.[322]   Lactating women should not use mugwort; it has a tendency to dry up breast milk, and could also pass through the milk to the nursing child. Mugwort should not to be used by women who have had a recent pelvic inflammation. People with seasonal allergies or asthma should avoid mugwort. People with an allergy to peaches may have a hypersensitivity to mugwort.[323]

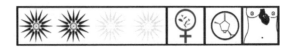

Mugwort Emmenagogual Dosage

Infusion (leaves): 3 tsp. (15 ml) to one cup (250 ml) water. Steep
15 -20 minutes, three times a day for up to seven days.

Tincture (fresh leaves): 1:5, 50% alcohol, 10 - 25 drops, four to six
times a day, for up to seven days.

Powdered Leaves: 5 - 7 #0 capsules four to six times a day, for up to
seven days.

Nutmeg
Myristica fragrans

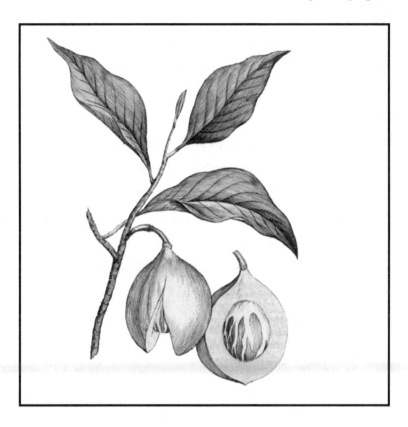

*In all cases of nutmeg poisoning there was prostration with
partial or complete coma. Most of them had vertigo, delirium,
chiefly hallucinations of sight, rapid, feeble pulse, and free
urination. In five instances the nutmegs were taken to produce
abortion, and in every case without accomplishing the desired result.*

-E. E. Hinman in *Northwestern Lancet,* January 15, 1902

217

Family Myristicaceae

AKA: Jaiphal and jawz at tiyb.

Part Used: Dried seed kernels.

Medicinal Properties: Gastro-intestinal stimulant, and oxytocic.

Effects on the Body: Narcotic hallucinogenic poison in large doses.

Abortifacient Action: Uterine contraction.

Contains: Myristicin.

Description: Nutmeg is a tropical tree with a round fruit that looks like a yellow apricot streaked with red and green. Upon maturity, the fruit splits open to release the seed, a brown ovoid seed having a scarlet covering (aril). The seed is dried and ground to become the nutmeg spice. The aril is dried and becomes the spice known as mace.

Nutmeg Herbal Lore and Historical Use[1]

Since it was first imported to Europe, nutmeg has been expensive and mysterious. During the medieval period, nutmeg cost as much as gold or silver. A gilded nutmeg was given as a Christmas present from those who could afford such luxury. Nutmeg was worn on a string or as a poultice to ward off the plague. Nutmeg was also used as a tranquilizer, a sleeping potion, and a medieval form of Viagra™. The profit potential for nutmeg, which was marked up above cost upwards of 30,000%, perhaps was reason enough for some to claim nutmeg as a cure for all ills. Medicinally, roasted nutmeg was applied internally as a remedy for leukorrhea and also was used to help

---

[1] The purpose of this book is to recapture information about historical approaches to self-induced abortion. Nutmeg has been included; however the reader must keep in mind that many deaths have resulted from overconsumption of nutmeg.

218

alleviate nausea. Perhaps once, while nutmeg was being used to cure morning sickness, a spontaneous miscarriage happened accidentally, and nutmeg became rumored as an agent to produce abortion.

Nutmeg became an 'abortifacient' during the Victorian age when women's rights were not acknowledged, abortion was criminalized, and common knowledge of herbal abortifacients had been censored for several centuries. Unfortunately, the dosage of nutmeg that was rumored to cause an abortion was very close to the lethal dose. Many deaths resulted from the use of nutmeg to try to induce abortion. Often psychotic effects of nutmeg preceded death. Nutmeg continued to be rumored as an agent to cause abortion into the 1950's in the United States.[324] Nutmeg was not documented as an abortifacient in antiquity, and nutmeg was not recorded as being used to induce abortion in its native habitat of the South East Asian Bandas Islands.

Preparation: For abortifacient purposes, nutmeg was often taken orally. Sometimes nutmeg was used internally as a pessary.[325]

Words to the Wise: In amounts of one gram or more, nutmeg is a mild to medium hallucinogen, producing visual distortions and a mild euphoria. Ingestion of as little as three grams may cause dry mouth, fast pulse, fever, flushing and possibly death. Large doses of seven grams or more are very dangerous, potentially inducing convulsions, palpitations, nausea, eventual dehydration, and generalized body pain. Onset of toxic effects from nutmeg can be delayed taking up to six hours after ingestion and may last for up to three days. Nutmeg can also cause liver damage when used in large quantities.

219

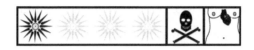

Watch for Signs of Toxicity Specific to Nutmeg: Delirium, hallucinations, excitement, thought disorder, a sense of impending death and agitation.

Nutmeg Dosage*

*Extreme caution! Nutmeg is ineffective, psychoactive, and possibly deadly when used as an abortifacient. Nutmeg does have a uterine contracting activity, however its effects on the hypothalamus and the pituitary only occur at life threatening doses of one to three nutmeg kernels.

Onion

Allium cepa

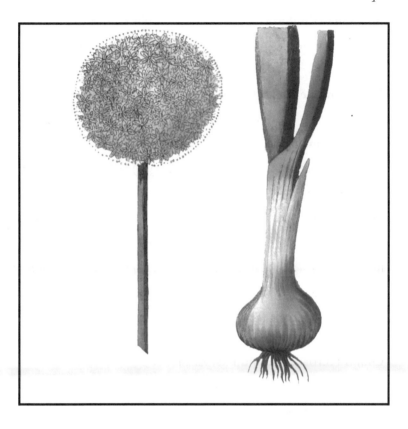

...the most common variety of [vaginal] suppository consists of a mixture of grilled (or boiled) onion and one of several varieties of the herb shih [Artemisia sp.]...

-Marcia Claire Inhorn in *Quest for Conception*, 1994

221

Family Alliaceae

AKA: Garden onion, bulb onion, and shallot.

Medicinal Properties: Externally, the bulb is hydragogue, stimulant and rubefacient, roasted it acts as a demulcent both internally and externally.

Effects on the Body: Expels water from the lower genital tract.

Abortifacient Action: Estrogenic, uterine contracting, inhibits prostaglandins, and stimulates release of fluids.

Contains: Beta-sitosterol (a phytoestrogen), allyl propyl disulphide, chromium, Vitamin C, and quercetin.

Description: *Allium cepa* is the common onion. There are white, yellow, and purple varieties. Onions are perennial, and they have hollow green stems that can reach 3 ft. (1 m) in height. Small flowers, usually white or purple appear in late summer. The large round fleshy bulb is harvested for food and medicinal purposes.

Onion Herbal Lore and Historical Use

The ancient Egyptians worshipped the onion, believing that its spherical shape and concentric rings symbolized eternal life. In the *Kahun Gynecological Papyrus*, 1900 BC, to test for pregnancy, an onion bulb was placed deep in the woman's vagina. The next morning, if the odor of onions appeared to her nose, a positive outcome was determined.[326] This 'test' may have served as a contraceptive measure in early pregnancy, for the knowledge of onion's menstrual promoting aspect was likely present. Only three hundred years later in the *Ebers Papyrus*, two recipes for onion abortifacients exist. One recipe calls for one part onions and one part wine, mixed together and used as a

222

vaginal pessary "for the extraction of woman's blood."[327] The other recipe includes onion along with other herbs as a vaginal suppository.[328]

Women, in many countries around the world, have used onion to regulate their fertility. In Europe,[329] India,[330] and Vietnam[331] the onion bulb is documented as being eaten with the intention of encouraging menstruation. In India, the hot water extract of onion bulb is drunk as an emmenagogue.[332] In Germany, the hot water extract of the bulb is taken orally to induce miscarriage.[333] In Egypt, roasted onion bulb is used as a contraceptive pessary, both before and after intercourse.[334] In the Middle East, Unani medicine utilizes the onion bulb in the form of a pessary as an emmenagogue.[335] As late as the 20th Century, Jewish women of New York City attempted to abort by sitting over a pot of steam (or hot stewed onions), a technique described in an 8th Century Sanskrit source.[336]

Onions are natural anti-clotting agents due to their sulfur content, and research has shown onion bulbs to have antifertility, estrogenic, prostaglandin inhibitory, and uterine contracting effects. Dried red onion bulb skin, at a concentration of 20% drinking water, injected into the abdomen was found to have abortive effects on pregnant mice.[337] The water extract of the fresh onion bulb, in cell culture, actively inhibited prostaglandins on platelets and rat aorta.[338] In one study, the water extract of the onion bulb produced strong uterine contracting effects in pregnant mice and rats.[339] In another study, the fresh bulb juice was found to have an active uterine stimulating effect on the rat uterus.[340]

Preparation: The onion is widely available for purchase. The most pungent onions have the most medicinal benefits, for it is said the same mechanism that causes the eyes to tear when cutting onions works to increase the fluid release from the uterus. When purchasing onions for medicinal use, avoid sweet varieties and look for unblemished firm bulbs. Sometimes onion is combined with honey, mugwort, or Asian ginger juice. When applied as an ointment to the abdomen, onion will increase urination.

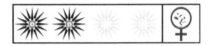

Words to the Wise: Consuming large quantities of onion can lead to stomach distress and gastrointestinal irritation that may result in nausea and diarrhea. Onion is estrogenic.

Onion Dosage

Uterine Cleansing Onion Pessary*: Bake onion for one hour at 350°F
(177°C). Cool. Baked onions left whole or mashed (as a
simple or in combination) may be wrapped in cheesecloth,
tied with string, and inserted. Replace pessary every eight to
twelve hours for up to six days.
* This pessary, usually worn overnight while sleeping on a
towel, tends to increase release of fluids cleansing the uterus
and vagina. Used in the week prior to menstruation, it helps
to encourage a menstrual flow. Used in the week after

menstruation, it helps to clear the uterus, leading to increased fertility.

Onion Decoction: Slice three or four onions (with their skins); boil for ten minutes in one quart (1 L) of water. Filter and sip throughout the day. Decoction can be used as fumigation and douche. Strained onions can be made into a pessary.

Onion Scale Infusion: 2 oz. (50 g) onion skins to one cup (250 ml) water, simmer for ten minutes, and sip throughout the day.

Papaya
Carica papaya

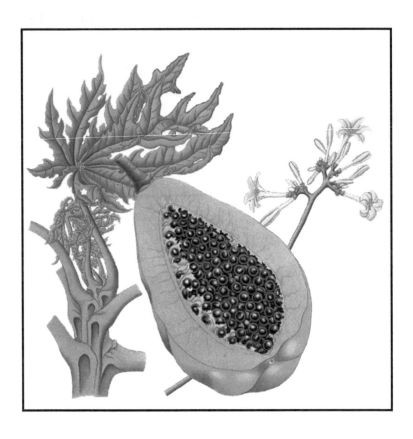

*A belief in [papaya's] powerfully emmenagogue properties prevails
amongst all classes of women in Southern India; so much so, that
they assert that if a woman partake of them, even in moderate
quantities, abortion will be the probable result. This popular belief is
noticed in many of the reports received from India. In them, it is stated that
the milky juice of the plant is applied locally to the os uteri with
the view of inducing abortion.*

-Dictionary of the Economic Plants of India, 1889

226

Family Caricaceae

AKA: Papaya, pawpaw, tree melon (China), lechoza (Puerto Rico), and fruta bomba (Cuba).

Parts Used: Green (unripe) fruit, latex, seeds, and root.

Medicinal Properties: Anodyne, stomachic, carminative, anthelmintic, styptic, demulcent, abortifacient, emmenagogue, and vermifuge.

Effects on the Body: The dried latex helps to digest protein, and is used as a food supplement. The fresh latex also has uterine contracting effects.

Abortifacient Action: Seeds are believed to contain chemicals which interfere with prostaglandin production and cause contraction of the uterus. The papain in papaya latex is known to effect progesterone.

Contains: BITC (benzyl isothiocyanate) and papain.

Description: Papaya is an erect, fast growing tree with usually a single trunk, up to 20 – 30 ft. (6 – 9 m) in height. Papaya's large leaves cluster near the top of the truck. Aromatic flowers and large green to yellow fruits often appear simultaneously under the leaves.

Papaya Medicinal and Herbal Lore

Papaya originated in Central and South America where it has been used for food and medicine for thousands of years. Papaya is now grown widely in tropical areas around the world where it is cultivated for its fruits and for the papain enzyme the unripe fruits contain. Papain is used as a digestive aid and meat tenderizer.

Women in many countries use papaya as a contraceptive and abortive. Papaya has gained a reputation as being the most effective and cheapest means of fertility regulation outside of clinical methods.[341] In East Africa, women drink the unripe fruit juice to induce abortion.[342] In India, unripe papaya latex[343] or the plant juice[344] is applied to the mouth of the uterus as an abortive, the seeds are considered an emmenagogue, unless eaten with ginger and honey whereby they become abortifacient,[345] and the unripe fruit is eaten including its seeds to cause abortion.[346] In South America, the Tikuna eat grated green papaya with two to six aspirin, inducing abortion in about two days.[347] In Ghana, the ground root of papaya is made into a decoction[348] or blended with salt water and used as a douche to cause abortion.[349] In Vanuatu, women eat four small unripe papayas together with four tablets Nivaquine (an anti-malarial medicine) and the juice of two limes to induce abortion.[350]

Scientific studies have suggested that papaya contains substances that have effects on the reproductive system. Although the unripe fruits are used most widely, extracts of the ripe dried fruits have also been shown to have abortifacient qualities.[351] The fruit[352] and the seed[353] have been shown to be embryotoxic. Anti-estrogenic effects have been noted as well.[354] Green papaya (unripe) can cause abortion due to the presence of a plant compound, benzyl isothiocyanate (BITC), found primarily in the latex of green papaya tissue.[355] The enzyme papain (made from latex of unripe fruit) interacts with progesterone. Crude papaya latex has been shown in laboratory studies to cause spasmodic contraction of the uterine muscles, similar to oxytocin and prostaglandin.[356]

Gathering: Papaya is endemic to the tropics. The fruits, both green and ripe, are available year round. Green (unripe) fruits can be harvested using a knife to cut the stem that attaches the fruit to the truck.

Purchasing: Papaya fruit is green when unripe and orange when ripe. In large cities around the world, Papaya fruit is available for purchase year round in both ripe and unripe forms in Asian food stores and larger supermarkets. Unripe fruits can range in size from a large orange to a cantaloupe and should be firm and unblemished. Some shopkeepers do not display unripe papaya, but will often have them boxed in storage. Papaya seeds sold for gardening are often treated with a fungicide.

Preparation: Papaya's abortifacient action is most effective if used in early pregnancy. The eating of one unripe papaya fruit a day in the week prior to menstruation is used as an emmenagogue in Asia. The seeds are well documented in folk medicine as having powerful abortifacient qualities. The application of the uterotonic papaya latex to the cervical os is considered to be one of the most effective herbal abortifacient preparations. One may chose to use just one preparation or a combination of them.

To harvest papaya latex: Wash one unripe fruit. Working a small section at a time, make long shallow scratches on the thin papaya fruit skin with a sharp knife. The milky papaya latex will immediately start to ooze and run out of the cuts. Collect the latex in a clean cup or receptacle. Papaya latex can be used immediately in a fresh state, made into a tincture, prepared into homeopathic potencies (See

229

Homeopathy), or dried to a powder at low temperature. The unripe fruit may be made into a juice or salad.

Words to the Wise: Papaya latex is an irritant and can cause blistering of skin exposed to it.[357] Although rare, some people are allergic to the papaya fruit and latex. Persons with a known latex allergy should avoid papaya latex. Papaya latex has shown prolonged anticoagulant activity.[358] Persons with clotting or blood disorders should not use papaya. The seeds, leaves, and latex of papaya contain small quantities of a toxic alkaloid called carpine. Carpine in large quantities can lower the pulse rate and depress the nervous system.[359] The seeds and pulp of papaya are known to contain benzyl isothiocyanate, which is known to induce glutathione transfer.[360] Glutathione is a master antioxidant present in every cell that transports toxins to the liver.

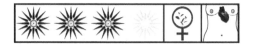

Watch for signs of Toxicity Specific to Papaya (*Carica papaya*): Decreased heart rate, heart palpitations, visual changes, and difficulty breathing when lying down.

Papaya Dosage

Abortifacient Papaya Os Ointment: Using a speculum, and a clean
paint brush, smear 1 tsp. (5 ml) fresh papaya latex on the
cervical os. Alternately, liquid latex can be collected into a
small plastic syringe (like the kind used to administer baby
medicines) and the syringe inserted into the vagina and

released at the cervix. Repeat two times a day, for up to three days.

Papaya Seeds: 1 - 2 Tbs. fresh papaya seeds or 1 tsp. dried powdered papaya seeds, mixed with water, taken two to three times a day for up to six days.

Green Papaya Salad, (also known as Som Tam or Tam mak hoong) According to a survey in Thailand, green papaya salad is the most popular food dish among Thai women.[361]

1 ½ Tbs. sugar

juice of 1 - 2 limes, to taste

2 cups shredded green papaya, peeled and grated

6 green beans, bruised

1 - 3 cloves garlic, minced, to taste

1 ½ Tbs. fish or soy sauce

1 or 2 fresh chili peppers, to taste

5 Roma tomatoes, roughly chopped

1 Tbs. dried shrimp or prawns (optional)

2 Tbs. peanuts, toasted (optional)

Peel the green papaya; and using a cheese grater, grate the flesh into a large bowl. Mix the dried shrimp, fish or soy sauce, lime juice and sugar, and add a little at a time to the grated papaya, to taste. Add the garlic, tomatoes, and green beans. Mix well. The salad is traditionally served with sticky rice, a sliver of cabbage, scallions, green beans, and Thai basil.

231

Parsley

Petroselinum sativum (Curled parsley)
Petroselinum neapolitanum (Italian parsley or flat leaf parsley)

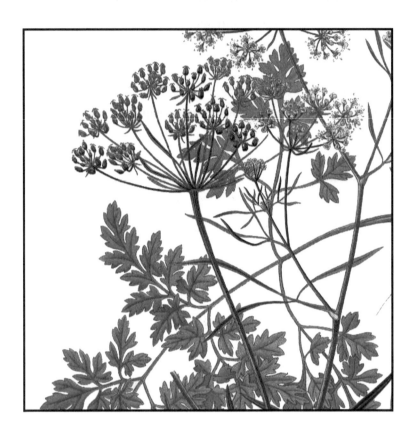

One of them handed out parsley,
the symbol of clandestine abortion,
which others put in their hair.
There were about four thousand of us, mostly women...

-Simone de Beauvoir in *All Said and Done*, 1974

Family Umbelliferae

Parts Used: Seeds and essential oil.

Medicinal Properties: Diuretic, prevents kidney stones, emmenagogue, and carminative.

Effects on the Body: Stimulates menstruation and increases urine output.

Abortifacient Action: Contracts uterus and is embryotoxic.

Contains: Apiol (uterine tonic), myristicin (embryotoxin), and unidentified water soluble uterine contractors.

Description: Widely cultivated and well-known culinary herb, parsley is a short-lived perennial with a smooth erect stem and shiny dark green compound leaves. Small ribbed oval seeds follow tiny white umbel flowers. The curly-leaf variety grows to 12 in. (30.5 cm) in height and is best known as a garnish and favored in Britain. The flat-leaf variety, preferred in Italy, has a stronger flavor, is used like a vegetable, and grows to 3 feet (1 m) in height.

Parsley Herbal Lore and Historical Use[m]

In ancient Greece, parsley was considered sacred. Parsley was dedicated to Persephone and used in funeral rites. Parsley was reputed to have sprung from the blood of an infant who was killed by the serpent that guarded the sacred grove of Zeus at Nemea. The baby was given immortality, renamed Archemorus, the forerunner of death. Homer related that chariot horses were fed by warriors with the leaves

---

[m] The purpose of this book is to recapture information about historical approaches to self-induced abortion. Parsley has been included; however the reader must keep in mind that some deaths have resulted from the ingestion of apiol (parsley essential oil).

of the parsley plant. Greek gardens were often bordered with parsley and rue, symbolizing respectively the edge of death and grace, and were planted to banish evil. Parsley was worn in wreathed crowns and put on graves. In the Middle Ages, parsley continued its sacred stance; it was consecrated to St. Peter.

Through the ages, parsley was also known for its emmenagogual and abortifacient qualities. Folkloric reports of parsley used as an abortifacient are numerous and widespread, reaching across the Atlantic from Europe and Africa to the Americas.[362] Hippocrates documented that parsley was used to cause an abortion. Pliny the Elder (AD 23-79) said parsley was used to cause sterility. In medieval times, parsley was used as an abortifacient; women used the seeds to bring out their menstruation, however parsley seeds were thought to be inferior to other emmenagogual herbs.[363] Infusion of the top and root of *Petroselinum crispum* was utilized by Native American Cherokee as an abortive for "female obstructions."[364]

The emmenagogual effect of parsley preparations is often attributed to a substance called apiol found in parsley seeds. Apiol is an organic chemical compound also known as parsley camphor. Apiol was discovered in 1715, by Heinrich Christoph Link who noticed greenish crystals forming while processing the essential oil of parsley. In 1855, Joret and Homolle documented the effectiveness of treatment of amenorrhea with apiol.[365] Apiol is thought to 'cause a relatively safe abortion' in pregnant women if taken in small quantities,[366] however the deaths of some women trying to induce an abortion is attributed to the toxic properties of apiol.[367]

234

In the United States, apiol prescription by doctors as an abortifacient was widespread in the early 1900's. The First World War spread the knowledge of the use of apiol for abortion into Europe. It is estimated by some scholars that millions of women took apiol to produce abortion with few negative side effects and only a handful of deaths reported.[368] The use of apiol stopped when a highly toxic adulterated product containing apiol and triorthocresyl phosphate was introduced to the American market in the 1920's.[369] Now that other methods of abortion are widely available, apiol is no longer available in the United States; but apiol was recently produced and sold as an abortifacient in the Middle East and Mexico.[370]

Other components in parsley, not yet identified, are likely to have abortifacient activity. Parsley is known to have an oxytocic effect, stimulating the pituitary via the hypothalamus. Researchers in Bulgaria reported that water based extracts of parsley, which would have little to no apiol present, still have significant uterine stimulating effects.[371] In Russia a drug called Supetin, derived from parsley juice, is used to stimulate labor.[372]

Gathering: A detailed field guide should be consulted to gather members of the Umbelliferae family. Parsley is easily confused with its poisonous sisters: fool's parsley *Aethusa cynapium* and poison hemlock *Conium maculate*. Parsley leaves may be gathered throughout the summer, as after they are cut back they readily grow back. Parsley seed is gathered when dry in late autumn. Parsley's roots are collected for medicinal purposes in the second year, in autumn or late summer when the plant has flowered.

235

Purchasing: Fresh organic parsley is available at some groceries and health food stores. Although any parsley can be used, flat leaf parsley has been shown to contain higher levels of essential oil than curly leaf parsley. Apiol is not widely available in the United States, but may be available in Mexico. Organic parsley essential oil is available for purchase at health food stores and online. The natural parsley essential oils in food have not shown abortifacient effects when eaten by pregnant women.[373] However, the German Commission E. cautions that larger doses of parsley seed oil than what is found in food preparations have the potential to produce uterine contractions.[374]

Preparation: Parsley is most effective when used as an emmenagogue in the first two weeks of gestation. Sometimes parsley tea is combined with the juice of lemon or high doses of Vitamin C (500 mg/ hour. up to 6000 mg per day, maximum six days). Vitamin C has been shown to have progesterone suppressive effects.[375] Parsley is occasionally combined with angelica. Parsley is sometimes combined with lemon and/or rue in abortifacient preparations.[376] Apiol is more effective when taken at small dosages. Apiol is most effective when used in the first eight weeks of pregnancy.

Words to the Wise: Parsley contains psorlens, which can damage DNA and blister the skin when it is exposed to sunlight. Parsley should not be used by women with inflammatory kidney conditions, for parsley is high in oxalic acid. Occasional allergic reactions, photosensitivity, or mucous membrane irritations have been reported, especially with the essential oil when used internally. Parsley essential oil, or apiol, is an irritant to the body systems. If apiol is given in too high a dose or for too long, it can cause liver and kidney damage. Parsley also contains myristicin which is very toxic and is also one of the toxic substances in nutmeg. Parsley oil can contain potentially dangerous amounts of myristicin. Parsley oil, like nutmeg, can cause hallucinations, paralysis, and liver and kidney degeneration if taken in too large a quantity.

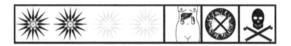

Watch for signs of Toxicity Specific to Parsley: Nausea, hallucinations, vomiting, vertigo, hives, paralysis, liver swollen and painful, urine scanty and darkly colored, and tremors.

Parsley Dosage

Emmenagogual Parsley Infusion: Take one bunch fresh parsley rinse clean, chop, and place in a glass container with a lid. Boil one quart of water, pour over herb. Cover and steep 20 - 30 minutes. Strain. Drink throughout the day. Parsley infusion can be taken for up to seven days.

Parsley Pessary: A few sprigs vaginally inserted, replace every 12 hours.

Parsley Root Tincture: 1:5, 60% alcohol, 30 – 60 drops, up to three times a day.

Parsley fresh seed essential oil (Apiol): 5 – 15 drops (0.2 - 0.6 ml), two to three times a day, for up to five days.

Pennyroyal

Hedeoma pulegioides (American)
Mentha pulegium (European)

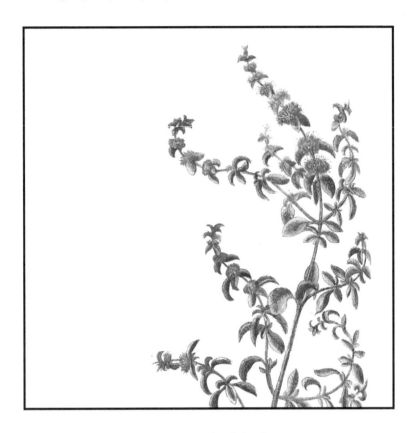

A very lovely land,
well cropped and trimmed,
and spruced with pennyroyal.

-Aristophanes (450-380 B.C)

It [pennyroyal infusion] will often bring on the menses nicely, and
combined with a gill [5 ounces] of brewer's yeast, it frequently acts well as
an abortivant, should the intended be not too late with her prescription.

-Charles F. Millspaugh in *Medicinal Plants,* 1887

Family Labiatae

AKA: Squaw mint, mosquito plant, flea bane, run-by-the-ground, lurk-in-the-ditch, tickweed, and pudding grass.

Parts Used: Leaves and flower tops.

Medicinal Properties: Aromatic, carminative, corrective, diaphoretic, diuretic, emmenagogue, expectorant, nervine, stimulant, and sudorific.

Effects on the Body: Soothes respiratory, reproductive, and digestive systems; stimulates elimination through kidneys and perspiration.

Abortifacient Action: Uterine contractor.

Contains: Hepatotoxic ketone pulegone and volatile oil.

Description: American pennyroyal, *Hedeoma pulegioides*, an indigenous annual, growing to a height of only 1 ft. (0.3 m), is one of the smallest of the mints. Square erect branching stems grow from a yellow fibrous root ball. Small ½ in. (1.3 cm) long dark green leaves are hairy on the bottom surface and appear opposite each other at regular intervals along the stems. From June to September, small light blue to lavender flowers circle the stems at the leaf axles. American Pennyroyal grows commonly in dry fields and woods and often in limestone country from the Atlantic coastal United States, west through to Minnesota and Arkansas.

European pennyroyal *Mentha pulegium*, native to Europe and Asia, grows a little higher 1 ½ - 2 ft. (0.5 m), but otherwise looks very similar to the American variety. The main difference in the two is their habitats and root formation. The American pennyroyal grows from a root ball and likes dry areas. European pennyroyal spreads in runners 'run-by-the-ground,' and it is most likely to be found in moist, rich areas. The European variety of pennyroyal is also found in North

239

America, having escaped to the wild from gardens, where it is commonly cultivated.

Pennyroyal Herbal Lore and Historical Use[n]

The ancients were aware of the power of some mints like pennyroyal to cause abortion, as Pliny (AD 23 - 79) and Dioscorides (40 - 90 BC) mention the abortifacient aspect of pennyroyal in their writings. Mints were interwoven in ancient historical myths of love, life, death, and the underworld. In Greek myth, Hades on a foray from the underworld spied the nymph Mintha and fell in love with her. Persephone, Hades wife, plotted revenge against Hades and turned the Nymph into the mint, which by its nature is attractive, fragrant, and also abortifacient (see Pomegranate). In ancient Rome, the most common word used for the penis was *mentula*, which is believed by scholars to be derived from *menta*, which means stem of mint.[377]

European pennyroyal, native to most parts of Europe and Asia, was valued as a medicinal as well as spiritual plant and was used in ancient ceremonies.[378] Pennyroyal was known in Europe as an emmenagogue and was known to have strong abortifacient qualities. Pennyroyal was also highly esteemed in Anglo-Saxon and Welsh medicine. When the European colonists first came to America, they brought European pennyroyal along to grow in their gardens for medicinal purposes. Early women colonists combined pennyroyal tea

---

[n] The purpose of this book is to recapture information about historical approaches to self-induced abortion. Pennyroyal has been included; however the reader must keep in mind that many deaths have resulted from the ingestion of pennyroyal oil.

with brewer's yeast to produce abortion.[379] The colonists found the Native American women had long been using the indigenous American pennyroyal for similar purposes. The women of the Rappahannock tribe drank a tea made of pennyroyal leaves to relieve menstrual cramps. For the same condition, the women of the Kiowa tribe combined pennyroyal leaves and dandelion blossoms to make a medicinal tea. Cherokee women took the infusion of the pennyroyal leaves for 'obstructed menses.'[380] A decoction of the entire pennyroyal plant has been used to assist in treatment of uterine tumors and uterine fibroids.[381] Susan Weed in her *Wise Woman Herbal* calls American pennyroyal a powerful menstrual promoter. She recommends limiting pennyroyal to no more than five days, as taking pennyroyal for longer can tax the woman.[382]

Gathering: Pennyroyal's leaves and flower tops should be gathered in full bloom in early to mid summer, in the morning of a warm day after the dew has dried.

Preparation: Pennyroyal is occasionally combined with blue cohosh or sometimes with mugwort in emmenagogual preparations. Pennyroyal was combined historically with brewer's yeast, which may help protect the liver. Some liver protective factors of brewer's yeast have been suggested in scientific testing.[383] Pennyroyal tea is sometimes used as a hot footbath to mildly encourage menstruation, and the tea may be added to the water of the bathtub for the same purpose.

Words to the Wise: Pennyroyal contains pulegone, which is a direct liver toxin (hepatotoxin). Pulegone depletes glutathione stores in the liver. Glutathione is required by the body to detoxify and to help neutralize free radicals. Without glutathione the immune system cannot function. Caution should be exercised when using pennyroyal. Anyone with any kidney disease or liver damage should not use pennyroyal. Pennyroyal can cause contact dermatitis in susceptible individuals. Pennyroyal is thought to cause placental adhesion among women who use it, fail to cause abortion, and then carry the pregnancy to term.

Do not use pennyroyal oil, internally! As little as 2 tsp. (10 ml) of the oil has caused fatalities. Pennyroyal oil is very concentrated. Avoid tincture of pennyroyal, for it may contain dangerous amounts of the essential oil. Although the essential oil and the tincture should be avoided, the infusion poses little risk of fatality, but even the infusion has health risks. University of Illinois pharmacognosist Norman Farnsworth, Ph.D. estimated that one would have to drink 50 - 75 gallons of pennyroyal leaf infusion to equal a fatal dosage of pennyroyal oil. [384] However, many women who have taken pennyroyal tea orally to cause abortion have suffered kidney and liver problems afterwards. If choosing to use pennyroyal infusion for abortifacient purposes, the user would be wise to combine pennyroyal with milk thistle, nettle, and/or brewer's yeast to help protect kidneys and liver. N-acetylcysteine, an antioxidant dietary supplement available online and in specialty health food stores, has been used successfully to prevent damage to the liver caused by pulegone in pennyroyal oil.[385] Limit use of pennyroyal infusion to five days.

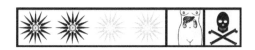

Watch for Signs of Toxicity Specific to Pennyroyal: Nausea, numbness in hands and legs, liver irritation, kidney and bladder irritation, and diarrhea.

Pennyroyal Dosage

Abortifacient Infusion (leaves and flowers): 3 – 4 tsp. (15 – 20 g)
    herb to 1 pint (500 ml) water. Steep 15 - 30 minutes, drink throughout the day, for up to five days.

Leaves and flowers: 3 - 8 #0 capsules, two to three times a day, for up to five days.

Pineapple
Ananas comosus

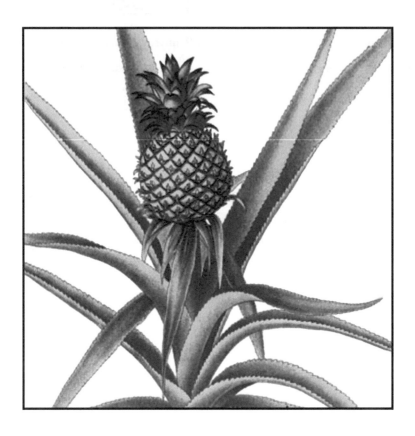

*The juice of the green pineapple, we are informed by an exchange, is
accredited in Java and throughout the Far East generally, with being a blood
poison of the most deadly nature. It is said to be the substance with which
the Malays poison the creeses and daggers and to be also
the finger-nail poison formerly in use among the aboriginal Javanese women
almost universally. These women cultivated a nail on each hand to a long
sharp point, and the least scratch from one of these was certain death.*

-Frank Kraft, M.D., ed. in *The American Homeopathist*, 1901

244

Family Bromeliaceae

AKA: Abacaxi (Brazil), komala, and anarosh (India).

Parts Used: Fruit and root.

Medicinal Properties: Digestive, anti-inflammatory, anthelmintic, labor inducer, and purgative.

Effects on the Body: Violently purges the bowels.

Abortifacient Action: Estrogenic, embryo toxic, and cathartic purgative.

Contains: 5-stigmastene – 3 Beta 7-alpha-diol dibenzoate (abortifacient), C7 epimer (abortifacient), and 5-hydroxy-tyrptamine (uterine stimulant).

Description: Pineapple is a tropical perennial bromeliad. Pineapple reaches 3 ft. (1 m) in height, with many thick trough-shaped leaves 1 – 3 ft. (0.3 – 1 m) in length spiraling around a thick stem. The flowers, 50 - 200 per plant, open in groups of 5 - 10 per day. The pineapple flowers spiral along the axis forming multiple pineapple fruit. The multiple fruits become pressed against the fruits of adjacent flowers, forming what appears to be a single large fruit.

Pineapple Herbal Lore and Historical Use[°]

In the West Indies, pineapples were planted around a village to keep out intruders. The spiky leaves of pineapple are sharp and cannot be walked through. After colonization, pineapple hung near a

---

[°] The purpose of this book is to recapture information about historical approaches to self-induced abortion. Pineapple has been included; however the reader must keep in mind that an occasional rare death has resulted from the ingestion of the juice of green pineapple.

245

doorway came to symbolize hospitality and abundance, a design theme that has continued to this day.

Around the world, women utilize the unripe pineapple for abortifacient purposes. The unripe fruit is eaten to produce abortion in French Guiana,[386] Indonesia,[387] Fiji,[388] and the West Indies.[389] The hot water decoction of the unripe pineapple fruit is taken orally to produce abortion in India,[390] South America,[391] and Trinidad.[392]

Scientific research has shown pineapple has abortifacient, implantation preventive, estrogenic, and embryotoxic effects. The juice of unripe pineapples, when given to pregnant mice, has an abortifacient effect in the first few days of pregnancy.[393] Pineapple has been shown to have an implantation prevention effect on rats at a dose of 100 mg/kg.[394] Pineapple is estrogenic;[395] and the ethanol extract of unripe pineapple fruit has shown an embryo toxic effect in rats.[396]

Gathering: Gathering pineapple is not usually feasible, as they rarely grow in the wild. Green pineapples are available in some tropical markets, like the Philippines and Hawaii.

Purchasing: Pineapple is usually shipped green and unripe to the continental United States and may be available at markets. An unripe pineapple is green and hard.

Preparation: Green pineapple is most effective if used in the first eight weeks of pregnancy.

Words to the Wise: Unripe pineapple is considered inedible and poisonous, irritating the throat and esophagus and acting as a drastic purgative on the bowels.[397] Consumption of unripe pineapple usually causes nausea, vomiting, and diarrhea. Sometimes excessive menstruation or skin rash occurs. Pineapple is estrogenic and may contribute to estrogen dependent tumors. People with a known allergy to pineapple should not use pineapple medicinally. Allergic reaction would be indicated by: skin rash, hives, swollen skin, chest pain, breathing problems, and tightness in throat or chest.

Phototoxicity can cause rashes in people who contact pineapple leaves or eat the fruit and then expose their skin to the sun.

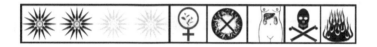

Watch for Signs of Toxicity Specific to Pineapple: Increased heart rate.

Pineapple Abortifacient Dosage

Upon waking in the morning, eat one fresh very young small-sized green pineapple (approximately 1 – 2 cups) with some honey to make it more palatable. Repeat for three days to cause an abortion.

Pomegranate

Punica granatum

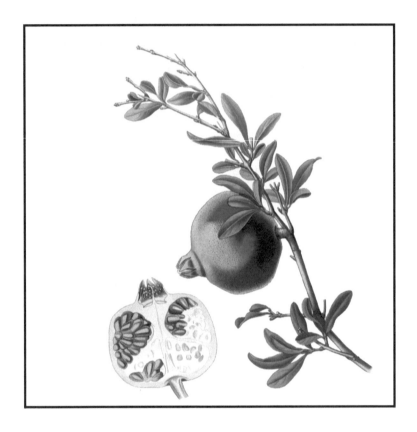

Juliet: Wilt thou be gone? It is not yet near day:
It was the nightingale, and not the lark,
That pierced the fearful hollow of thine ear;
Nightly she sings on yond pomegranate-tree:
Believe me love, it was the nightingale.

Romeo: It was the lark, the herald of the morn,
No nightingale: look, love, what envious streaks
Do lace the severing clouds in yonder east:

-William Shakespeare, *Romeo and Juliet*, 1595

Family Punicaceae

AKA: Granada (Spanish), grenade (French), and granatapfel (German).

Parts Used: Fruit rind and root bark.

Medicinal Properties: Fruit rind: Abortifacient and astringent. Root bark: Abortifacient, anthelmintic, emmenagogue, and purgative. Seeds: Estrogenic.

Effects on the Body: Fruit rind: Powerful astringent used for stomachache, colitis, dysentery, and diarrhea, leukorrhea, and abortifacient. Root bark: Purgative for tape worms and abortifacient.

Abortifacient Action: Seeds are estrogenic. Root bark is a gastrointestinal irritant. Fruit rind has unidentified action.

Contains: Fruit rind: gallotannic acid. Root bark: Ellagic acid. Seeds: Estrone (1.7 mg estrone per 1 kg ripe dried seeds).

Description: Pomegranate is a large shrub to a small tree, up to 15 ft. (4.5 m) tall. Pomegranate trees lose their leaves if growing in cool temperate regions, but when growing in their native sub-tropical climate pomegranate trees are nearly evergreen. Pomegranate has spiny tipped branches with opposite or alternate 2 in. (5 cm) long leaves: bright green, shiny, and lance-shaped. Out of the axils of some of the leaves arise short stalks and protective thick fleshy bell-shaped calyxes, which give birth to pomegranate's beautiful flowers. Pomegranate flowers are large crimson blooms, up to 2 in. (5 cm) wide, with 5 - 7 petals surrounding a circle of very numerous slender stamens. Standing in the center of the pollen-covered stamens is a single female stigma, which leads to a complex many-chambered ovary. The fruit, ripening in 5 - 7 months, grows to a size of a large orange and has a hard yellow-red leathery rind. Inside, each of the many encapsulated seed-

249

crystals is filled with refreshing sweetish-acid pink pomegranate juice. Pomegranates are grown in their place of origin, the Middle East, but also Africa, India, Malaysia, Italy, Spain and the Americas.

Pomegranate Herbal Lore and Historical Use

Pomegranate was considered sacred to the ancient worshippers of Cybele-Rhea (the Original Mother - Mother of all Gods - Mother of Zeus). From the earliest times, pomegranate has been a symbol of fertility. With its infinite seed-crystals and its blood red color, pomegranate's fruit symbolized the goddess's infinite 'yoni', pouring forth all life. An early name for 'Pomegranate' was Rimmon, a biblical name for the goddess's sacred genital shrine.[398] Pomegranate was said to have formed from the union of the great mother's yoni and the Babylonian phallic deity Nabu-Rimmani, who is credited with instituting the menstrual-lunar calendar.[399] With its abortifacient and fertility powers, pomegranate was held symbolic of the dual-fold cycle of life and death of the mother Earth. In one aspect, pomegranate with its infinite seed crystals was the most fertile of all fruit; and in another aspect, pomegranate had the power to promote infertility.

Pomegranate's abortifacient powers (held in the seed, fruit rind, and root) have been used since ancient times. Four thousand years ago, in Egypt, pomegranate seeds were ground into a powder and mixed with wax to form a vaginal pessary. This pessary was shaped into a pyramid, a symbol of the axis of the world and ascension to the afterlife. In Arab countries, the pomegranate fruit peel was used as a contraceptive pessary in Unani medicine.[400] In India, the dried root of the pomegranate tree was used as an abortifacient.[401] The

250

decoction of the root bark was used to induce menstruation in Europe and also in Ethiopia.[402]   In Indonesia, a decoction of the dried pomegranate fruit peel was taken orally as an abortifacient.[403]

Abortifacient qualities of pomegranate have been confirmed by scientific testing. The water extract of the pomegranate fruit peel was shown to be a stimulant to the uterus of non-pregnant rats.[404] The dried seed is estrogenic with up to 17 mg oestrone/kg.[405]   The seed oil is estrogenic[406] and has uterine relaxant properties.[407]   The oil was shown to have the ability to inhibit prostaglandins.[408]   A dose of 0.4ml pomegranate seed oil equals the effect of 0.1μg of oestradiol.[409]

Pomegranate, with its strong powers of woman principle, may have been the forbidden apple in the Garden of Eden. The early Latin name for pomegranate was *malum punicum*, meaning 'the apple of Carthage.' Pomegranate's name evolved to *poma granata*, meaning apples with many seeds.

In Turkey, a bride throws a pomegranate to the earth, and the number of seeds that fall out indicates the number of children she will have. In Chinese mythology the pomegranate signifies fertility. Women who wish to have children offer pomegranate to the Goddess of Mercy. The seed crystals of pomegranate may have been the original symbol in the modern suit of diamonds or pentacles in a deck of cards.[410] The diamond suit, today, is believed to represent courage and energy.

One of the best known stories in mythology follows, indicating the symbolic significance of pomegranate's abortive powers.

Note: Many of the Goddesses in this myth are deities that existed long before most of the male figures. Cybele or Rhea was the

251

original mother, Mother of all the gods, mother of Zeus.'[411] Demeter was the triangular form of the Goddess: Virgin, Mother, and Crone. Demeter, Mother of all creatures, was known to the earliest Egyptians and Sumerians.[412] Persephone was worshipped as the Queen of the Underworld, the crone aspect of Demeter, who existed long before the gods Zeus and Hades.[413] Even Hades, also called Pluto, was originally a female whose riches poured out of her breasts onto the world.[414]

Persephone

Hades, lord of the underworld and brother to Zeus, longed for a wife and was becoming more and more frustrated as every woman he asked refused to go into the dark underworld where there was no growth, no flowers, none of the beautiful life that abounded on the surface. Zeus, seeing his brother's plight, called into being a magenta and silver narcissus (the sacred magenta color of menstrual blood and silver color of the moon). The flower was so beautiful no woman would be able to resist coming closer once they saw it.

On sunny days when Persephone was not busy with her duties of tending to spring, she could be found with her sisters, care-free and happy, picking flowers on the fields of Sicily. Persephone wandered through the fields of flowers laughing with joy, picking flowers that especially caught her eye. When Persephone wandered past the magenta and silver narcissus, she was awe struck. She had never seen anything so beautiful. She swept toward it as the narcissus's fragrance enveloped her.

Instantly, the ground began to rumble, the earth fell, and in shock, Persephone watched Hades ride out of a chasm driving his coal black horses. Hades grabbed Persephone and plunged down into the chasm from which he came, into the black depths of the underworld. The earth's surface closed over them choking off Persephone's screams.

Demeter, who had been away from Sicily when Hades kidnapped Persephone, had no idea what had become of her daughter. For nine days and nights Demeter (carrying a lighted torch, an ancient symbol of anger) combed the earth and fasted, and took no part in the pleasures of bathing or eating. Finally after combing the entire earth, Demeter went to the sun.

The sun, which had seen what had happened, told Demeter the whole story. Learning that Zeus was involved, Demeter withheld her gifts to the earth, and the land became barren, icebound, and lifeless. Demeter's tears turned into crystal snow, and the land was covered with a blanket of sadness. That year was the worst year for all the creatures of the earth. Nothing grew from the grieving soil, no seeds, and no flowers. The earth was dry and lifeless. Zeus began to fear that the whole race of men would die of famine and sent god after god to Demeter to try to turn her from her anger, but she would listen to none of them. Never would she allow a single plant on the entire earth to bear fruit, until Persephone was returned to her.

Zeus sent Hermes, messenger to the Gods, to the underworld to bid his brother Hades return Persephone. Before Persephone could leave, Hades made Persephone eat some pomegranate seeds. When Persephone appeared at the surface with Hermes, there was much rejoicing by all the people and creatures of the land. Demeter and Persephone were so happy to see one another again. When Demeter heard of the pomegranate seeds Persephone was forced to eat, which would keep her daughter, the virgin Spring Goddess infertile, she cried in anger fearing she would not be able to keep her daughter with her.

Demeter, angry at the injustice done to the women of her family, retreated to her temple and wept. Rhea, the mother of Zeus (also known as Cybele), drove her winged chariot to Demeter's temple to comfort her.

'Come, my daughter. Come once again to where you will have your desire, your daughter Persephone, to comfort your sorrow. ...Peace now: Give men life, which comes alone from your giving.'[415]

Gathering: Pomegranate trees usually bear fruit after five to seven years of growth and continue for at least thrity years. Fruit should be snipped from the stem with clippers so not to damage the fruit bearing nodes, which have the capacity to bear fruit for many years. Harvest pomegranate fruit when the rind becomes yellow to red brown and when pressing on the rind gives the sound of grains crackling.[416] Root bark is best gathered at the end of the fruiting season just after the leaves turn brilliant yellow.

Purchasing: Choose a pomegranate heavy for its size with a bright and shiny skin.

Preparation: Slice the pomegranate as an orange, removing the top, bottom, and scoring the rind every few inches around the fruit. Peel fruit in a bowl of water, separating the peel from the fruit crystals (arils). Discard any discolored arils. Place the arils in a piece of cheesecloth and tighten to extract the juice into a container. Stir the fresh seeds into a jar of honey and store in the refrigerator. Seeds may be used contraceptively. (See Appendix J).

Words to the Wise: Pomegranate seeds are estrogenic and may cause estrogen-like side effects: abnormal blood clotting, liver problems, and may encourage the growth of estrogen-dependent tumors. Pomegranate roots have caused blindness in some people who have used them medicinally. The blindness caused by pomegranate roots is usually temporary but occasionally is permanent and is thought to be due to inflammation of the optic nerve.[417] Use Caution.

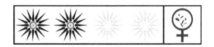

Watch for Specific Signs of Toxicity for Pomegranate Root Bark: muscle weakness, dizziness, nausea, vomiting, prolonged and abnormal dilation of the eye, dimness of vision, and loss of vision.

Pomegranate Dosage

Pomegranate Abortifacient Infusion (root bark): Soak 2 oz. (57 g) of
   root bark in 1½ cup (375 ml) water overnight. Boil gently to
   1 cup (250 ml). Pour into glass thermos. Give lukewarm in
   three doses, at intervals of one hour.

Pomegranate Abortifacient Pessary: Grind the inside of fresh
   pomegranate peel with water and apply to the cervix.[418]

Queen Anne's Lace

Daucus carota

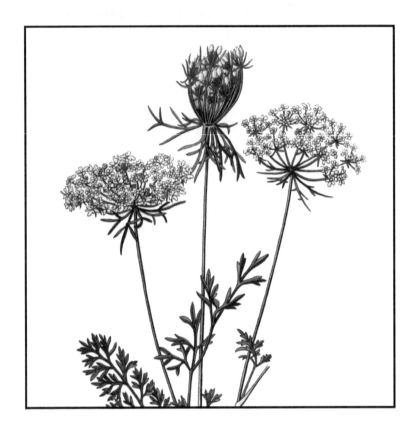

In India, the seeds (Daucus carota) are
popularly supposed to cause abortion, and
are kept by all the native druggists.

-William Dymock in *Pharmacographia Indica*, 1891

256

Family Umbelliferae

AKA: Queen Anne's lace, wild carrot, bird's nest, lace flower, devil's-plague, parsnip, and rantipole.

Part Used: Seed.

Medicinal Properties: Emmenagogue, estrogenic, also traditionally used as a deobstruent.

Effects on Body: Effects fertility, either positively or negatively, depending on dosage. Also removes calculi, kidney stones, and gall stones.

Abortifacient Action: Estrogenic and blocks progesterone synthesis.

Contains: Betaine (an abortifacient), beta-sitosterol (a phytoestrogen), and diosgenin (a phytoestrogen).

Description: Queen Anne's lace has erect, 1 – 3 ft. (0.3 – 1 m) high, hollow, ridged, bristly stems which bear alternate or basal leaves made up of feather-like segments. In late summer, tiny white flowers crowd flat-topped umbels, which mature to concave seed filled cups. One to several tiny flowers in the center of the umbel is deeper colored than all the rest, usually deep pink to purple. Introduced from Eurasia, Queen Anne's lace has spread to every state in the continental United States, with the possible exception of North Dakota. Queen Anne's lace is a very common weed found in dry fields, old meadows, pastures, and waste places.

Queen Anne's Lace Herbal Lore and Historical Use

Queen Anne's lace's abortifacient powers have been known since ancient times. Dioscorides (1st or 2nd century A.D.) noted in his *Materia medica* that *Daucus carota* had emmenagogual and abortifacient powers, "To bring forth the menses and abort the embryo, take Queen Anne's lace seed." The ancient Greeks called Queen Anne's lace 'Phileon' and noted a connection with affairs of love.[419]   In North America, women living in the Appalachian Mountains have used Queen Anne's lace seeds to regulate their fertility for hundreds of years. In the autumn, when the seeds are ripe, Appalachian women gather enough seed for their use throughout the following year. The day after sexual intercourse, women who do not want to be pregnant stir one teaspoon of the dried seeds into a glass of water and drink the mixture.[420] In India, women in Rajasthan, take the same seed in water mixture or chew on the dried seeds of Queen Anne's lace to reduce fertility.

The terpenoids in Queen Anne's lace seeds have been shown in Chinese laboratory tests to block progesterone synthesis in pregnant animals.[421]   When progesterone receptor sites in the uterine lining are blocked, the uterus cannot make a nutritive bed for the fertilized ovum, thus preventing implantation. The terpenoids in Queen Anne's lace's seed are recorded as having been studied as a promising substance in the development of a postcoital antifertility agent.[422]

Queen Anne's lace seeds' antifertility effects were recorded in a New York City study on 13 women from March 1992 to February 1993. The study was conducted by Robin Bennett, a woman with eight years of experience harvesting and using Queen Anne's lace seeds for contraception. The study showed a 98% success rate in contraceptive action.[423]

258

Gathering: One should always use an accurate field guide when gathering Queen Anne's lace; many poisonous look-alikes exist in the carrot family. Queen Anne's laces' mature seeds are gathered when ripe in the fall. The leaves of Queen Anne's lace have been used in the treatment of urinary stones. Leaves are traditionally gathered prior to flowering. Dry both seeds and leaves thoroughly, out of direct sunlight and not by artificial heat. Store in airtight containers.

Purchasing: Queen Anne's lace seeds should be organic. Beware of non-organic seed which may be treated with chemicals to increase germination rates.

Preparation: Queen Anne's lace seed prevents implantation and interferes with proper development of the endometrium (uterine lining), thus causing abortion. Queen Anne's lace is usually used as a simple in the first two weeks of pregnancy.

Words to the Wise: Some women who have used Queen Anne's lace seeds have noticed an occasional side effect of constipation. This side effect may be remedied by increased water consumption. Women with a history of kidney or gall stones should not use Queen Anne's lace seeds. Queen Anne's lace seeds are estrogenic. Estrogenic herbs contain estrogen-like substances, which act to produce the effects of the female sex hormone estrogen. Estrogenic herbs can cause estrogen-like side effects: abnormal blood clotting, liver problems, and may encourage the growth of estrogen-dependent tumors. Estrogenic herbs should be avoided by anyone taking birth control pills, estrogen medications, or blood pressure medications. Estrogenic herbs may not be as effective for premenopausal women.

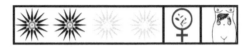

Queen Anne's Lace Dosage

Implantation Inhibiting Queen Anne's Lace Seed: Stir 1 tsp. (3 g) Queen Anne's lace seeds into a glass of water and drink the day after unprotected sex to inhibit implantation. OR One teaspoon (3 g) can also be chewed daily during ovulation or for up to one week to inhibit implantation.

Tincture (dried seeds): 1:5, 60% alcohol, 20 - 60 drops of tincture are taken once or twice the day after unprotected sex to inhibit implantation.

Rosemary
Rosmarinus officinalis

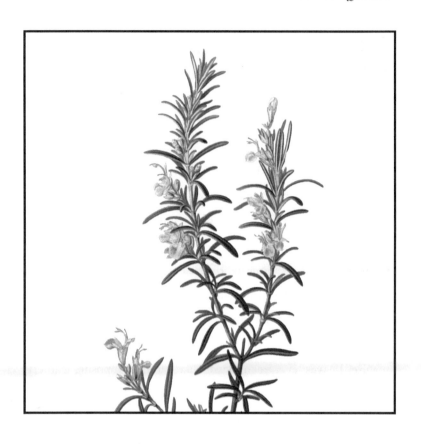

*...the oil of rosemary and a strong tea of the leaves
are among the numerous devices in
all large cities for inducing abortions.*

-Thomas Duché Mitchell in *Materia Medica and Therapeutics*, 1857

Family Labiatae

AKA: Rosemary, rosemarine, polar plant, compass plant, and incensier (Old French).

Parts Used: Leaves and flowers.

Medicinal Properties: Antispasmodic, aromatic, antimutagenic, astringent, carminative, cephalic, chologogue, diaphoretic, emmenagogue, expectorant, nervine, and tonic.

Effects on the Body: Soothing to digestive and respiratory system, stimulating to heart and uterus, strengthens nervous system, promotes liver function and the production of bile.

Abortifacient Action: Contains uterine contracting thujone. Estrogenic.

Contains: Alpha-thujone (abortifacient), beta-thujone (abortifacient), oleanolic acid (hepatoprotectant), and beta-sitosterol (phytoestrogen).

Description: Perennial aromatic rosemary grows in the form of a shrub, usually around 3 ft. (1 m) tall. Branches become woody as they mature. Leaves: evergreen, needle-like, simple, opposite, leathery, ½ - 1 in. (1.3 - 2.5 cm) long, smooth, dark green on top with tiny, soft, silvery-green hairs underneath. Small flowers, late spring to early summer, are pale blue, occasionally pink or white. In North America, rosemary is cultivated in gardens in mild regions.

Rosemary History and Medicinal Use

Rosemary, in the language of flowers, represents the power of rekindling lost energy. The French name for rosemary, 'incensier,' indicates the use of rosemary as incense when expensive imported incenses were not available. Spiritually, shamans have inhaled the burning rosemary smoke or chewed on the root to produce trances in which they prophesy and heal the sick.[424] The people of Spain held that rosemary was one of the bushes that sheltered and protected the Virgin Mary on her flight into Egypt.[425] The old Sicilian belief that young fairies, taking the form of snakes, could be found lying in branches of rosemary is reminiscent of the Biblical myth of the snake in the tree of knowledge. To the Europeans, rosemary's aromatic enduring scent was equated with remembrance. Rosemary was valued for its protective powers against insects, evil spirits, and sickness.

Rosemary branches were burned or steamed as an antibacterial vapor in sick rooms or carried at funerals. Rosemary has long been held as having protective powers against evil. For protection, rosemary was planted around one's home, used in spells to ward off black magic, worn as a charm against the evil eye, or placed in a pillow to dispel bad dreams. As a love charm during the middle ages, if a person tapped someone with a rosemary twig containing an open blossom, it was believed they would fall in love. In European weddings, rosemary was traditionally worn in the bride's wreath, and the bridal bed was decked with flowering rosemary twigs.[426] In Europe during the Middle Ages, protective emmenagogual rosemary became symbolic of the powers of women and came to be despised by the patriarchy. People said that where rosemary flourishes, the lady rules. During the 1500's, men were known to tear out rosemary bushes around the home to prove that they, not the women ruled.[427]

The French historian, L. Ruetter, reported in 1923, that a decoction of rosemary leaves, 10 - 20 grams in 200 grains (½ ounce) of water, was administered in Mexico as a carminative and an

263

abortive.[428]   James A. Duke in *Handbook of Medicinal Plants* notes Central American folk healers used rosemary and *Artemisia maritima* (related to mugwort and contains thujone) in combination for fertility control. A decoction of rosemary in combination with *Artemisia maritima* is also recorded as being used by Native Americans of the Opata tribe to produce abortion in combination with vigorous abdominal massage until contractions occur. Then, "they place her on her knees, take position before her, and holding her by the hips shake her back and forth with all their force, as in normal labor."[429] Rosemary oil is also noted as being used to promote menstruation.[430] Studies on rosemary extract on pregnant rats indicate that rosemary inhibits implantation, and rosemary shows no teratogenic effects on the fetus when the extract is given after implantation.[431]   Studies of rosemary extract on male rats showed decreased spermatogenesis.[432]

Gathering: The sprigs or leaves of rosemary are gathered from well-established plants ideally when they are just about to flower or during flowering. Tinctures are immediately processed or flowering branches are hung in the shade to dry.

Preparation: Rosemary's abortifacient properties are historically derived from the ingestion of rosemary's leaf decoction during early pregnancy. Rosemary is used as a simple or sometimes combined with mugwort and rue, or as a carminative with aloe. One source suggests rosemary be combined with a few lavender flowers, and maybe a slice of lemon and some honey.[433]

Words to the Wise: Contact dermatitis has occurred occasionally with rosemary. Rosemary's essential oil can cause psychoactive, inebriated effects. Rosemary is estrogenic and may cause estrogen-like side effects: abnormal blood clotting, liver problems, and may encourage the growth of estrogen-dependent tumors. Estrogenic herbs may not be as effective for premenopausal women.

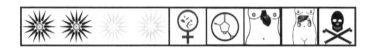

Watch for Signs of Toxicity Specific to Rosemary Essential Oil: Changes in personality, stupor, gastrointestinal irritation, nausea, and vomiting.

Rosemary Dosage

Emmenagogual Decoction (leaves): 1 oz. (28 g) herb to 2 cups
(500 ml) water. Simmer covered at least 1 hour, 2 – 3 Tbs., to
three to four times a day, for up to seven days.

Powder: 4 - 10 #0 capsules, three - four times a day, for up to
seven days.

Rue

Ruta graveolens

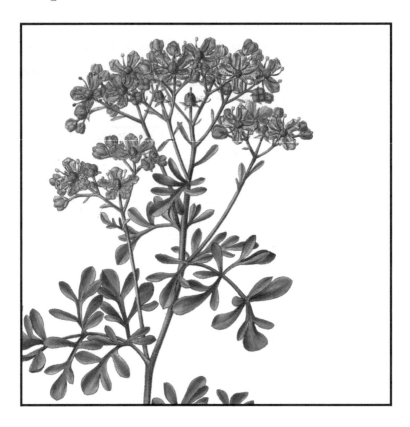

Here did she fall a tear; here, in this place,
I'll set a bank of rue, sour herb of grace;
Rue, even for Ruth, here shortly shall be seen,
In the remembrance of a weeping Queen.

-William Shakespeare, *Richard II*, 1595

266

Family Rutaceae

AKA: Rue, herb of grace, herbygrass, southern countryman's treacle, and garden rue.

Parts Used: Leaves and new shoots.

Medicinal Properties: Abortifacient, anthelmintic, antispasmodic, aromatic, emetic, emmenagogue, rubefacient, stimulant, and tonic.

Effects on the Body: Improves appetite and digestion, stimulates nervous and uterine systems, expels worms, and used as an antidote to poisonous snake and insect bites.

Abortifacient Action: Uterine contractor and contains rutin.

Contains: Rutin and the oxytocic alkaloids arborinine, graveolininine, skimmianine and pilocarpine.

Description: Rue is a bush-like aromatic perennial shrub that reaches heights of 2 – 3 ft. (0.6 – 1 m). Rue's stem is woody in its lower section. Aromatic bluish-green leaves are alternate and pinnately divided, 3 – 5 in. (7.5 - 12.5 cm) long, often having a whitish cast. Yellow flowers, ½ inch (1.3 cm) wide, with yellow, toothed petals and green centers, appear in summer to early autumn, forming in loose clusters at the top of the plant. Naturalized from Europe, rue is found in North America in old fields, roadsides and waste places from Newfoundland south to Virginia and west to Missouri.

Rue Herbal Lore and Historical Use[p]

Rue, 'herb of grace,' was the model for the suit of clubs. The symbol of the suit of clubs is not a club but a trefoil, meaning a plant that has compound leaves with three leaflets. Trefoil rue has long been associated with the three-fold Roman goddess Diana. Diana was the Triple Goddess: Virgin Moon, Mother of all Creatures, and the Crone Destroyer, as well. The name Rue is thought to be derived from the Greek *reuo,* meaning 'to set free.' The orgiastic followers of Diana are known to have used the abortifacient rue as a love charm.' [434] Respect and worship of the triple feminine aspect of the Earth Mother was so widespread, the Christians saw the Roman goddess Diana as their competitor and called her the "Queen of Witches."[435] Rue, powerful gynecological medicine, was associated with the wise-woman midwives who were brutally harassed as witches and declared by Christians "to use rue to brew magical drinks for causing harm." [436] In the North American Voodoo religion, rue is sacred to Erzulie, loa (goddess) of love. Sensual, pleasure loving, and a protector of women, Erzulie (sometimes compared to Aphrodite) represents the power of seduction and fertility.[437] Rue, when carried in a red flannel bag, is believed by the Voodoo worshippers of Erzulie to "help protect the virginity of a female and protect the wearer against all poisons."[438] Rue is a traditional abortifacient of the Hispanic people of New Mexico,[439]

---

[p] The purpose of this book is to recapture information about historical approaches to self-induced abortion. Rue has been included; however the reader must keep in mind that many deaths have resulted from the ingestion of rue.

and rue infusion has been documented as being used as an abortifacient throughout Latin America.[440]

Rue contains a chemical substance called philocarpine, which is used in veterinary medicine as an abortifacient for horses.[441] Rue also contains a substance called rutin, or Vitamin P. Rutin, present in many plants, is one of the essential bioflavonoids that serves to help the body strengthen arteries and veins and harden bones and teeth. Rutin is also known to have the power to prevent pregnancy. In large doses, rutin prolongs the action of the adrenal hormone adrenaline and decreases capillary permeability in the uterine tissues.[442] Decreased capillary permeability in the uterine tissues causes the endometrium to become non-nutritive to the fertilized egg. The egg does not implant, and abortion occurs. Chinese research on a related species in the Rutaceae family, *Murraya paniculata*, has shown the active substance, named yuehckukene, at a dose of 3 mg/per kg of body weight on the day after coitus, to be 100% successful in preventing pregnancies in female rats. The yuehckukene extract of this rue-sister is said to look promising as a future postcoital interceptor.[443] Some tests on pregnant mice have shown that rue has the ability to interfere with embryo development and interfere with fallopian tube transport and implantation.[444] However, another test of *Ruta graveolens* on pregnant mice showed no anti-implantation effects, only fetal death.[445]

Gathering: A mature rue plant may be harvested several times a year if each time the leaves or shoots are harvested, a top-dressing of rich compost is added to stimulate new growth.[446] The best time to gather rue's green shoots is right before the flowers open in the morning after

269

the dew has dried. Shoots are immediately processed into tinctures or dried in the shade. Dried rue is stored in airtight containers.

Preparation: Rue and rutin have strong implantation inhibiting abilities in the first three weeks of pregnancy. Rue should not be taken before eating, for rue has a tendency to cause vomiting due to its emetic properties. Rue is used as a simple or sometimes in combination with rosemary or pennyroyal infusion. Rue should not be boiled.

Words to the Wise: Multiple cases of death and multiple organ system failure have occurred in women using rue to induce abortion.[447] Anyone with heart, kidney, or liver damage *or* on heart medications should not take rue. Rue, in excess, can cause kidney irritation and liver degeneration.[448] Rue is known to cause contact dermatitis in susceptible individuals. Rue is also phototoxic, meaning rue can cause rashes and blistering in people who take rue and subsequently expose themselves to sunlight. Rutin, because it prolongs the action of the 'fight or flight' hormone adrenaline, may cause the physiological expression of anxiety or fear. Rutin, available in capsule form in the vitamin section at most health food stores, is usually taken as a single.

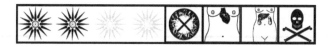

Watch for Signs of Toxicity Specific to Rue Essential Oil: Confusion, exhaustion, severe stomach pain, vomiting, convulsions, and fatality.

Rue Dosage*

Rue Abortifacient Infusion: ½ oz. (14 g) herb to 1 cup (250 ml) water.
    Steep 10 minutes, 1 – 3 Tbs. (15 - 45 ml), three - four times a
    day.

Abortifacient Tincture (fresh leaves and flowers): 1:5, 65% alcohol,
    5 - 20 drops, two to three times a day.

Powdered herb: 1 - 4 #0 capsules, three - four times a day.

*Extreme Caution! Many deaths reported!

Saffron
Crocus sativus

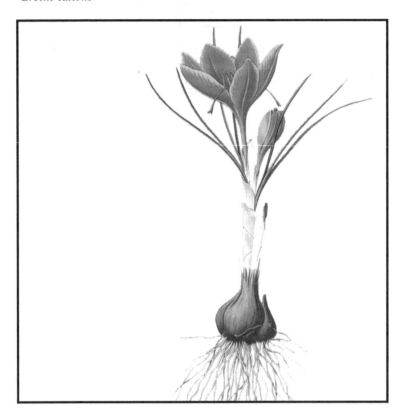

Crocus has the power of producing great venous congestion of the uterus, with passive uterine hemorrhage, and a feeling in the abdomen as of something alive. The emmenagogue action of crocus, though ignored by most old-school writers, has been abundantly confirmed by our proving. On the blood, it has a peculiar action, making it dark and stringy.
-William H. Burt in *Physiological Materia Medica*, 1881

A Japanese informed me that the abortifacient drugs contained saffron, which grows prolifically on Hokkaido, and is a very safe abortifacient. Ainu women have great faith in Japanese abortifacients but seldom betray their secret, because they receive these drugs under secrecy due to prohibitions in Japan.
-Bronisław Piłsudski, 1909

Family Iridaceae

AKA: Crocus, keshar, tree saffron, and Spanish saffron.

Medicinal Properties: Anodyne, antispasmodic, aphrodisiac, cardiotonic, diaphoretic, diuretic, ecbolic, emmenagogue, expectorant, laxative, nervine, stimulant, stomachic, and sudorific.

Effects on the Body: Soothes pains, releases toxins through sweat and urine, regulates menses, excites sexual instincts, soothes digestive and uterine muscle, soothes nerves, and stimulates the heart.

Abortifacient Action: Estrogenic and embryo toxic.

Contains: Unidentified substances.

Description: Perennial saffron grows from a corm and reaches a height of 1ft. (0.3 m). At the top of saffron's stem-like corollas, flowers bloom briefly in the early spring or early fall. Lily-like flowers have six violet petals with three dark orange to red stigmas and a pistil. The three-pronged dark orange stigmas have been collected by hand for centuries for their medicinal, culinary, as well as color-dye properties. Saffron is grown in gardens throughout the United States.

Saffron Herbal Lore and Historical Use[q]

Saffron, with its deep yellow die properties, was named the herb of the sun. Ancient Egyptian and Greek goddesses and gods were often described as clothed in deep yellow flowing robes dyed with saffron. Worn as an amulet, saffron protected against evil spirits and disease, and saffron was mixed into incense used spiritually and

---

[q] The purpose of this book is to recapture information about historical approaches to self-induced abortion. Saffron has been included; however the reader must keep in mind that deaths have resulted from the ingestion of this herb.

273

medicinally. Saffron was used to sooth the nerves, as a kidney and liver remedy, a menstruation promoter, and an aphrodisiac. As an aphrodisiac, saffron was said to excite a woman's libido and was used in magical love rituals.[449] Saffron stigmas are often enlisted in folk medicine in the treatment of tumors and cancer.[450] Saffron is commercially grown in Spain. Each saffron stigma must be handpicked, and it takes over 70,000 flowers to produce one pound of saffron. The 'Golden Spice,' is literally worth its weight in gold; one pound of saffron stigmas sells for a retail price of around $8000.00 USD. Studies of saffron have shown efficacy in the treatment of premenstrual syndrome.[451]

Gathering: Saffron stigmas are carefully gathered with a tweezers when the plant is in full bloom. Stigmas are dried thoroughly and stored in an airtight container.

Preparation: Saffron stigmas may have emmenagogual and abortifacient qualities in early pregnancy, but because saffron stigmas are so expensive to purchase and because of the potential danger of using saffron as an abortifacient, saffron is rarely used for that purpose.

Words to the Wise: Saffron is estrogenic. Estrogenic herbs may encourage estrogen-dependent tumors, liver problems, and abnormal blood clotting. The crocetin in saffron stigmas is toxic in large amounts. Some women have died attempting abortion with saffron. A dose of ½ ounce (9 grams) or more can be toxic. Overdoses of saffron are narcotic, causing changes in personality, often excessive gaiety and laughter. Saffron has cause death at a dose of 20 g.

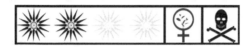

Watch for Signs of Toxicity Specific to Saffron: Flush of redness to the skin; nosebleed; heaviness in the head; changes in personality: stupor, excessive gaiety, convulsive laughter; sleepiness; vertigo; vomiting; loss of muscular control; and loss of consciousness. As always, reduce dosage at first sign of toxicity.

Saffron Dosage*

Abortifacient Saffron Stigma Dosage: 10 g. May be taken orally or made into an infusion by steeping covered 10 - 20 minutes.

*Extreme Caution! Abortifacient dose is toxic.

Squirting Cucumber

Ecballium elaterium

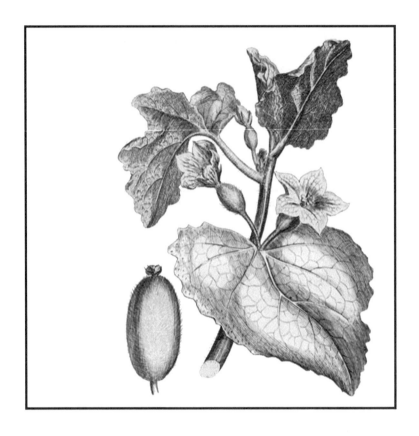

It is from that preparation of the juice, which
is admitted into our pharmacopœia,
under the title of Extract of Elaterium, that we may
expect to meet with mischief…it destroys life by its local action.

-J.A. Paris and J.S.M. Fonblanque Esq. in *Medical Jurisprudence, 1823*

Family Cucurbitaceae

AKA: Wild balsam apple and pikragouro.

Part Used: The dried fruit juice.

Medicinal Properties: Abortifacient, analgesic, anti-cancer, cathartic, emetic, nephritic, and purgative.

Effects on the Body:

Abortifacient Action: Gastrointestinal irritant.

Contains: Elaterin (a resin).

Description: This native to southern Europe and the Mediterranean is a trailing bushy perennial with palm-like bristly leaves. Male and female funnel-shaped yellow flowers appear separately on the same plant. Fruits are green, oblong, and bristly like cucumbers on the end of long stalks. When ripe the fruits explode, shooting mucilaginous liquid and seeds up to 18 feet (6 m).

Squirting Cucumber Herbal Lore and Historical Use[r]

Squirting cucumber has been used as a medicinal plant for 2000 years. Hippocrates in *Diseases of Women* says that the preferred drug for abortion is *Ecballium elaterium*. Squirting cucumber is a very powerful purgative that produces watery stools, griping, and sometimes vomiting. Squirting cucumber is one of the strongest herbal purgatives known, and for this reason is rarely used Squirting cucumber has no specific action on the uterus. Squirting cucumber has caused deaths in women who have taken it.[452]

---

[r] The purpose of this book is to recapture information about historical approaches to self-induced abortion. Squirting cucumber has been included; however the reader must keep in mind that many deaths have resulted from the ingestion of this herb.

277

Gathering: The fruit is collected just before it ripens and is left until it matures and ejects the seeds and juice. This must not be artificially hastened or the medicinal product will be affected. The juice is dried in flakes.

Preparation: Elaterium is usually made into pills or sometimes into tinctures. Elaterium is not widely available, as it has fallen out of use.

Words to the Wise: Elaterium can vary greatly in strength, use extreme caution. Juice can cause dermatitis. Exposure to the juice if inhaled can cause irritation or obstruction of the mucous membranes. Eyes should be promptly irrigated if exposed to prevent injury. Elaterium has caused the death of some women who have used it in an attempt to cause abortion.

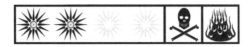

Watch for signs of Toxicity Specific to Squirting Cucumber: Violent gastroenteritis, circulation system and nervous system depression, cardiac failure, and renal failure.[453]

Squirting Cucumber Dosage*
Elaterin: 1/40 - 1/10 grain, taken every three to four hours until abortion commences.

* Extreme caution. Elaterin (the concentrated juice of squirting cucumber) is not used in modern medicine because it is so dangerous!

Stoneseed

Lithospermum ruderale

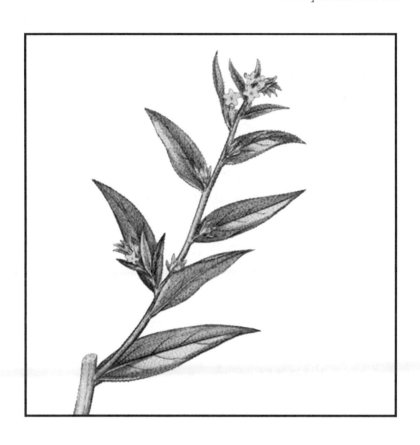

I know of a woman who used it, but
it worked too well. She could never have children after using it.
The Crow word for stone seed, eldocxabio, means
'miscarriage plant'... The wrong dose can leave a woman sterile.

-Alma Hogan Snell in *A Taste of Heritage, 2006*

Family Boraginaceae

AKA: Woolly gromwell and western puccoon.

Medicinal Properties: Antigonadotropic, antithyroidal, contraceptive, and diuretic.

Effects on the Body: Reduces gonadotropic hormone, reduces estrogen, mimics progesterone, and inhibits thyroid stimulating hormone.

Abortifacient Action: Inhibits progesterone.

Contains: Lithospermic acid. Seems to suppress lactate dehydrogenase leakage particularly in renal cells.

Description: Stoneseed grows in open dry places from the valleys up to the lower sub alpine forests in western North America, from Colorado to California and north to British Columbia. Stoneseed's narrow lance-shaped leaves, with small pale yellow to orange tubular flowers (March – July), spiral around the upper stems. It can reach 2 ft. (0.6 m) in height. In late summer, the seeds (like little stones) are seen, four seeds inside each calyx.

Stoneseed Medicinal Use and Herbal Lore

Native Americans from the Shoshoni and Navajo also are documented as utilizing the stoneseed plant as an oral contraceptive.[454] Decoctions of stoneseed are known for their pronounced contraceptive action, and its use by the Native Americans provided inspiration for the development of oral contraceptives.[455] Six months of continued use was believed to cause sterility.[456]

Like many abortifacient herbs, stoneseed was associated with the goddess, and in stoneseed's case, the herb was associated with a

280

living goddess in the Native American Blackfoot tribe. Stems of stoneseed were used by children of the Native American Blackfoot tribe to make headdresses for acting and playing out the affairs of the Holy Woman.[457] Blackfoot women were known among Native American tribes for their fierce independence and for the respect they were given within their tribe. The Holy Woman of the Blackfoot tribe presided over the Sun Dance, which could not be held if the Holy Woman was not there praying for the tribe and its continued connection to the Sun Deity.[458] The Sun Dance, held on or near the summer solstice, was the coming of age ceremony which allowed a young man the unquestioned right to the title of warrior. In other Native American tribes, stoneseed was believed to have magical powers to make it rain or to stop a thunderstorm.[459]

Scientific testing of stoneseed has confirmed the antifertility effects of stoneseed. Stoneseed has been found to inhibit progesterone hormone due to a direct effect on the hypothalamus. Extract of stoneseed was found to decrease the gonadotropic activity in the pituitary glands of female mice.[460] Extract of stoneseed root impaired the development of the gonads and accessory sex organs in female rats.[461]

Gathering: For the best medicinal qualities, the root of stoneseed should be gathered after sunset. The seeds of stoneseed are gathered in the late summer.

Preparation: Stoneseed is used in the week preceding a woman's period to inhibit implantation. If used every day of the menstrual cycle, stoneseed acts to permanently reduce estrogen levels. Stoneseed used daily for over six months is reported to induce permanent sterility. Stoneseed is not documented as being combined with any other herbs.

Words to the Wise: Some plants in the Lithospermum genus contain pyrrolizidine alkaloids. Pyrrolizidine alkaloids are known to be toxic to the liver.

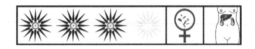

Stoneseed Dosage*

Contraceptive/ Implantation Inhibiting Stoneseed Decoction: 1oz.
(28 g) dry root to two cups (500 ml) of water, infused cold overnight, 1 tsp. (5 ml) every three hours, for up to five days.
Contraceptive/ Implantation Inhibiting Powdered Seed: ½ tsp. (1 g) every four - five hours, for up to five days.

*Extreme caution! Stoneseed is known to cause sterility.

Tansy
Tanacetum vulgare

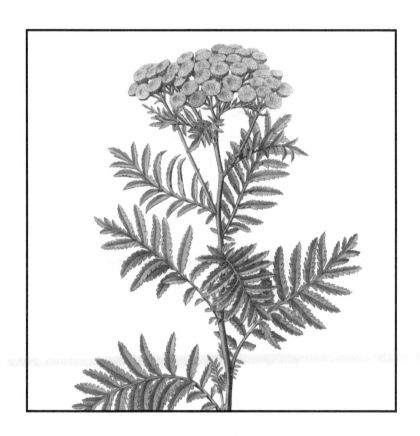

Dr. Caton's Tansy Pills!
The most reliable remedy for ladies.
Always safe, effectual, and
the only guaranteed women's salvation.
Price $1.
Second advice free.
R. F. Caton, Boston, Mass.

-Turn of the 20th century newspaper classified

283

Family Compositae

AKA: Tansy, bitter-buttons, hindheal, ginger plant, and parsley fern.

Parts Used: Flowers, leaves, seeds, and root.

Medicinal Properties: Abortifacient, anthelmintic, emmenagogue, stimulant, and tonic.

Effects on the Body: Uterine stimulant, menstrual regulator, and expels worms.

Abortifacient Action: Contracts uterus.

Contains: Beta-thujone.

Description: Tansy is an aromatic perennial with strong erect stems reaching 2 - 3 ft. (0.6 - 1 m) in height. Alternate 3 - 4 in. (7.5 – 10 cm) long leaves, deep-green, lance-shaped, with alternate deeply toothed leaflets, give tansy a feathery appearance. Golden-yellow flower 'buttons', late summer to mid-autumn, appear tightly grouped together in flat-topped flower-clusters. Found on wastelands, wood clearings, and undisturbed nitrogen-rich soils in North America from Nova Scotia to British Columbia, from Nevada to North Carolina.

Tansy Herbal Lore and Historical Use[s]

Tansy has been known since ancient times as a meat preservative and insect repellant. The leaves and flowers were rubbed on meats to help preserve them, and mattresses and pillows were stuffed with tansy to keep bugs away. Compared with most of the

---

[s] The purpose of this book is to recapture information about historical approaches to self-induced abortion. Tansy has been included; however the reader must keep in mind that deaths have resulted from the ingestion of this tansy essential oil.

herbs featured in this book, it has only been relatively recently that tansy has been used as an emmenagogue.

Hildegard of Bingen (AD 1098 - 1117), a remarkable mystic and pioneer in science, sometimes mentioned as the first European woman doctor, was the first to mention tansy as having emmenagogual powers.[462] A strong wise-woman, Hildegard was chosen to represent her convent as the abbess. Hildegard's achievements include: *Scivias*, twenty-six of her visions about the relationship between God, man, and creation; two books of medicine and natural history; hymns and canicles of which she wrote both words and music; a play; and a language of her own composed of 900 words and an alphabet of 23 letters. Hildegard regularly traveled throughout Germany and parts of Gaul speaking to people of all classes and walks of life. Hildegard was endeared to the people, many of whom still refer to her as Saint Hildegard. To this day, tansy is used throughout Europe to induce menstruation.

The abortifacient use of tansy is also documented in North America. The decoction of tansy leaf was taken by young Native American Chippewa girls for "stoppage of period."[463] The infusion of tansy was taken to prevent pregnancy by the Malecite tribe.[464]

Gathering: Leaves and flowers of tansy are gathered when in full bloom. The root of tansy may be gathered when the above-ground portions of the plant begin to die back in late fall. Tansy seeds are gathered when mature. Gathered material is immediately processed into tinctures or dried in the shade and stored in airtight containers.

Preparation: Tansy's emmenagogual and abortifacient properties are mainly derived from the infusion or tincture. Tansy is taken as a simple or sometimes combined with blue cohosh and pennyroyal infusion.

Words to the Wise: Do not confuse Tansy *Tanacetum vulgare* with Tansy Ragwort *Senecio jacobea*, found in the Northeastern United States and known to produce irreversible liver damage when taken internally. Compared to other abortifacient herbs, tansy has been used for abortifacient and emmenagogual purposes only in the recent past. Tansy is a very strong herb and can cause side effects even at therapeutic doses. Use caution. Tansy has been known to cause temporary lumps in the breasts of women who use it to promote menstruation, and tansy can cause hemorrhage in women who normally menstruate heavily.[465]   Tansy contains the uterine contracting and possibly toxic thujone. The amount of thujone in tansy varies widely from plant to plant, some plants contain no thujone; other plants may have up to 95% thujone in their oil.[466] Because of tansy's chemical variability, use extreme caution. Stay out of the sun when taking tansy. Tansy is phototoxic; it can produce a skin rash or blistering in individuals who have taken it and then expose themselves to sunlight. Tansy's essential oil is very concentrated. As little as 4 ml (less than 1 tsp!) of the oil has caused death.

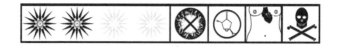

Watch for Signs of Toxicity Specific to Tansy: Nausea, vomiting, inflammation of the stomach lining, dilated pupils, weakened and/or rapid pulse, convulsions, and coma.

Tansy Dosage*

Abortifacient Infusion (dried flowering tops): One handful (4-8 teaspoons) of the dried aerial parts of tansy to 1 quart (1 L). Simmer 15 minutes. Sip throughout the day. Take no longer than five days.

Tansy Emmenagogue: Drink one cup (250 ml) the night before expected menstruation, and then one cup (250 ml) in the morning if menstruation has not already started.

Tincture (flowering tops): 1:5, 95% alcohol, 20 – 30 drops, three to four times a day for no longer than five days.

*Extreme Caution! Tansy's inherent chemical variability is extremely dangerous.

Wild Ginger

Asarum canadense

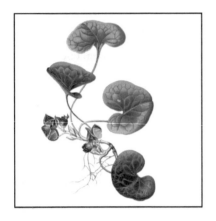

In the night of December 9th I was called to see Mary W., aged seventeen years, unmarried...I suspected she might be pregnant, and questioned her concerning her catamenia in the presence of her mother. She assured me that she had her 'menses regular,' that she was slightly unwell then, and her mother did not contradict her story...Early next morning, her father called on me, stated that she had given birth to a child, and desired me to see her at once. I found that she had given birth to a three month's embryo, without calling any of the family...she [admitted she] had been using a strong tea, and chewing a root...she said the girls use it, and that one of her female companions had used it for the same purpose, and with the same results. For the past few days [she] had taken a strong tea of the root. Her mother, on searching her pockets, found some of the root, which she gave ...the root as Asarum canadense...having my doubts about the matter, I asked where she got the so-called root. I called at the drug-store designated, and asked the proprietor to show me some...He assured me that...large quantities of the Asarum canadense are sold to women, especially to girls.

-Dr. P. R. Palm in *Transactions of the Medical Society of Pennsylvania*, 1874

288

Family Aristolochiaceae

AKA: Canada black snake root, catfoot, broad-leafed sarabacca, Indian ginger, colicroot, and coltsfoot.

Part Used: Root.

Medicinal Properties: Abortifacient, aromatic, carminative, diaphoretic, diuretic, emmenagogue and purgative, and stimulant.

Effects on the Body: Soothes stomach, stimulates circulatory system, relieves joint and muscle pain, cleans out intestines, and promotes menstruation.

Abortifacient Action: Estrogenic and may reduce luteinizing hormone.

Contains: Aristolochic acid (abortifacient) and beta-sitosterol (a phytoestrogen).

Description: Wild ginger, *Asarum canadense*, is a native North American perennial herb with heart-shaped, velvety, 5 – 6 in. (12.5 – 15 cm) wide leaves arising on whitish hairy stalks from a tan to brown rhizome. In spring, tiny dark reddish-brown triangular bell-shaped flowers appear hidden under the leaves at the fork between the two leafstalks. The stems and rhizome have a spicy ginger-like odor. Wild ginger is found in rich woodlands growing in cool shaded areas often by streams from Quebec to Ontario, south to Florida, and west to Minnesota, also found west of the Rockies, northern California to Canada. Wild ginger is often used in shaded landscapes as a slowly spreading ground cover.

Wild Ginger Herbal Lore and Historical Use[t]

Wild ginger was used by the Native Americans for heart palpitations, as a condiment, and to induce menstruation. It was used specifically by Cherokee women to start their periods. The practitioners of the American Physic Medical School maintained that wild ginger root has a direct influence on the uterus.[467] Herbalists have used wild ginger for centuries to induce perspiration, menstruation, and to aid in elimination of waste matter and gas. Powdered wild ginger root, inhaled like snuff, has been used relieve aching head and eyes.

Wild ginger contains aristolochic acid. Aristolochic acid stimulates contractions of the uterus; it is 100% effective in blocking pregnancy in mice after a single oral dose (100 mg/kg) on the 6th or 7th day after coitus. A dose of 20 - 90 mg/kg was sufficient to block implantation, and a dose of 30 mg/kg interrupted midterm pregnancy.[468] Aristolochic acid inhibits phospholipase hydrolysis, which checks inflammation and may alter release of luteinizing and growth hormones from the pituitary.[469]

Gathering: The root may be gathered when the leaves begin die back. It should be dried thoroughly and stored in an airtight container.

---

[t] The purpose of this book is to recapture information about historical approaches to self-induced abortion. Wild Ginger has been included; however the reader must keep in mind that deaths have resulted from the ingestion of wild ginger.

Preparation: Wild ginger tea should be taken in small doses, as large doses tend to nauseate the stomach. Wild ginger is most effective as an emmenagogue if taken in early pregnancy.

Words to the Wise: A related Asarum plant *Asarum Europoem* has caused death in women who tried to use it to induce miscarriage in the second trimester.[470] Modern science has shown a strong correlation between consumption of herbal products containing aristolochic acid with delayed onset renal failure and cancer. Carcinogenic doses of aristolochic acid have been noted at long-term low doses or short-term high doses, and thus herbs containing aristolochic acid have been relegated to the back of the shelf because of safety issues.[471] Wild ginger is also estrogenic and may contribute to estrogen-dependent cancers or interfere with normal blood clotting.

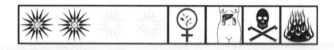

Watch for Signs of Toxicity specific to Wild Ginger: Vomiting, pains in the abdomen, and convulsions.

Wild Ginger Dosage

Abortifacient Decoction (root): 1 tsp. (5 g) macerated root to 2 cups (500 ml) boiling water. Simmer 5 -10 minutes. 1 – 2 Tbs. (15 – 45 ml), four to six times a day.

Tincture (fresh root): 1:2, 65% alcohol, 20 - 40 drops, two to three times a day.

Powdered Root: 2 - 4 #0 capsules, four to six times a day.

Homeopathy

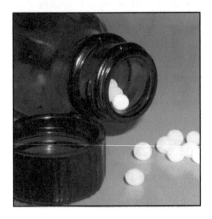

The adherents of the old school of medicine assail the body with large, often protracted and rapidly repeated doses of strong medicine, whose long-lasting, not infrequently terrible effects they do not know, and which they apparently make purposely unrecognizable through the commixture of more such unknown substances into one medicinal formula...
With the medical art of homeopathy, it is entirely different.

-Samuel Hahnemann, 1833

Homeopathy is an alternative form of medicine created in the late 1700's by German physician Samuel Hahnemann. Hahnemann saw the harm done by traditional medicine and sought to develop a medicinal art where the medicine would do no harm, and the disease would be cured. A homeopathic remedy is made from an individual substance that in undiluted form, given to a healthy individual, causes symptoms that are similar to the disease that the homeopathic remedy is intended to treat. The substance intended as a homeopathic remedy is extracted into a tincture (called the mother tincture) and then diluted

292

repeatedly and dymatized (moved) at each dilution. Dymatization, through shaking or spinning, is believed to increase the power and vitality of the remedy to act on an energetic level by inducing a temporary weightless vortex which excites the molecules of the diluted substance. Dymatization has been likened to the increased magnetism produced in a steel rod when it is rubbed repeatedly.

Homeopathy is founded on the ancient principle of the law of similars, *similia similibus curantur*, which holds that a substance of natural origin that produces certain symptoms in a healthy person will cure those same symptoms in a sick person. Hippocrates, in his work *On the Place of Things which Regard Man,* commented on the ancient understanding "Disease is born of like things, and by the attack of like things people are healed – vomiting ends through vomiting."

Homeopathy is sometimes described as quantum medicine, for the particles of medicinal substances are so small that they are believed to influence the cells of the body at the molecular level. Often a homeopathic remedy will have no scientifically discernable molecules of the original active ingredient in the final dilution. In homeopathy, it is believed the more diluted the remedy the more powerful the biological effects. Hahnemann said, "Homeopathic medicine's goal is to provide a gentle permanent cure to disease without significant side effects." This is in contrast to pharmaceutical medicines which are thought by those who believe in homeopathy to negatively affect the life force.

It is widely known that pharmaceutical drugs can have significant negative side effects to the liver, kidneys, and reproductive systems, even at the appropriate doses. Homeopathy remains controversial, because it is directly opposed to medical and pharmaceutical knowledge founded on observed dose-response relationships of conventional drugs.

Homeopathic abortion holds the promise of having a simple, natural form of abortion with few side effects. If homeopathic abortion proves itself to be safe and effective, all other self-induced abortion methods may be deemed inferior. Unfortunately, no scientific testing has been undertaken to evaluate homeopathic abortion methods.

Inducing abortion with homeopathic preparations is a controversial subject even among homeopathic doctors. Some homeopathic doctors believe that inducing miscarriage is not possible via homeopathic preparations. Pregnancy is a natural human function, and homeopathic drugs are intended to promote natural processes of the human body. Homeopathic abortion in some literature is shown to be generally ineffective. One study in rural Bangladesh found that only 4 out of 29 attempts to induce abortion with homeopathy succeeded.[472] However, certain homeopathic prescriptions in a double-blind trial have been shown in childbirth studies to impact pregnancy by reducing labor time and decreasing abnormal labor.[473] In India, one homeopathic medicine, Abroma radix, has developed a reputation among homeopathic doctors for its effectiveness at inducing abortion; one homeopathic physician has claimed Abroma radix "may be used for easy abortion, minimizing the scope of D&C operations."[474]

Homeopathic medicines used to induce abortion are often in the LM (also called Q) potency. LM is the term used to describe one of the most diluted potencies available; it is serially diluted at a 1:50,000 dilution ratio and vigorously shaken at each dilution. LM potencies are believed to have a strong curative action without causing therapeutic aggravation when prescribed according to the homeopathic principle of similar disease symptoms.

When using homeopathic medicines:
1. Utilize the assistance of a trained homeopathic physician.
2. Remember that less is more. Taking more of the medicine will not be more effective.
3. Contraceptive pills and prescribed drugs can negatively affect homeopathic medicine.
4. Do not eat, drink, or use toothpaste 15 minutes before or after using the homeopathic remedy.
5. Avoid strong smelling substances, like menthol or camphor.
6. Avoid drinking caffeinated coffee. Decaf is okay, and tea is okay.
7. Record and make notes.

Words to the Wise: Homeopathic abortion has all of the risks of abortion, but may have additional risks as well. There are few studies that document the effectiveness of homeopathic remedies.

It is possible that a woman may have sensitivity to a homeopathic abortion medicine, and that balancing hormones with additional individualized prescriptions and herbal remedies may be necessary. Being advised by a homeopath, trained with Hahnemann's 6th edition of *Organon*, would be advisable during and after a homeopathic induced abortion.

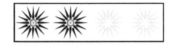

Step by Step: Taking Homeopathic LM1 Remedy

1. Without touching the granule, as hand oils can interfere with the medicinal effect, place one LM1 granule or liquid drop in a sterilized 4 oz. glass bottle filled with 3 oz. distilled water and 3 tsp. 95% alcohol to make a liquid homeopathic.

2. Knock the bottle containing liquid homeopathic 1-10 times on a book or wooden table. (As if dropped from a height of one foot onto a firm dense surface like a book.) A person sensitive to medicines should knock the bottle one time. A person over forty years old should knock the bottle five times. A healthy and young person should knock the bottle ten times.

3. Place one teaspoon of the liquid homeopathic into half a cup of water. Stir vigorously for ten seconds. Take one teaspoon into the mouth and hold it for a few seconds before swallowing. Throw the rest of the contents of the cup away.

4. Liquid homeopathic, created in step one, may be stored for several days in a cool dry place. Homeopathic granules can be kept for decades without loss of medicinal qualities if stored in a sealed container in a cool dry place.

Homeopathic Remedies Used to Induce Abortion:

Abroma radix (LM) is derived from the fresh juice of the root bark of

the tropical Asian plant *Abroma augusta* with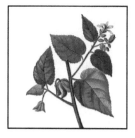
the common names olat kambal or devil's
cotton. The root of *Abroma augusta* has a long
history of being used in Ayurvedic medicine as
an effective emmenagogue for dysmenorrhea
and as an oxytocic uterine tonic.

Abroma radix LM Dosage: Repeat every 2 hours until bleeding is
underway.

Carica papaya (LM) is used topically on the uterine os to cause

softening of the os and uterine contractions.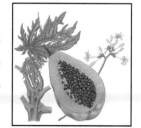
Carica papaya LM Dosage: Use liquid
homeopathic as a topical application to the
cervical os or as a vaginal douche. Repeat every
two hours until bleeding is underway.

Gossypium forte (LM), a homeopathic preparation made from the

fresh green root of cotton *Gossypium herbaceum*,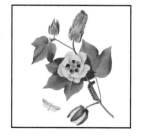
is used as a strong emmenagogue and labor
promoter. Gossypium forte (LM) has been
used by midwives to release retained
placentas.[475] Homeopathic Gossypium is
considered a powerful emmenagogue.[476]

Gossypium forte LM Dosage: Repeat every two hours until bleeding is
underway.

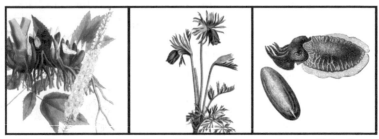

Cimicifuga racemosa　　*Pulsatilla pratensis*　　*Sepia officinalis*

Humphrey's 11™ is a commercial homeopathic medicine advertised for delayed or irregular menses. Humphrey's 11™ is known to cause the cervix to soften and has a reputation of inducing abortion in very early pregnancy in some women. However, Humphrey's 11™ can cause potential problems. If it is not effective and a woman seeks a vacuum aspiration abortion, the softened cervix may be more vulnerable to injury during a vacuum aspiration abortion procedure.[477] Humphreys 11™ Contains: Black cohosh (*Cimicifuga racemosa*), Wind flower *Pulsatilla pratensis*), and Cuttlefish (*Sepia officinalis*). Follow dosage directions on packaging.

Macrotinum (LM), a homeopathic preparation made from the resin of
the root of black cohosh *(Cimicifuga racemosa)* is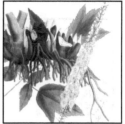
used to encourage overdue menstruation.
Macrotinum is sometimes combined with
Gossypium forte and Carica papaya.

Macrotinum LM Dosage: 3 pills or 5 drops,
three times a day.

Pulsatilla (LM), a homeopathic preparation made from wind flower
Pulsatilla pratensis, is used to encourage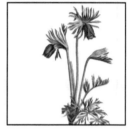
suppressed menstruation.

Pulsatilla LM Dosage: 3 pills or 5 drops, three
times a day.

Acupuncture

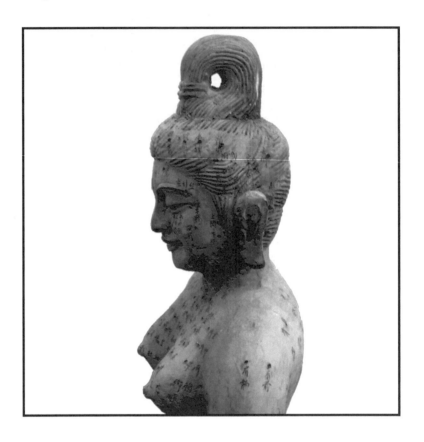

An empress laid a wager with Xu Wenbei, a physician, about
the effectiveness of his abortion techniques, for
attempts to abort with acupuncture were far from certain.
Xu employed acupuncture on a pregnant woman, and
the fetus was successfully aborted.

- from Nanshi (Official History of the Southern Dynasties),
AD 420-589

It is generally believed acupuncture originated in China 2500 years ago. However, recent archeological discoveries may predate the existence of acupuncture in China. Ötzi the Iceman, the natural mummy found in the Italian Alps in glacial ice in AD 1991 and dated to around 3300 BC, had 57 simple dot and line tattoos on his body of which 80% have been found to correspond to acupuncture points used today.[478] Where acupuncture originated is unknown, but there is some evidence that it may have originated in Sri Lanka and spread through trading merchants to the rest of the world.[479]

Acupuncture gradually developed and was refined in China over the last 2500 years. The Yellow Emperor's Classic of Internal Medicine (300 BC) outlines the philosophy of the natural flow and movements of life: yin and yang, the Five Elements, the organ system and the meridian network along which acupuncture points are located. The 50-volume Compendium of Materia Media was published during the Ming Dynasty (AD 1368-1644) by the Li Shi Zen herbalists/acupuncturists. After the Ming Dynasty, a decline in traditional medicine occurred, coinciding with the increase of Western ideas and influence on China. This decline in traditional medicine continued up until the mid 20th century when the Cultural Revolution brought traditional Chinese herbal medicines and acupuncture back to the forefront.

In the mid 1960's, China's Chairman Mao issued an edict proclaiming no married couple could have more than one child. Women who already had one child and became pregnant were forced to undergo abortion. Many of these abortions were performed in hospitals or clinics using acupuncture.[480]

301

Trained acupuncturists are aware of the acupuncture points that are generally avoided or needled only with great care during pregnancy. Strong needling of these points during pregnancy is widely known to cause strong uterine contractions and expulsion of the fetus.[481] Manipulation of points contraindicated in pregnancy can cause abortion in the first trimester or induce birth from 19 weeks of pregnancy onwards.[482]

Locating Acupuncture Points

There are over 2000 known acupuncture points on the human body. Acupuncture points are located on channels of energy that run through the body. These channels are called meridians. Stimulation of an acupuncture point can change the energy or qi (chi or ki) through the meridian associated with that acupuncture point and through the body energy meridians as a whole.

Cun measurement, qi sensing/awareness, and an electrical acupuncture point locator are used, often in conjunction, to accurately locate acupuncture points. Cun measurement is a system of measurement that is unique for each individual. The width of the patient's thumb is used to measure and find the approximate location of an acupuncture point. The sensing on the qi energy moving from the acupuncture point further pinpoints the point location. Further, a handheld acupuncture point location device may be used to accurately locate the point. Acupuncture points are fluid moving energy points on the body. Points are known to move, sometimes significantly, depending on the health and well being on the individual.

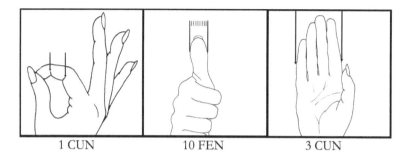

| 1 CUN | 10 FEN | 3 CUN |

Cun is the standard unit of measurement of the body used in acupuncture. As every human body is unique in its dimensions, cun is defined according to the person whose body is being treated. Like one centimeter is divided into ten millimeters, one cun is divided into ten fen.

1 cun= width of thumb, in the middle, at the crease.

3 cun= combined breadth of the four fingers, at the level of the pinky fingers' first joint above the palm of the hand.

10 fen = 1 cun

Qi Awareness

The ability to locate acupuncture points with qi (or energy) awareness requires calm relaxation, (meditation), and attention (focused awareness).

Sensing Qi:

1. Calm yourself, breathe slowly and deeply until a state of deep relaxation and peace is reached.

2. Close your eyes. Relax the mind and body. Hold your hands apart in front of you, palms facing each other. Move your palms toward each other, sensing the space between. Focus on the space between your hands. Abide in calm awareness – sensing. For each person the sensation of qi energy will be unique. Some describe the sensation as a pressure, pulling, tingling, heat, or coolness.

3. Sensing meridians: Hold your finger two inches above the body surface near a meridian. Move your finger perpendicular back and forth across the meridian area (like plucking a guitar string). Feathers are useful tools to sense energy. Hold the feather above the meridian and move it back and forth. Open yourself to the sensation of the subtle energy. If you find your hands getting tense, shake your hands for a few seconds to release any excess qi that may have accumulated at your fingertips.

4. Sensing Acupuncture Points: Using cun measurements, and acupuncture point diagrams, roughly locate a particular acupuncture point. In a state of non-expectation with open

calm awareness, point your finger at the acupuncture point approximately two inches away from the surface of the skin. Move your finger slowly back and forth in a diameter of a couple inches. The place where you feel the strongest sensation is the center of the point.

Using an Electric Acupoint Locator

Small hand-held devices, called electrical acupuncture point locators, utilize the electrical resistance near the skin at the points to indicate the correct location of an acupuncture point. An electric acupoint locator can greatly assist in finding particular acupuncture points, however because the body contains over 2000 acupuncture points, the use of an electric acupoint locator is best reserved for reading the difference in electrical resistance in a small radius at a defined location where a major acupuncture point is believed to be located on the body.

There is no one single documented method of inducing the uterus to empty its contents with acupuncture. Each individual is unique and would require a unique approach; a trained TCM acupuncturist's assistance is vital. The following are examples of documented acupuncture methods used to induce menstruation, abortion, or full term labor:

- One method suggests the use of four acupuncture points once daily for two to three days: LI4 is mildly stimulated. SP6 is strongly stimulated where the needle is directed slightly upwards so a sensation extends into the lower abdomen. GV1 is inserted to a depth of three fen and the needle is directed upwards so that a sensation is felt in the sacrum. SP9 is directed upwards so a sensation is felt in the lower abdomen. LI4 and SP6 are considered the principal points, while GV1 and SP9 are supplementary, and the principal and supplementary points are used in rotation.[483]

- Another method of inducing abortion with acupuncture is the combined acupuncture of LI4, LR3, SP6, BL67, and BL54 using the reducing method which includes: quick insertion of the needle tip against the direction of the channel at the moment of exhalation, then strongly lifting, softly thrusting, and rapidly rotating the needle clockwise six times, and then slow withdrawal of the needle without pressing on the point afterwards. Sometimes electrical stimulation is used.[484]

- One point specifically used to terminate pregnancy, Jueyun, is named after its function. Jueyun is located two cun and three fen below the umbilicus. Using acupuncture needling on this point is believed to bring about induced infertility. This point, when used with moxa, is used to induce labor at term.[485]

- Rina Nissim, founder of the women's health center in Geneva, Switzerland and author of *Natural Healing in Gynecology*, documents her use of acupuncture stimulation in combination with emmenagogual herbs and abortive massage to induce menstruation up to ten days past missed menses. Acupuncture needles are inserted at SP6 and LI4 for thirty minutes (rotated clockwise every two minutes until they jam).[486]

- Andrew Orr worked in Guangxi, China and observed labor induction via daily acupuncture stimulation for three hours with an electro muscle stimulator at 3Hz. Orr, later an acupuncturist at the Natural Birthing Center at the Royal Women's Hospital in Brisbane, Australia, utilized acupuncture points LI4, SP6, GB21, and KI6 to induce labor in women whose pregnancies were at 40 weeks and over. First, the needles were stimulated by hand rotation, and then the needles were attached to electro stimulation for 1.5 hours at 1.5 Hz. Labor was induced in 88% of cases after the first treatment. The time frame for the beginning of labor after the treatment varied from 2 ½ to 26 hours.[487]

- Acupressure of the points that are used in acupuncture to induce miscarriage are also used by some women to help bring on menstruation. Jeanne Elizabeth Blum in *Woman Heal Thyself* documents a detailed regime to stimulate menstruation including strong acupressure massage of LI4, SP6, SP1, SP2, SP4, SP9, ST36, KI1, KI6, and GB41.[488]

Words to the Wise: Acupuncture treatment is intimately designed for the individual. Seeking the advice, assistance, and support of a trained acupuncture specialist is advised. Acupuncture is a medicinal art which takes years of study and practice to become proficient. An acupuncturist will often look at the tongue and ask a patient many questions to help determine the extent of yin and yang balance within the body, as an imbalance of yin or yang will cause the qi to move in opposite directions when an acupuncture point is stimulated.

To induce an abortion using acupuncture, strong needling and stimulation is usually necessary, for utilizing forbidden acupuncture points with prudence during pregnancy has been found to be safe and non abortive.[489] It is believed by some that causing an abortion with acupuncture is more related to the degree of stimulation to the point than the selection of the appropriate point.[490] All of the examples of acupuncture methods documented above include the retention of the needles for durations ten to sixty times longer than the normal duration of only three to seven exhalations, and often include manually stimulation by turning the needles and/or electrical stimulation.

Acupuncture complications are rare in the hands of a skilled practitioner. However they do occur; the most common problems being bruised skin at acupuncture point, pain, burns, bleeding, and contact dermatitis.[491] A very rare complication is an acupuncture needle breaking off in the skin. This requires removal with pliers or emergency surgery.

The effectiveness of using acupuncture to induce abortion is debated. Although there are many historical accounts of acupuncture being used to induce abortion, there is little evidence from medical literature that stimulation of the forbidden pregnancy points during pregnancy results in abortion. It is widely believed by medical experts that inducing abortion with acupuncture is not effective.[492]

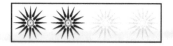

1. Use only properly sterilized needles. Needles may be purchased with tubes which help guide the needle for insertion.
2. Locate points.
3. Wash hands.
4. Carefully clean skin with alcohol.
5. Do not allow the needle to touch anything prior to insertion.
6. Carefully insert the needles at the points.
7. Rotate the needle to and fro to stimulate the acupuncture point.
8. If using electrical stimulation, attach electrodes to needles.
9. If using moxa (specially prepared balls of mugwort burned on the ends of acupuncture needles) place a protective shield of aluminum foil under and around the needle to protect the skin from loose and falling ash. If the heat becomes uncomfortable, remove moxa. If moxa is used incorrectly, redness or a heat blister may appear on the skin.
10. Remove needles by carefully grasping the handle and pulling in the direction the needle was inserted, usually perpendicular to the skin. Gloves may be worn to help protect from disease transfer.
11. Using a cotton ball dipped in alcohol, each point may be dabbed immediately after removal of the needle to help prevent infection.
12. Carefully dispose of needles in a protective container or sterilize for future use.

BL54 - Zhi Bian – Gives strength to the lumbar region.
Location: On the buttock, three cun lateral to the midline, at the level of the fourth sacral foramen.
Moxa: 3 cones.
Needling depth: 1.5 – 2 cun.
Method: Perpendicular.

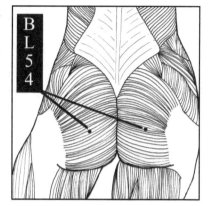

BL67 - Zhi Yin - Used to address difficult labor and retention of placenta.
Location: 0.1 cun posterior to the corner of the nail on the lateral side of the little toe on both feet.
Moxa: 3 cones.
Needling Depth: 1 fen.
Method: Perpendicular.

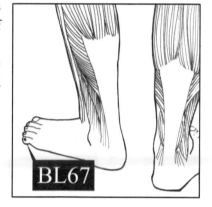

GB21 - Jian Jing - Promotes oxytocin. Expels retained placenta.
Location: Halfway between the spine at C7 and the outer edge of the shoulder.
Moxa: 3-5 cones.
Needling Depth: 3 - 5 fen.
Method: Perpendicular

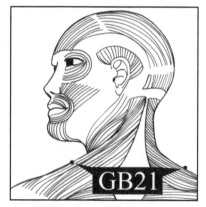

311

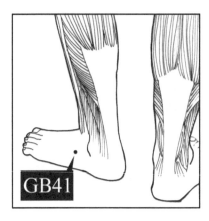

GB41 - Zu Lin Qi - Used for breast pain and swelling, irregular menses.
Location: On the top of the foot, in the depression between the fourth and fifth metatarsals on both feet.
Moxa: 3 cones.
Needling depth: 3 fen.
Method: Perpendicular

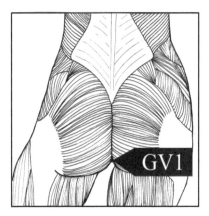

GV1 - Chang Qiang - Used to regulate the menstrual periods.
Location: Midway between the anus and the tip of the coccyx.
Moxa: 3 cones.
Needling depth: 1 fen.
Method: Perpendicular

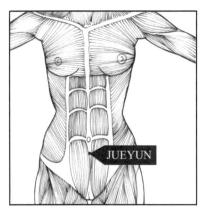

Jueyun - Terminating Pregnancy Point - Used to interrupt pregnancy and induce labor.
Location: 2 cun and 3 fen below the umbilicus.
Moxa: 7 cones.
Needling depth: 2 – 5 fen.
Method: perpendicular.

KI1 - Yong Quan – Moves excess qi downward.
Location: One third of the way between the webs of the toes and the heel of the foot, between the second and third metatarsal bones.
Moxa: 3 cones.
Needling depth: 3 - 5 fen.
Method: Perpendicular

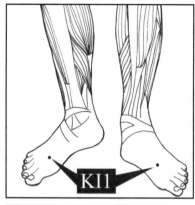

KI3 - Tai Xi - Used for irregular menses.
Location: At the midpoint between the prominence of the medial malleolus and Achilles' tendon on both ankles.
Moxa: 3 cones.
Needling depth: 3 – 5 fen.
Method: Perpendicular

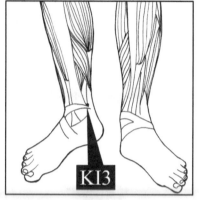

KI6 – Zhanohai - Used for amenorrhea and uterine prolapse.
Location: One cun below the medial malleolus at the junction of the red and white skin.
Moxa: 3 cones.
Needling depth: 3 - 5 fen.
Method: Perpendicular

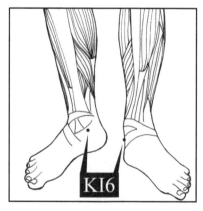

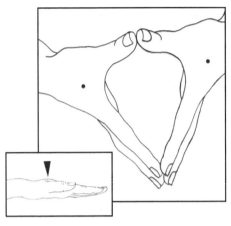

LI4 - He Gu - Used for inducing labor, amenorrhea, and retention of a dead fetus.

Location: At the summit of the hill formed when the thumb and index finger are pressed together.

Moxa: 3 cones.

Needling Depth: 3 - 8 fen.

Method: Perpendicular

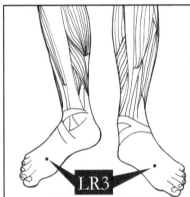

LR3 – Tai Chong – Used to regulate menstruation.

Location: Top of the foot, 2 cun towards the body from the webbing between the big toe and second toe.

Moxa: 3 – 7 cones.

Needling Depth: 5 fen – 1 cun.

Method: Perpendicular

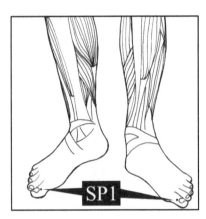

SP1 - Yin Bai - Used in combination with SP 6 for irregular menstruation.

Location: On the medial side of the big toe, .01 cun from the corner of the nail bed.

Moxa: 3 cones

Needling depth: 1 fen.

Method: Perpendicular

SP2 - Da Du – Used for constipation and abdominal distention.
Location: On the medial big toe, in the depression distal to the metatarsophalangeal joint, at dorsal plantar junction.
Moxa: 3 cones.
Needling depth: 2 fen.
Method: Perpendicular

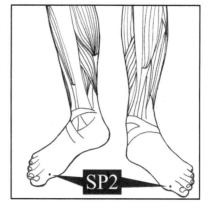

SP4 - Gong Sun - Used for irregular menstruation, vomiting, abdominal pain, diarrhea, and endometriosis.
Location: On the medial foot, in the depression distal to the base of the first metatarsal bone.
Moxa: 3 cones.
Needling depth: 4 - 8 fen.
Method: Perpendicular

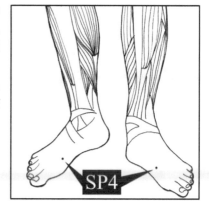

SP6 - San Yin Jiao - Used for amenorrhea, retained placenta, and expelling a dead fetus.
Location: On the medial leg, 3 cun superior to the medial malleolus, on the posterior border of the tibia.
Moxa: 3 cones.
Needling Depth: 1 - 3 fen.
Method: Perpendicular

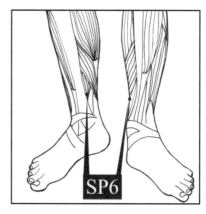

315

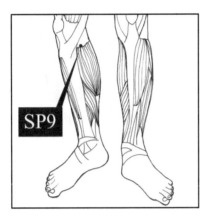

SP9 - Yin Ling Quan – Used for irregular menstruation.
Location: Inside of the leg in the depression at the meeting of the posterior tibia and the gastocnemius muscle on both legs.
Moxa: 3 cones.
Needling depth: 5 - 8 fen.
Method: Perpendicular

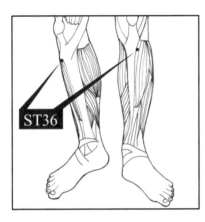

ST36 - Zu San Li – Nourishes blood circulation and used for reproductive system disorder - a special command point for the abdomen.
Location: With the knee flexed, 3 cun below the patella and one cun lateral to the tibia's anterior crest.
Moxa: 3 cones.
Needling depth: 1.5 cun.
Method: Perpendicular.

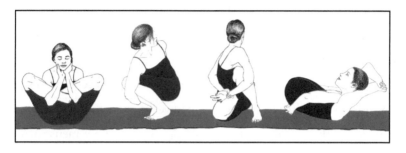

Give the order positively and firmly, telling the organ just what you wish it to perform, repeating the command sharply several times. A tapping or mild slapping of the part, or the part of the body over the affected part, will act to attract the attention of the cell group just as does the tapping of a man on the shoulder cause him to stop, turn around and listen to what you have to say...Irregular menstruation may be regulated, and normal habits acquired in just a few months by marking the proper date on the calendar and then each day giving oneself a gentle treatment along the lines, above mentioned, telling the cell groups controlling the function that it is now so many days before the expected time and that you wish them to get ready and do their work, and that when the time arrives everything will be normal. As you near the time, call the [cell] group's attention that the time is growing shorter and that it must attend to its business. Do not give the commands in a trifling manner but as if you really mean them — and you must mean them — and they will be obeyed. We have seen many cases of irregular menstruation relieved in this way in from one to three months. This may sound ridiculous to you, but all we can say is try it for yourself.

-Yogi Ramacharaka in *Hatha Yoga*, 1904

317

Yoga has a long history in the Indus Valley civilization spanning back to 3000 BC. The word yoga stems from the Sanskrit root yuj, meaning union. Yoga is a system of healing based on practices that encourage the union of the body, mind, emotions, and intellect. Yoga, as a religious practice, does not accept the use of posture for abortifacient purposes. However, women practicing yoga have found that certain postures can help to bring about menstruation, and that eliminating certain postures can assist a woman in getting pregnant.[493] Some postures in yoga can constrict internal pelvic organs, and may interfere with fallopian tube transport of the ovum or the ability of the uterus to provide a nurturing environment for the fertilized egg.[494]

Words to the Wise: The following yoga postures are advanced postures and require flexibility established through regular practice. The woman should be realistic in her assessment of her body and its limitations, listen to her body, and choose a qualified yoga teacher. Yoga instructors will adjust for medical conditions that may make certain postures problematic and will help to modify poses to work for the individual. Contraindications for yoga are high or low blood pressure, headache, diarrhea, insomnia, and back injury.

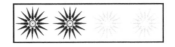

318

Nidraasana

\NEE-drah-AHS-anna\

Nidraasana is especially demanding of hip and sacroiliac flexibility. To test if the flexibility to attempt this posture is present, a woman can lie on her back and bring her legs up to her chest. Then, she can attempt to bring her arms between her knees and with 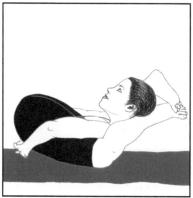 her elbows press her knees to the floor on either side her chest.

Benefits: Massages abdominal organs, energetically awakens spine, and benefits the immune system, thyroid, and parathyroid gland.

Nidraasana Step by Step:

Lie down on your back in relaxation.

Exhale. Bring legs up to chest.

Inhale. Bring left leg behind shoulder. Secure left foot behind neck. Bring right leg behind shoulder. Secure right foot over left. Crossing ankles.

Exhale. Clasp hands behind hips.

Remain in posture for five breaths.

Gently release to lie again on your back in relaxation.

Nidraasana Props:

Wall: Rest buttocks on the wall first to get a feel for the pose.

319

Marichiasana D

\mar-ee-chee-AHS-anna\

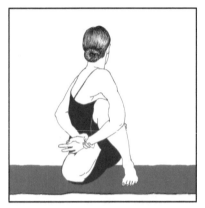

Marichiasana D is considered by many to be the most difficult twisting posture in yoga.

Benefits: Massages abdominal organs, places direct pressure on uterus, stretches spine, and stimulates the brain.

Contraindications: High or low blood pressure, migraine, diarrhea, headache, and insomnia.

Marichiasana D Step by step:

> While sitting, bring right foot into half lotus, centering the heel of your right foot just above your pubic bone. Bend the left knee and put the left foot on the floor, with the heel as close to the left sitting bone as possible. Press the inner left foot actively into the floor. Grounding the left foot will help you lengthen and rotate your spine.

> Exhale. Rotate your torso to the left, sweeping your right arm around the leg and notch the left shin in the crook of the right elbow.

> Inhale. Bring the back of the right hand to the outside of the right hip.

320

Exhale. Complete the twist by swinging your left arm around the back and clasping the left wrist in your right hand. Rotate your head in the same direction as your torso.

Stay in the pose for 30 seconds to one minute. Then release with an exhalation, reverse the legs and twist to the right for an equal amount of time.

Marichiasana D Props:

Wall: Set up the pose with your back approximately one foot away from the wall. Use your hands to press against the wall and push your torso up and forward.

Strap: Have a strap ready to use if your hands do not touch behind your back.

Bolster: Sit on a thick blanket or bolster to help keep your spine straight and pelvis forward.

Garbhasana

\garb HA-AHS-anna\

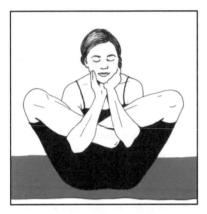

Garbhasana is called the 'Child of the Womb,' as it is thought to resemble a fetus's position in the womb.

Benefits: Massages blood supply and stretches spine.

Garbhasana Step by Step:

Inhale. In a sitting position, bring your feet into full lotus. Right foot first. Lift your knees and balance on your sitting bones.

Exhale. Weave your right hand and arm palm down through the triangle space formed by your right calf, your right thigh, and your left ankle. When your elbow passes through, bend your arm palm up.

Inhale. Repeat on left side.

Exhale. Bring your hands to your ears and balance. Look at your nose. Hold for five breaths.

Garbhaasana Props:

Clothing: Wear shorts and sleeveless tops.

Lubrication: Use water to lubricate arms and legs.

Pasasana

Pasasana means snare. The arms loop around the legs to trap them.

Benefits: Stimulates abdominal organs, stretches ankles, thighs, groin, and spine. Improves digestion.

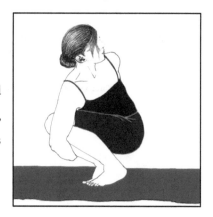

Pasasana Step by Step:

Exhale. Squat with feet together and knees together.

Inhale. Twist, rotating the navel and the ribs to the right.

Exhale. Deepen the twist, bending your left elbow and reaching with the left shoulder with the goal of getting your left armpit to the outside of the right knee.

Inhale. Straighten, rotate, and wrap the left forearm around the front of the shins and reach for the left hip. Stretch your right arm behind you and clasp the left hand. Rotate your head in the same direction as the twist.

Hold this posture for several breaths.

With an exhale, release hands and the twist returning to a squat. Slowly lift the sitting bones up to the sky for a relaxing pause in a standing forward bend.

Repeat on the left side.

Pasasana Props:

Wall: Attempting this posture next to a wall will allow one to use the wall for support and get a feel for the posture.

Bolster: For those who have difficulty squatting, a rolled blanket or small sandbag under the heels is advised.

Strap: A strap can be used to help inch the hands closer together into a full clasp.

Nauli kriya, when practiced intensively several times a day, may assist in bringing on an overdue menstruation. Nauli (meaning ocean wave) is best learned in several stages over several weeks, so one can learn how to isolate the central, left and right side of the abdomen. Benefits: Nauli removes toxins, eliminates constipation, destroys diseases, and strengthens the liver, kidneys, and pancreas.

Stage I: Uddiyana Bandha (practice at least for one week before proceeding).

Stand with legs one foot apart. Lower the chin. Forcefully exhale through the mouth to completely empty the lungs. Allow the relaxed abdominal muscles to draw up and back towards the spine. Hold for several seconds. Relax the sides of the 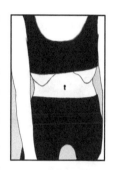 chest, then relax the neck and the chin to inhale without gasping. Repeat several times, exercising and strengthening the muscles used in nauli kriya.

Stage II. Madhyama Nauli (practice for several days, before proceeding).

After doing Uddiyana Bandha (Stage I), allow the center of the abdomen to relax by contracting the left and right side of the abdomen. When performed correctly, all the muscles of the abdomen will be in the center of the abdomen in a 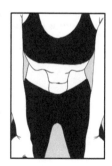 vertical line. Hold for as long as you can comfortably.

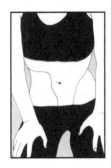

Stage III: Vama Nauli and Dakshina Nauli (practice for one week before proceeding).

Bend slightly to the right side. While contracting the right side of the abdomen, leave the left side free (Vama Nauli). Hold the contraction for as long as you can with comfort. Then while bending slightly towards the left side, contract the left side of the abdomen, leaving the right side free (Dakshina Nauli). Hold for as long as you comfortably can.

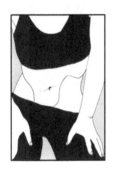

Stage IV: Madhyama Nauli (Advanced) (Practice up to 8 times a day).

In Stage IV (Madhyama Nauli) slowly bring the centerline of the muscles to the right side of the abdomen and then back to the left side in a circular way. Practice this movement several times and then reverse the movement, going from the left side to the right side. Practice this movement several times focusing on slowly moving the muscles in a circular motion. In this final stage of Nauli, the muscles of the abdomen will appear to churn like a wave.

326

Massage

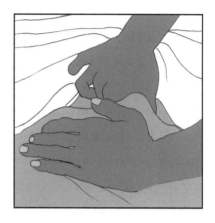

...frequently is massage used for the purpose of producing abortion. Among some of our own Indians, the Piutes among others, many of the natives of Australia, the inhabitants of the Sierra Leone, and of the interior of Africa, the Loango Negros, and others, produce abortion, either by firmly kneading and rubbing the abdomen with the hands, or pounding and working it with their fists. Many do it for criminal purposes, others because they dread the often fatal labor with half-breed children. This is a somewhat remarkable circumstance, but true among our own Indians upon the Pacific Coast and in the interior, in Australia, and in India, that labor following intercourse with whites is always tedious and dangerous, frequently ending in the death of both mother and child. Hence they produce abortion in preference to undergoing this ordeal. In India and in Africa, abortion is often produced when the mother is suckling one infant and finds herself pregnant with another.

-George Julius Engelmann in *Labor Among Primitive Peoples, 1883*

Massage, as a method of abortion, has a long history all over the world. Abdominal massage abortion is still practiced by traditional folk medicine practitioners in Burma, Thailand, Malaysia, the Philippines, and Indonesia.[495] The oldest sculpture believed to show an abortion is in Angkor Wat, Cambodia and has been dated to 1150 AD; it shows a pregnant woman receiving a massage with an implement on the lower abdomen. In Taiwan, prior to westernization, massage abortion was used to terminate all pregnancies until a woman was in her late thirties, when her husband ended his active participation in hunting and war activities.[496]

In modern Cambodia, massage abortion is practiced in the second trimester. The woman receiving the massage lies on her back on a mat and resting her feet on the mat brings her knees up to relax her stomach muscles as much as possible. The traditional birth attendant uses one hand to steady the uterus, while pressing as hard as possible with the fingers of the other hand, or possibly the bare heel of her foot, or sometimes the pestle from the mortar used to grind rice[497]

In North America, the Pima Native Americans were documented as using massage, pressure and a heated stone on the lower abdomen to cause abortion.[498] The White Mountain Apache were known to use a stick, a rock, or manual pressure applied to the fundus of the uterus to cause abortion.[499] The Zuni Native American female healers were known to grasp the uterus thorough the abdominal wall and use twisting and squeezing massage to detach the fetal connections.[500]

The Opata Native Americans had a method of combining herbs and massage that they believed to be infallible. First, the woman would be given rosemary and ocean artemisia (a plant related to mugwort). Then, on her back, her lower abdomen would be kneaded until cramping pains were brought on. Then, the woman would turn and take a position on her hands and knees. She would be shaken back and forth by her hips with all the healers' strength. If this was unsuccessful the first time, it was repeated.[501]

Words to the Wise: It is estimated that 300,000 massage abortions are performed annually in Thailand alone.[502] The majority of massage abortions do not have serious complications. However, women can die from internal bleeding resulting from massage abortion. Women who have bleeding or clotting disorders should not use massage abortion. Women who seek care at medical facilities after massage abortion often present symptoms similar to appendicitis: abdominal rigidity, a low fever, and rebound tenderness.[503]

Massage abortion is usually used after the uterus is able to be felt above the pubic bone (second trimester), but can be used in early pregnancy, too. Just as in other abortion techniques, the later the procedure is attempted the more difficult.[504] Generally, massage abortion is considered "a very painful procedure," [505] where the uterus is bruised by extreme pressure. It is easier to have assistance with massage; however women can utilize the self massage techniques of leaning on a stick, or laying on a rock to try to achieve the desired amount of pressure.

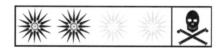

Massage Abortion: Step by Step

1. To help moderate pain, a pain medication may be used 30 minutes prior to procedure. Acetaminophen is preferred as it is less likely to thin the blood than aspirin.

2. The woman having the massage may choose to combine massage with herbs, acupuncture, yoga, or hydrotherapy. Smooth rocks for massage may be heated to 120 - 140°F. Woman should empty bladder prior to massage.

3. The woman lies down on a hard surface with a rolled towel under her lower back, exposing the lower belly. Apply a lotion or oil to allow for less friction. In early pregnancy, the uterus is located through external or bimanual palpitation by an assistant. Then the uterus is pulled and pressed with the fingers to dislodge the fetal mass. Then the area above the fetal mass is massaged with a rotating motion using the palm or thumb.

4. In the second trimester, the fingers of one hand reach into the lower abdomen just above the pubic bone to attempt to steady and fix the uterus. The other hand is placed just above the pubic bone where it deeply massages the abdomen in a circular clockwise direction. In the case of self massage, you may use your fist or elbow to go deeper with pressure-or use a smooth rock as a massage tool. If the massage becomes too painful, stop and wait a few days before reattempting.

5. More rarely bimanual massage (see Appendix C) is used to isolate pressure on the uterus. Occasionally, in the first trimester, the heel of a foot is used to raise the uterus by

pressing the heel into the area below the vagina. When bimanual massage is used, fingers placed against the cervix should be very clean and nails trimmed, and should be held still while the opposite hand applies pressure and force in circular movements.

6. Massaging in the uterine area is thought to sometimes bring up past psychological issues, as some believe trauma is stored in muscle memory.[506]

7. Massage is ceased when vaginal bleeding is observed.

Hyperthermia

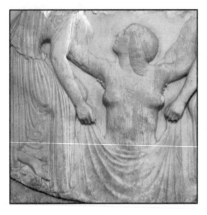

...hot baths... can cause miscarriage, especially during the first three months.

-Mary Lillian Reed in
The Mothercraft Manual, 1921

Hyperthermia is a condition where the body absorbs more heat than it can dissipate. The intentional use of heated objects to induce abortion by increasing the temperature and circulation of the uterus is widespread. In Southeast Asia, women are documented as having utilized a heated coconut shell or rock to lie on top of to cause an abortion.[507] Native Americans of the Yurok tribe are documented as using hot stones on the abdomen to induce abortion.[508] The Buin, of Papua New Guinea, are also documented as using hot stones to induce abortion.[509] The women of the Manja of the Congo were known to induce abortion by making a big fire and, when the earth was very hot, cleaning away the fireplace, sprinkling the earth with water and lying down on their belly on the hot steaming earth.[510]

The use of hot water baths has a long history as an abortive method. Soranus (AD 98-138) prescribed an abortive regime that included hot baths, which became more protracted as the woman moved into the second trimester of pregnancy.[511] In the mid 1800's, a method of hydrotherapy abortion inserted a tube into the vagina in order to apply a warm, strong, pressured douche to the uterus twice a day. The method was said to be "safe and efficient."[512] More commonly in the 20th century was 'a steaming hot bath and a bottle of gin,' a folk recipe for inducing miscarriage which has been handed down via word of mouth to the modern-day.[513]

In early pregnancy if a woman gets an infection and develops a fever increasing her body temperature, often a spontaneous abortion will occur, as increased heat has a teratogenic effect on the growing fetus.[514] Hyperthermia was found to be a teratogenic element in many animals, and its link as a teratogen in humans was researched and confirmed.[515]

Modern studies have found an association between hot tub use and increased risk of miscarriage in early pregnancy.[516] The miscarriage rate has been shown to increase with frequent use of a hot tub in the first four weeks of pregnancy and with higher water temperature settings. Studies on elevated body temperature during pregnancy have shown a possible association between extended hot tub, bath, or sauna use during the first six weeks of pregnancy and neural tube defects and miscarriage.[517] If the temperature of the body is raised to above 101° F (38°C) for an extended period of time during the first six weeks of pregnancy there is a significantly higher chance of miscarriage or neural tube defects in the baby if the pregnancy is brought to term.[518]

Words to the Wise: Monitor body temperature with a thermometer. Women with diabetes, anemia, tuberculosis, cancer, weakness, heart

333

disease, or kidney damage should not use hyperthermia as a method of abortion. Utilizing hyperthermia as a means to induce abortion entails the rare risk of scalds, burns, brain damage, and death. Body temperatures above 104°F (40°C) are life threatening. At 106°F (41°C), brain damage begins. Hyperthermia during pregnancy is a known teratogen.

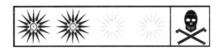

Hyperthermia Abortion Step by Step

To utilize hot baths as part of an abortive regime, set the temperature of the bath to 102° F (39°C) and stay in the bath for at least twenty minutes. The longer a woman can keep her body temperature elevated above 102°F, the greater the chance that the woman will have an abortion.

Rocks may be heated for 30 minutes in a 140°F (60°C) oven or water bath. Place a towel on the belly, and place the wet hot rock on the towel, allowing the heat to slowly penetrate into the abdomen. Laying on the hot rock intensifies the temperature. If using the rock for direct massage on the skin, apply olive oil (and perhaps a drop of essential oil) to the rock before massage.

The first experiences of connecting will often be visceral in nature – the parents-to-be will know, feel, or sense something which will be difficult to put into words. They will know that it is true in their bodies, not in their heads. After validation of that experience they will start to see colors or hear words.
-Teresa Robertson, Birth Intuitive

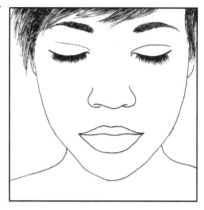

Throughout human history, nearly all traditional societies recognized the existence of entities that had no defined physical form. One of Ayurveda's medicinal branches, Bhuta-vidya, was devoted to the science of spiritual entities. In traditional Chinese medicine, the word kuei (meaning discarnate spirit) makes up part of the secondary name of at least seventeen acupuncture points, evidence of the ancient belief that spirit is vitality important in the health and well-being of the body. Ancient Egypt had one of the most advanced medical systems of the time, however spells and incantations are believed to have been regarded by the ancient Egyptians as an even more effective means of medical treatment on all levels of being: mind, body, and spirit.

Ancient cultures are documented as having believed to have utilized psychic abortion to induce miscarriage, however the anthropological record is limited. The Hopi Native Americans are documented to have believed that a girl could induce abortion by simply wishing it to happen.[519] Magic being used to induce abortion is

335

hinted at by a female Native American Aleut, however when questioned further she refused to speak about it and would talk only about basketry.[520] The Native American Mohave claimed that witchcraft could be used to affect abortion without the woman's knowledge.[521] George Devereux's extensive anthropological work on abortion indicates that many cultures utilized religious or magical rituals in combination with herbs and massage to induce abortion.[522]

Modern accounts of psychically induced abortion come from women who believe to have self-induced psychically and through psychics who have assisted in the process of inducing abortion.

One woman writes:

> I didn't want a baby, in fact didn't want kids at all, but I wanted *him*. I didn't want to be pregnant. I didn't want to have to be dealing with it! What kind of idiot was I, getting pregnant again?

> And I could feel him there, hanging out with me, sweet and mine. I agonized over it.

> But one night I decided, and the next evening I walked to a nearby park and sat on a swing. I thought, *Hey, baby. You need to go. I can't have you now, but you can come back later. I can't care for you properly. You have to go.* And I felt such sadness, but also a certain amount of pragmatism in myself. I thought, *There's more than one door, baby. If you have to come in now, pick another woman. Or if you wait, maybe I can be your mother later. But not now. Please, not now, can't you see?*

> And it was sunset, and cars drove by, and I sat on the swing. By and by I couldn't feel him any more. I walked slowly home. When I got there I started bleeding.[523]

Teresa Robertson, a Colorado certified nurse midwife and intuitive counselor who offers pre and post abortion support services, comments on how she became involved in communicating with unborn souls. "During 1987-89 I worked as a clinical coordinator for a first trimester abortion clinic...Many times while witnessing an abortion procedure I would see or sense the spirit of the baby leave. Early on I had a patient who needed a repeat procedure. What she shared with me dramatically changed my counseling approach. She said, in reference to her pregnancy, 'I just wasn't ready to let go of that part of me and my boyfriend last week.' From that moment on, I have talked to women who are considering terminating a pregnancy or who are miscarrying, advising them to connect with the baby and say goodbye in order to let go."[524]

Linda Baker, a spiritual hypnotherapist and author of the book *Soul Contracts*, says, "Doing this work requires a commitment to self-healing. It is an inner process that requires courage and the willingness to explore individual truth. It is a spiritual process and not a simple command ordering a spirit to leave. This work does not encourage abortion but allows for the spiritual healing of mother, father, and child when abortion is the choice."

Baker comments on the nature of healing in psychic abortion: "Some of the most common lessons the spirit comes to teach are about healing the inner child, bringing forth creative energy, empowering the self, healing relationship issues, and healing from past abortions or miscarriages so that the mother can choose a healthy new pregnancy. Sometimes the connection between a mother and the unborn child runs very deep and the mother experiences feelings of great love and pain in letting go. It is important to remember that pain does not equal bad or wrong. A right choice in our lives can bring

337

feelings of loss, grief, or loneliness and still be the right choice for us. For example, leaving an abusive relationship can bring up many painful feelings and still be the best, healthy choice for us. The love Spirit has for us is so strong that I have had many clients burst into tears when they feel this energy. It is the purest love they have ever felt. There is no demand, no desire, and no judgment. There is only love...By its very nature spirit is alive, so we cannot deny a spirit life...Through the work I have done, I have felt and seen how loving and forgiving spirit is, how connected the physical and spiritual world are, and how important it is for each one of us to honor our highest truth."[525]

Sometimes a request to the child/soul to depart will not be honored. "I have been asked if there are times when a spirit does not agree to leave. The answer is yes, this does happen. But the only times I have experienced this were with women who had issues of not taking their own power and wanting to please others. I remember three cases like this when the spirit came forth with, *"No, I will not go."* Each of these times the client had to work on being willing to make the right choice for herself. Each time the woman took the power, and demanded, *"This is my body. The timing is not right and you must leave."* The spirit was joyful and expressed this was the lesson to be learned."[526]

Abortion due to psychic or spiritual communication has been attributed by women to be successful as a self-induced abortion technique; however the assistance of a psychic healer may be necessary, at least initially. Robertson comments: "I strongly believe and promote this field of my work to be self empowering -- so that someone doesn't need to seek someone outside of themselves to talk to their unborn baby. However, it really depends on who is trying to connect, why, and what state of being they are in. Also, if someone has a block or a blind spot it is often useful to have an outside person to help clear any blockages and facilitate the communication. We are raised and immersed within a culture which tells us that only 'crazy' or special 'psychic' people are able to hear or see spirits. Clients often use the time I spend with them to learn how they receive this information -- do they know it, sense it, smell it, hear it or see it?"[527]

Learning to intuit psychic information may prove difficult for many women who have no experience, yet once it is experienced, the knowledge gained may be profound. Robertson writes, "It is a knowing within their heart, body, soul that this is true. They may sense a vibration of hot or cold, may hear the baby's voice or (if already pregnant) the baby may start to move or kick. It is a visceral, gut knowing and understanding. They will know from every cell of who they are that this is true."[528]

A woman, who may wish to abort, must set her own desires aside and open herself to the ever-changing movement of the mind and the spirit. Through the process of psychic communication, a woman may gain a new understanding or may even change her mind regarding her pregnancy. Robertson writes, "It is essential to approach this experience and techniques with an open mind and heart and with the quality of neutrality. It is also important to communicate in a manner which is cooperative and in which negotiations are made on both sides so that each party (parent and unborn child) is fully seen and heard. Trying to connect in order to orchestrate or engineer a

339

certain fertility or birthing experience will evoke more of controlling energy and probably will not prove to be satisfying."[529]

For more information on birth intuitives, councelors, and psychics, see Resources.

Words to the Wise: The effectiveness of psychic abortion is unknown. There may never be scientific proof of the phenomenon of psychic abortion, and it may never be completely understood. Western science largely discounts psychic abortion as magical thinking.

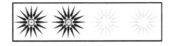

Part IV - Post-Abortion Care

Following an abortion, it would be considered normal to experience one or more of the following:

- Spotting or continuous bleeding for up to three weeks.
- No bleeding at all.
- Passing black, brown or red clots.
- Cramping (abdominal or back pain).*
- Emotional changes (unusually happy or depressed) for no apparent reason.
- Discharge from the nipples.
- Disappearance of most pregnancy symptoms in less than one week.

*Deeply massage downward toward the public bone to help pass clots. A hot water bottle also usually helps.

Anytime a woman has an abortion, whether induced or spontaneous, there are risks of infection and hemorrhage, both of which can potentially lead to death. For this reason, women should carefully monitor temperature, blood pressure, and blood loss throughout an abortion and seek medical care if needed.

Do	Do Not
• Monitor blood loss: Soaking three thick pads in three hours or less requires medical attention.	• Do not put anything in the vagina for three weeks after your abortion. No tampons, no vaginal intercourse, no douching, no baths, and no swimming.
• Monitor temperature: Take your temperature two times a day for one full week following abortion. Fever of 101°F (38°C) or more indicates infection and requires immediate medical attention or to start immediately on an antibiotic regime. (See Appendix I).	• No aspirin, no marijuana, and no alcohol for three weeks. These act as blood thinners and muscle relaxants and may cause heavier bleeding.
• Rest often, especially during the first 48 hours, give your body time to begin healing.	• No strenuous activity for three weeks. This includes exercise, heavy lifting, walking long distances, or being on the feet for long stretches of time, which may cause heavier bleeding and cramping.
• Use pads and change them often to keep harmful bacteria at bay.	
• Utilize uterine massage to help your uterus contract and slow bleeding. Push down as hard as you can above your pubic bone. (Passing clots while doing uterine massage is normal).	• Do not stimulate your breasts for two weeks following abortion. Breast stimulation encourages lactation.
	• Do not sit in a bathtub to bathe. Instead, take showers or stand in the tub to wash down for three weeks after the abortion.
• Plan to use contraceptives immediately after your abortion, as it is possible to become pregnant before your next period.	• Do not stop antibiotics until the entire course is finished.

Always Seek Immediate Emergency Medical Care, if you have:

- Heavy persistent bleeding - soaking through 3 or more thick pads in 3 hours or less.
- Fever of 101° F (38°C) or more.
- A sudden drop in blood pressure (which can indicate systemic infection).
- Unusually severe cramping where you cannot stand up.

Call a doctor, if you have:

- Longer than expected bleeding (over three weeks).
- Severe or increased pain.
- Chills or fainting.
- Unusual or foul smelling vaginal discharge.
- Continued pregnancy symptoms after two weeks.
- Severe psychological distress.
- No menstruation for more than three months.

Words to the Wise: A woman should never hesitate to seek emergency medical care, if needed. A woman may say, "I am having a miscarriage," as the treatment and care is the same whether a women has complications arising from an induced abortion or a spontaneous miscarriage. Refusing to tell medical professionals that you are having a miscarriage or abortion may delay treatment or lead to a misdiagnosis. Miscarriages are very common in pregnancy. Up to 31% of all conceptions end in spontaneous miscarriage; a majority of miscarriages happen during the first trimester, and up to 20% of miscarriages occur in the second trimester.[530]

Although Roe v. Wade made clinical abortion services legal throughout the United States, self-induced abortion may be viewed as fetal homicide in states that have made recent changes in fetal homicide laws. In nearly all states in the United States, a person outside of the medical system who assists a woman in an abortion may be arrested for practicing medicine without a license or homicide, but a woman's right to terminate her pregnancy by herself without assistance has been repeatedly upheld in case law. However, endangering one's own life or the life of others may trump doctor/patient confidentiality, and the doctor may feel required to report a woman's actions to authorities under threat of loss of medical license. If a woman chooses to tell medical personnel about how she attempted or succeeded at a self-induced abortion, she may be arrested. Recently, women in the United States have spent time in jail for self-induced abortion and even unintentional abortion related to drug abuse.[531]

The terrorist tactics of the Pro-Life movement should never deter a woman from seeking emergency medical care if she is in need. Remove any abortifacient medications from the vagina before submitting to a vaginal exam, and exercise the Fifth Amendment to refuse to answer questions which may incriminate.

344

Homeopathic Post-Abortion Care

Several homeopathic remedies can be used to help finalize and balance after an abortion. Utilizing the assistance of a trained homeopathic doctor is advised. Multiple factors will influence the choice of the correct remedy, and a trained homeopath's assistance in determining the correct remedy for your particular situation is essential.

Some homeopathic remedies traditionally utilized to care for an aborting woman:

Arsenicum Album – For feelings of guilt after an abortion.

Cinchona Officinalis- Weakness due to excessive bleeding.*

Kalium Carbonicum - General weakness after an abortion.

Natrium Muriaticum - For feelings of guilt after an abortion.

Nux Vomica – Hemorrhage* after abortion with intestinal griping.

Pyrogenium 200 - Fever.*

Sabina – Genital soreness and/or low back pain.

Sepia – Suspected placental adhesion.*

Trillium Pend. Q – Prolonged bleeding.*

*In the event of hemorrhage or fever, a woman should not rely solely on homeopathy remedies, but should always secure immediate emergency medical services.

Traditional Chinese Medicine (TCM) Post-Abortion Care

In Chinese medicine, it is believed that any abortion, whether spontaneous or induced, may cause either blood statis in the uterus or kidney damage. The kidney in Chinese medicine not only refers to the organ but also to the body's regulation of hormones, fluid balance, and energy metabolism. TCM individual herbs or formulas are used to help bring the body back into balance. Acupuncture can also be utilized after an abortion to help balance energy levels. Contracting the services of a TCM doctor is vital if you are interested in TCM herbal formulas or acupuncture to balance the systems of the body after an abortion, as these treatments are formulated for the unique characteristics and sensitivities of the individual. TCM formulas are available by prescription or sometimes through Asian specialty stores or online (see Resources). A formula for menstrual irregularities are taken in the week prior to menstruation but not during menstruation, as it is believed that taking the formula during menstruation weakens the woman's health. The herbs and formulas used in TCM to treat menstrual irregularities are numerous, some of the more common ones are:

TCM individual herbs:

Tao Ren (Semen Persicae), made from the pit of a peach fruit, quickens the blood and dispels stasis, breaks the blood and moves it downward, moistens the intestines and frees the flow of the stool.

Hong Hua (Flos Carthami), made from the safflower, a common spice, quickens the blood and frees the flow of menstruation, dispels stasis, disperses concretions, and stops pain. Hong Hua and Tao Ren are sometimes combined to increase their power to quicken the blood and free the flow of menstruation.

Dang Gui Wei (Extremitias Radicis Angelicae Sinensis) supplements and quickens the blood, regulates menstruation and stops pain.

Da Huang (Radix Et Rhizoma Rhei - uncooked) quickens the blood, cools the blood, and transforms stasis.

Ji Xue Teng (Caulis Spatholobi) quickens and nourishes the blood, stops bleeding and regulates menstruation.

TCM formulas:

Tao Hong Siwu Tang –
A TCM formula for when there is irregular menstrual cycle, premenstrual stress, abdominal pain and distention just before or during menstruation and sometimes excessive bleeding.

You Gui Wan - Tonify Yang
A TCM formula for when a period is irregular, cycles are long, or amenorrhea with small amount of light red or light brown watery flow with no clots. There may be a low sexual drive and/or a low body basal temperature after ovulation when it should go up. There may be

347

ringing in the ears, dizziness, dark circles under the eyes, and aversion to cold with cold extremities and possibly a cold lower abdomen.

Si Wu Tang- Nourish Blood

A TCM formula for when abortion occurred with heavy bleeding, and now experiencing irregular light period, no period, or heavy period with dark purple blood, clots, and painful cramping. Pain is better when clots discharge. There may be dizziness or blurred vision.

Gui Zhi Fu Ling Wan (also known as Keishibukuryogan)

A traditional Chinese medicine formula containing equal parts of five herbs: Gui Zhi, Fu Ling, Bai Shao Yao, Mu Dan Pi, and Tao Ren. Used for a few days, according to the directions on the packaging, this TCM is used when women have suffered psychological and physical effects of abortion, which may present as abdominal pain, irregular bleeding, acne or skin conditions associated with menstruation, anxiety, depression, and/or uncontrolled crying. Also used for uterine fibroids and ovarian cysts.

Liang Di Tang – Clear Deficient Heat

This is a TCM formula for menstruation that lasts too long. Women may be irritable with fluctuating emotions of anger and sadness. Menstruation may be accompanied by fever. Blood is very thick red with a relatively small amount.

abortifacient - an agent or action that induces abortion.

abortion – the removal or expulsion of a fetus from the uterus, may be spontaneous or induced.

acupuncture – an ancient healing practice of inserting fine needles through the skin at specific points to alter the energetic balance of the body.

adjuvant – agents that have few or limited effects when given by themselves, however when given in combination with another agent enhances its effects on the body.

albaspidin – an anthelmintic compound extracted from aspidium.

albuminuria - the presence of albumin (a protein) in the urine which can be an indicator of kidney damage.

alexiteric – a substance used against poisoning or snake venom.

alion – a bitter yellow compound isolated from the aloe plant, which is used as a laxative to induce intestinal peristalsis.

alkaloid - any of numerous organic substances (such as nicotine or caffeine) containing nitrogen that are often physiologically active.

allopathic – a term coined by Hahnemann, founder of homeopathy, to describe the western medical system that aims to combat disease by the use of surgery or drugs which directly counter a patient's symptoms.

aloe emodin – a variety of purgative anthraquinone resin found in socotrine, barbados, and zanzibar aloes.

alterative – traditionally known as blood cleansers, these herbs gradually restore proper function in the body, thus improving health and increasing vitality.

alternate - growing at alternating intervals on either side of the stem.

amenorrhea - abnormal absence or suppression of menstruation.

annual – a plant that completes a life cycle in one year or growing cycle.

anodyne – a substance, usually applied externally, that serves to ease pain.

anthelmintic – kills and/or expels parasitic worms especially of the intestine.

anthraquinone - *a* substance found in many plants, lichens, fungi, and insects which serves as a basic skeleton for their pigments, used in the commercial manufacture of pigments and dyes and used medicinally as a laxative.

antibacterial – a substance or process used against bacteria.

anticancer – a substance or process used against cancer.

anticoagulant - a substance that interferes in coagulation of the blood.

anti-inflammatory – a substance that relieves inflammation.

antimetabolite - a substance with structure similar enough to a metabolite to function for normal biochemical reactions, however different enough to inhibit the function of cells. antimetabolites are used in cancer treatment, antibiotics, and sulfa drugs.

antimicrobial – a substance that destroys or inhibits the growth of pathogenic microbes, like bacteria, fungi, and viruses.

antioxidant – a substance that can slow or prevent the oxidation of other molecules.

antimutagenic – a substance that reduces the rate of mutation of cells.

antiparalytic – a substance that helps to relieve the symptoms of paralysis.

antiperiodic – a substance used to prevent the periodic return of illness, such as malaria.

antiprogesterone – a substance which interferes in the production of progesterone, a steroid produced by the adrenal glands, brain, and during early pregnancy the corpus luteum and then later the placenta. Progesterone, which has a symbiotic relationship with estrogen, helps the uterus provide a fertile bed for the fetus and is integral to fetal development.

antiseptic – a substance applied externally to the body to help prevent infection.

antispasmodic – a substance that suppresses the contraction of smooth muscles, like the uterus, stomach, intestine, and urinary bladder.

antitussive – a substance used to suppress coughing, used with dry coughs.

antiviral – a substance used to treat viral infections.

aphrodisiac – a substance believed to excite sexual desire.

apiol – an organic chemical compound found in parsley seeds and essential oil.

aromatic – a volatile substance which has a detectible smell or odor.

astringent – a substance used externally to shrink mucous membranes.

bacteria – single celled microorganisms that do not have a nucleus, and are vital in the recycling of nutrients in the ecosystem. some bacteria are beneficial to humans, while some are pathogenic.

balsamic - an aromatic and usually oily and resinous substance flowing from several trees and shrubs, containing benzoic or cinnamic acid, and used as a base for botanical medicines.

biannual – a plant which completes two growing cycles in one year.

biennial – a plant which blooms every two years.

bilirubinuria - excretion of bilirubin in the urine, which can be a sign of liver damage.

bilirubin - a reddish yellow pigment that occurs naturally in bile and blood and causes jaundice if accumulated in excess.

buccal – the area between the cheek and the gum.

bulb - a modified underground stem with scales containing stored food for the undeveloped shoots at its center.

calyx - a flower's protective outer covering, composed of green segments called sepias.

cambium – a layer of tissue from which the plant grows found inside the roots and stems of a plant.

carcinogen – a substance which promotes or facilitates the growth of cancerous cells.

cardiotonic – a substance which has a favorable effect on the tone of the heart muscle.

carminative – a substance that induces the expulsion of gas from the stomach or intestines so as to relieve flatulence or abdominal pain or distension.

carposide – a glycoside found in papaya.

catamenia – monthly menstrual cycle.

cathartic – a substance which causes vigorous evacuation of the intestines.

cephalic – a substance used to treat diseases of the head: headaches, sinus congestion, etc.

cervical os – in the center of the cervix the hole which leads to the uterus.

cervical os mucous plug – a mucilaginous substance that plugs the os and serves as a barrier against bacteria entering the uterus during pregnancy.

cervix – the lower narrow portion of the uterus which joins to the vagina.

chorionic villi – little fingers of tissue that sprout from the chorion to give the maximum contact of surface area to the maternal blood. eventually some of the chorionic villi anchor into the uterine wall and form into a placenta.

Chorionic Gonadotropin (CG) - hormone secreted around the second week of pregnancy by the chorionic villi, hormone detected in urine in pregnancy tests.

cocarcinogen – a substance that alone causes no growth of cancer, but when combined with a carcinogenic substance can increase the carcinogenic action of that substance.

colostrum – yellowish colored milk secreted for a few days after birth and characterized by high protein and antibody content.

combinations - two or more herbs taken at the same time.

conception – union of egg and sperm.

contact dermatitis - inflammation of the skin caused by skin contact with a substance.

contraception – intentional prevention of conception through the use of various devices: drugs, condoms, sexual practices, or surgical procedures.

contraindications - something that makes a particular treatment or procedure inadvisable.

corm - an underground stem, differing from a bulb only in that it has no scales.

corolla - outer envelope of a flower, petals.

corpus luteum - a yellowish mass of progesterone-secreting endocrine tissue in the ovary that forms immediately after ovulation. The corpus luteum regresses rather quickly if the ovum is not fertilized, but if the ovum is fertilized the corpus luteum persists throughout the pregnancy.

courses – *Middle English* meaning monthly menstrual cycle.

decoction – a medicinal substance made by simmering herbs in water to extract the medicinal components.

demulcent – a substance used to sooth and relieve pain in inflamed tissues.

desaspidin – a substance derived from a Finnish fern, used to help eliminate tapeworm.

diaphoretic – a substance capable of inducing sweating.

digestant - a substance aids in digestion.

diuretic - a substance that increases the excretion of urine.

dysmenorrhea - painful menstruation.

ecbolic - a substance that tends to increase uterine contractions and that can be used to facilitate delivery.

ectopic pregnancy – implantation and gestation of the ovum elsewhere than in the uterus, most often in a fallopian tube, but can also be in the peritoneal cavity.

embryo – the developing human from the time of implantation until the eighth week after conception.

emesis – vomiting.

emetic – a substance that induces vomiting.

emmenagogue - an agent that promotes menstruation.

endometriosis - the presence and growth of functioning endometrial tissue in places other than the uterus.

endometrium - the mucous membrane lining the uterus.

essential oil – the concentrated oil obtained from a plant by steam distillation, expression, or extraction.

estrogen – a group of steroids, named after the female estrous cycle, which function as the primary female sex hormone. All estrogens in the body are produced from androgens through the actions of enzymes.

estrogen-dependent tumors- cancerous growths that increase abnormal cell division when estrogen is present.

estrogenic – a substance that promotes ovulation.

expectorant – a substance that promotes the discharge or expulsion of mucus from the respiratory tract.

extra amniotically – not within the amniotic fluid, usually indicates the space between the gestational sac and the uterine wall

fallopian tube - muscular hollow arms of the uterus that seek out, find, and usher the ovum to the uterus.

fetus – the developing human in the womb is considered a fetus once the basic structure is attainted, usually 48 days after conception until birth.

fibroid cyst – benign tumors that can grow usually in the uterus or breasts.

filicin - an active principle obtained from male fern.

flavaspidic acid – an acid obtained from male fern that inhibits bilirubin.

follicle cells - a protective group of spherical cells surrounding and containing the egg at ovulation.

formulation - the process of preparing and combining certain substances to create a final medicinal product.

fumigant - a substance used in fumigation.

fumigation - to smoke, vapor, or gas certain substances and direct the resulting smoke, steam, or aromatic toward the body for medicinal purposes.

Fungus – a member of the kingdom fungi, characteristically lacking chlorophyll including: molds, rusts, mildews, mushrooms, and yeasts.

gastritis - inflammation of the stomach.

glycoside – a series of molecules where a sugar is bound another molecule.

In plants, glycosides are often stored for use. If the glycoside is needed by the plant, the glycosides are brought in contact with water and an enzyme, the sugar is broken off, and the chemical is thus made available to use. Many plant glycosides are used in medicine.

habitual abortion - spontaneous abortion occurring in three pregnancies in a row.

hemorrhage – bleeding in excess, can lead to fatalities. In abortion, hemorrhage is roughly defined as soaking through 3 or more thick pads in 3 hours or less. Hemorrhage may be caused by inadequate evacuation of tissue from the uterus, and requires MVA and immediate medical attention.

hepatic - remedy specifically for diseases of the liver.

hepatotoxic – causing injury to the liver.

hydragogue – causing the discharge of watery fluid.

hypotensive - reduces blood pressure.

HRT - hormone replacement therapy.

hydrotherapy - the therapeutic use of water.

hyper catharsis – excessive purging of the intestines.

hypotensive - causing low blood pressure or a lowering of blood pressure.

implantation - the process of attachment of the embryo to the wall of the uterus.

infusion - the soaking in water of an herb or combination of herbs in order to extract its soluble constituents or principles.

intra amniotic – the space within the gestational sac, which is filled with amniotic fluid.

irritant - tending to produce inflammation.

isobarbalion – an aloin compound found in the aloe plant.

IUD - a device (as a spiral of plastic and copper) inserted and left in the uterus as a contraceptive device.

ketone – chemical compound that contains a carbonyl group.

lactagogue – a substance that promotes the secretion of milk.

LMP – the first day of the last menstrual period before conception.

lanceolate - narrow leaves, tapering at each end.

laxative – a substance used to loosen or relax the bowels and used to relieve constipation.

leukorrhea – thick, whitish vaginal discharge.

lithotriptic – a substance that dissolves or helps to release kidney and gall bladder stones.

lunar cycle – the 27.32 day orbit of the moon around the earth.

malaise – a feeling of lack of health often indicative of the onset of an illness.

massage - manipulation of tissues (as by rubbing, stroking, kneading, or tapping) with the hand or an instrument for therapeutic purposes.

menorrhagia - abnormally heavy menstrual flow.

menstruation - monthly cyclic release of the uterine lining and the blood of the-uterine vessels in women.

metabolite - a product of metabolism.

miscarriage - spontaneous expulsion of a human fetus before it is viable, also known as spontaneous abortion.

molar pregnancy – A rare form of disorder in pregnancy, occurring in approx.1 in 1500 pregnancies, possibly caused by a nutritional deficiency, where a hydratiform mole forms in the uterus. Uterus may seem larger than normal for gestational age. There is no placenta, there may be bleeding into the vagina. hCG levels increase often rapidly. Molar pregnancies usually end in spontaneous miscarriage where grape like forms are passed.

Montgomery's tubercles or glands – small bumps in the outer areola of the nipple that appear during pregnancy.

moon cycle – the 27.32 day orbit of the moon around the earth.

multiparous – having had two or more children.

myrosin - an enzyme occurring in various plants of the mustard family (Cruciferae) that hydrolyzes the glucoside sinigrin.

nervine – a substance used to soothe nervous excitement.

nocturnal - occurring at night.

oleanolic acid - a triterpenoid found in many plants (raisins, olive leaves, etc.), and found to have many healing properties.

oleoresin - a natural plant product containing chiefly essential oil and resin.

opposite - leaves that grow in pairs on either side of a stem.

ovary - one of the pair of female reproductive glands that produce ovum (eggs), in a flower, the part of the pistil containing the ovules (eggs).

ovum - a mature egg that is ready for fertilization.

oxytocin - a hormone secreted by the pituitary gland that stimulates the contraction of uterine muscle and the secretion of milk.

panicles – a branched of cluster of flowers, where each branch is a raceme.

parturient – in labor, about to give birth.

parturifacient – a substance given to induce or stimulate labor. **pelvic inflammatory disease (PID)** - infection of the female reproductive tract that can happen after abortion if microorganisms enter the uterus, characterized by lower abdominal pain, an abnormal vaginal discharge, and fever, and is a leading cause of infertility in women.

perennial – a plant that lives for more than two years.

pessary - a suppository placed in the vagina for therapeutic purposes.

petrochemical – chemical products made from raw materials of petroleum or other hydrocarbon origin.

philocarpine – a drug used for glaucoma, has a constricting effect on the pupils and helps to reduce eye pressure.

phototoxity - a phenomenon where the skin becomes abnormally sensitive to sunlight after the ingestion of certain plant substances.

phototoxic – a substance which becomes toxic when exposed to light, thus increasing the susceptibility of the skin to sunburn and blisters if exposed to sunlight.

photochemical alterations – abnormal changes in cells due to exposure to ultraviolet radiation from the sun.

placenta – the vascular organ attached to the uterine wall, designed to filter and transform the nutrients in the mothers blood to the fetus without direct contact between the fetal and maternal blood supply.

plaster - a medicated or protective dressing that consists of a film spread with a usually medicated substance.

PMS - premenstrual syndrome, a varying constellation of symptoms manifested by some women prior to menstruation that may include emotional instability, insomnia, fatigue, headache, edema, and abdominal pain.

PMS acne – skin eruptions manifesting prior to menstruation.

post-coital interceptor – a substance taken soon after unprotected intercourse to prevent fertilization or implantation.

poultice - a soft usually heated and sometimes medicated mass spread on cloth and applied to inflammations to supply moist warmth, relieve pain, or act as a counterirritant.

progesterone - a female steroid secreted by the corpus luteum to prepare the endometrium for implantation and later by the placenta during pregnancy to prevent rejection of the developing embryo or fetus.

progestin - a naturally occurring or synthetic progestational steroid.

prolactin - a protein hormone produced in the pituitary gland that induces and maintains breast milk.

prostaglandins – lipid compounds found in nearly all tissues and organs which perform a variety of hormone like actions on the cells from which they are synthesized: blood pressure regulation regulates intraocular pressure, control hormone regulation, and influences cell growth).

protozoa – single celled organism.

purgative – a substance given to induce bowel evacuation.

pyrogenic – a substance given to produce fever.

raceme – a type of flower cluster, where the flowers spiral along an unbranched stem as the flower spike grows.

resin - a secretion of coniferous trees, used in incense.

rhizome - horizontal underground stem of a plant.

RU486 – the designation given to mifepristone during clinical trials.

rubefacient - a substance used on the skin to increase circulation, **sea sponge** – natural sponge harvested from the ocean.

sedative – a substance used to calm the nerves.

simple – herbal medicine having only one ingredient.

sitz bath - a bath in which the hips and buttocks are immersed in hot water for the therapeutic effect of moist heat.

solstice – when the tip of the earth's axis is at its furthest and closest points to the sun, occurs twice a year.

sori – small dots of spores on the underside of fern fronds.

spermicide - a preparation or substance inserted in the vagina used to kill sperm.

stigma - apex of the pistil of a flower, on which pollen is deposited at pollination.

stimulant – a substance that temporary produces an increase in the activity of an organism or any of its parts.

stomachic – a substance taken to tone the stomach, increasing digestion and appetite.

stupor - a condition of greatly dulled senses.

styptic – a substance that stops bleeding when applied to a wound.

succulent - a plant that has fleshy leaves that store water.

sudorific – a substance that induces sweating.

suppository - a solid medicinal molded cylinder inserted into a body cavity, where it melts releasing the medicinal components.

syrup - a thick sticky sweet liquid.

teratogen - a substance that can cause the development of abnormal structures in the embryo or fetus.

thujone - a fragrant oily ketone that can affect the GABA receptors in the brain.

tincture - a medicinal preparation made by soaking herbs in alcohol and straining off the resulting liquid.

tampon - a wad of absorbent material introduced into the vagina to absorb menstrual blood.

tonic - a substance that increases body tone

toxicity - the quality, state, or relative degree of being poisonous.

umbilical cord - a cord arising from the navel that connects the fetus with the placenta.

umbel - flat or curved top flower cluster.

urticaria – hives, the raised edematous red patch of skin or mucous membrane characteristic of hives.

uterine contractor – a substance taken to induce or increase uterine contractions.

vasoconstrictor – a substance taken to constrict the muscular walls of the blood vessels.

vermifuge- a substance taken to expel or destroy intestinal worms.

vesicant - an agent that induces blistering.

volatile oil - rapidly evaporating oil, an essential oil.

whorls - an arrangement of 3 or more parts (leaves, petals) radiating from a central point.

yoga - a system of physical postures, breathing techniques, and meditation to promote bodily or mental control and well-being, and ultimately enlightenment.

Appendixes

Appendix A: Rh Factor and RhoGam®

Accompanying each blood type is a positive or negative symbol which indicates the Rh factor. The Rh factor is an antigen (a substance that evokes an immune response) present in red blood cells. If one has a positive Rh factor (Rh+), one has the antigen. If one has a negative Rh factor (Rh-), one does not have the antigen. The majority of women are Rh+. Only around 15% of Caucasian women, 6% of African American women, and 1% of Native American and Asian women, are Rh-. If a woman who is Rh- becomes pregnant with a baby that is Rh+, and if a minute amount of the Rh+ fetal blood mixes into the Rh- blood of the woman (due to intrauterine trauma, premature separation of the placenta, placenta previa, abortion, or miscarriage), a dangerous action called isoimmunization will occur.

In isoimmunization, the mother's immune system reacts to the fetal Rh+ blood as a foreign invader and produces antibodies that attack the Rh+ cells of the fetus. This can lead to severe anemia in the unborn child and increasingly intense reactions if the mother has future Rh+ fetuses. In the future, if the Rh- woman becomes pregnant again with an Rh+ fetus, her immune system remembers how to create the antibodies against Rh+ blood because of prior sensitization. Immediately, the woman's immune system will react, attacking the blood of the fetus, treating the blood of the fetus as an invading virus. With constant attacks on its blood cells, the fetus can become severely anemic.

359

If an Rh- mother delivers an Rh+ baby, a hospital will administer a shot of RhoGam® to ensure that future Rh+ fetuses are protected. A RhoGam® shot makes a woman's system believe it has already produced the antibody, and that it is not necessary to continue to produce more antibodies. With the RhoGam® shot, the Rh- woman does not produce any antibodies herself, and in the future, her immune system will have no memory of how to produce the antibodies. It is standard hospital procedure to give RhoGam® to every Rh- woman after an abortion. For women who are less than 12 weeks pregnant, a Mini-Gam (300 mg dose) is usually given, and for women over 12 weeks pregnancy, a full RhoGam® (1 ml dose) is given.

If an Rh- woman has conducted a self-induced abortion, to protect against isoimmunization, she should get a RhoGam® shot. The RhoGam® shot must be given within 72 hours of the beginning of bleeding. Planned Parenthood will generally give RhoGam® shots to women who are current patients. Women without health care providers should go to an emergency room or an immediate care center and describe their condition as having just had a miscarriage and say they are Rh- and need to receive RhoGam®.

Appendix B: Breastfeeding and Abortion

A woman who is breastfeeding faces a set of unique conditions that affect her situation if she becomes pregnant and desires an abortion:

❖ Obtaining a sonogram will help to determine accurate gestational age. A lactating woman may be unaware that she has become pregnant, as her menstruation may not resume for six to eighteen months after the birth of her child.

❖ Breastfeeding immediately before taking medicine and/or 'pumping and dumping' her breast milk will help prevent contaminated breast milk being passed to her baby.

  ➢ Abortion methods, listed in this book, which may be most suitable for women who are breastfeeding include:

  Clinical Abortion
  Medical Abortion
  Menstrual Extraction
  Herbal: Papaya Latex Pessary
  Homeopathy
  Acupuncture
  Hyperthermia
  Yoga

Appendix C: Bimanual Pelvic Examination

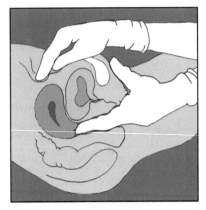

Selecting the most appropriate method of abortion depends on an accurate assessment of gestational age. Bimanual pelvic examination is one tool that is often combined with ultrasound, pregnancy test, and detailed menstrual history to determine the gestational age of the fetus.

1. The woman to be examined should empty her bladder prior to the exam. The person performing the exam should have washed hands in latex gloves. A water based sexual lubricant can be used on the tip of the index and middle fingers of one hand (usually the left) to ease insertion.

2. Woman lies down on back, knees up, and feet placed comfortably 2 - 3 (1 m) feet apart.

3. The woman's assistant gently inserts the two lubricated fingers of one hand, seeking the nose like form of the cervix.

4. Holding her fingers steady under the cervix, the assistant uses her other hand to press down on the lower abdomen with firm pressure.

5. The assistant estimates position and the size of the uterus. The majority of women have a uterus that is anteverted, its long axis points forwards, and the cervix points backwards.

One in five women has a uterus that is retroverted or retroflexed; in this case, determining the size of the uterus can be difficult.

In a pregnant anteverted uterus:

- Five weeks LMP feels like a small unripe pear.
- Six weeks LMP feels like a small juice orange.
- Eight weeks LMP feels like a large navel orange.
- Twelve weeks LMP feels like a grapefruit.
- After 12 weeks LMP, the top of the uterus begins to be palpable above the pubic bone.

6. With hands in the same position the woman's assistant sweeps the fingers gently to one side to feel the ovaries, which feel like almonds. Sweep to both sides. The woman will probably feel a twinge when the fingers pass gently over each ovary. The fallopian tubes are not usually felt; but if they are felt, they should be soft and about the thickness of a pencil. If they are hard or enlarged or if she experiences pain, this may indicate an ectopic pregnancy. Although rare, it is possible to rupture an ectopic pregnancy during a bimanual exam. Ectopic pregnancies are characterized by doubled over pain. Immediate medical attention must be sought if an ectopic pregnancy is suspected. A ruptured ectopic pregnancy can cause hemorrhaging.

Moving the Uterus Hurts the Woman (Get Medical Help)	• may have ectopic pregnancy • may have an infection • may have endometriosis
Lumps or Growths Felt on the Womb (Get Medical Help)	• may have fibroids • may have cancer
Uterus Feels Smaller Than Expected	• pregnancy may not be as advanced as previously thought • may have a missed abortion, where the fetus ceased to grow during gestation • may have an ectopic pregnancy (get medical help)
Uterus Feels Larger than Expected	• pregnancy may be more advanced than expected • may have multiple pregnancy • may have uterine fibroids • may have a molar pregnancy
Unable to feel the Womb	• strong abdominal muscles • large amount of belly fat • uterus may be retroverted • try moving hand around lower belly and pressing down in different places

Appendix D: Speculum Insertion

1. Speculum should be cleaned and sterilized. The vagina is not a sterile environment, but sterilization will help prevent infection and disease transfer.

2. With the speculum locked in a closed position, separate the labia with one hand while gently inserting speculum with the other hand. Often it is more comfortable if the speculum is rotated at about 45 degrees (so the blades are oblique-not horizontal). Once past the entrance of the vagina, the speculum can be rotated to its normal horizontal position.

3. Once the speculum is inserted, slowly open the speculum and lock it into an open position.

4. Shining a flashlight into a hand mirror (held with the other hand between the legs, will allow the woman to see if the cervix is visible.

5. Often times the cervix will not present on the first attempt. As the speculum is inserted it may help to point the speculum to the left or right and then bring the point of the speculum to the center. This action will often free a cervix that is resting on the top of the speculum.

Appendix E: Cervical Dilation

The benefits of adequate cervical dilation are reduced time to complete abortion, more effective evacuation of the embryo, and reduced bleeding. Menstrual extraction often requires cervical dilation. For a woman who has never given birth vaginally, careful dilation will usually be required, especially after 9 weeks LMP. For a multiparous woman, often cervical dilation is not needed until 12 weeks LMP, as the cervical os will naturally be more open.

In menstrual extraction, often an entire set of plastic cannulas, ranging in size from 3 mm – 14 mm, are sterilized so they may be used as dilators, if needed. Then, the smallest cannulas are introduced into the os to gradually accustom the cervix to a greater diameter, up to required cannula size based on a woman's estimated gestational age. (The required size of cannula in millimeters roughly corresponds to the number of weeks LMP.[532])

Menstrual extraction has been shown to be most effective at around seven weeks gestation. At seven weeks LMP, the required cannula diameter is approximately 7 mm. Often the cervical os will accommodate the 7 mm cannula, if the os has been gradually opened with the smaller cannulas before the insertion of the 7 mm.

For menstrual extractions over seven weeks gestation, more gradual dilation with cannulas and pharmaceutical cervical dilation may be necessary. According to the World Health Organization, menstrual extraction can be used up through 12 weeks LMP, and possibly up to 15 weeks LMP, if the necessary sized cannulas can be secured and adequate cervical dilation achieved, and one study indicated that manual vacuum aspiration is as effective as electric vacuum aspiration between 14 to 18 weeks of pregnancy.[533]

Pharmaceutical Cervical Dilation

Taking care to adequately dilate the cervix prior to any second trimester abortion procedure will help to reduce side effects and increase the effectiveness of the procedure. Natural prostaglandins in the body cause the cervix to dilate; synthetic prostaglandins can also be used to artificially cause the cervix to dilate.

Misoprostol has been found to be effective in dilating the cervix in early second trimester abortion.[534] Misoprostol, a synthetic prostaglandin at a single dose of 600 mcg, taken orally or placed in the back of the vagina for six hours, results in approximately 6 to 8 mm of cervical dilation. Mifepristone 200 mg administered 48 hours before the misoprostol resulted in approximately 12.5 mm dilation in weeks 12 – 20 LMP.[535]

Misoprostol and mifepristone are contraindicated for some women (see Medical Abortion).

Ear Acupuncture Cervical Dilation

Auriculotherapy is an ancient form of acupuncture that focuses treatment on the ears. Auricular acupuncture has been found to be useful for dilating the cervix in preparation for an abortion.[536] The use of ear acupuncture to dilate the cervix has been shown to be upwards of 98% effective in studies on women who were unable to undergo a vacuum aspiration abortion because of the tightness of the cervical os. When the points are correctly located and needled, increased circulation and a feeling of warmth was often felt.[537]

Words to the Wise: The cartilage of the ear is not fed by blood vessels, thus any injury or infection may be difficult to treat and may result in serious consequences. Some auriculotherapy schools use cartilage penetration and some forbid it. When cartilage penetration is used, the treatment time is greatly reduced. To open the cervix, when cartilage penetration is used, the time that the needles are retained is about 5 minutes, whereas when only skin penetration is used, the time that the needles are retained is about thirty minutes to one hour.

Step by Step Ear Acupuncture

1. Woman must be calm with no anxiety. If anxiety exists during the application, the possibility exists that the ear acupuncture point stimulation may cause unconsciousness.[538]

2. Clean the ear well before acupuncturing.

3. Do not allow the needle to touch anything before insertion. Insert size ½ in. or size 23 - 30 needles which have been properly cleaned and sterilized into acupuncture points.

4. Rotate the needle to and fro to stimulate the point.

5. Needles inserted into the ear cartilage are retained for approximately five minutes. Needles inserted into the skin are retained for approximately thirty minutes to one hour.

6. Needles are removed once the desired relaxation of the cervical os is achieved. The woman usually feels warmth and a relaxation sensation when the stimulation of the points takes effect.

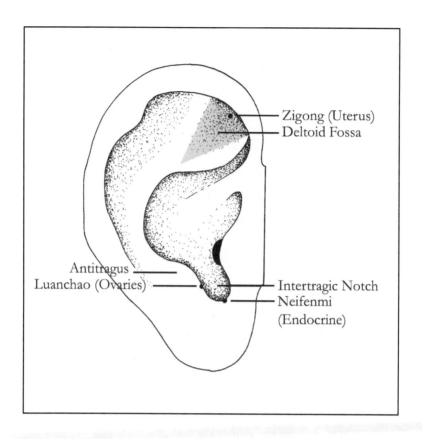

Zigong (Uterus) — Deltoid Fossa

Antitragus
Luanchao (Ovaries) —

Intertragic Notch
Neifenmi
(Endocrine)

Zigong (Uterus) - On the triangular area known as the deltoid fossa, with the point of the triangle pointing to the back of the head, the uterus point is found at the midpoint of the line between the two points of the triangle towards the front of the head.

Luanchao (Ovaries) - On the lower part of the medial wall of the antitragus.

Neifenmi (Endocrine) - This point is found at the very bottom of the intertragic notch.

Appendix F: Sterilizing Equipment

Sterilization is any process that effectively kills or eliminates microorganisms. All instruments that enter an already sterile part of the body or which may touch an instrument that will enter a sterile part of the body must be sterilized prior to use. The importance of sterilizing equipment to prevent infection cannot be stressed enough. Infection of the uterus can lead to maternal sepsis and death. The vagina is not sterile, but the interior of the uterus is.

Wet Heat Sterilization

- Pressure Cooker

    A pressure cooker, when used correctly, is like an autoclave. Thirty minutes in a pressure cooker or autoclave at 250°F (120°C) at twenty pounds per square inch (psi) will inactivate all fungi, bacteria, viruses, and spores. Nitrile gloves (not latex) may be sterilized in a pressure cooker.

- Boiling and Hydrogen Peroxide Soak

    Boiling instruments in tap water for thirty minutes will kill most bacteria and viruses; however this will not kill spores. Hydrogen peroxide is a chemical sterilizing agent which kills spores and may be used in addition to boiling in water. However, hydrogen peroxide must not be boiled, as the vapors from boiling hydrogen peroxide can explode.

    If you are concerned about spore based diseases, like anthrax, after boiling instruments in water for thirty minutes,

370

carefully transfer instruments with sterile tools to a hydrogen peroxide soak for one hour. Hydrogen peroxide is relatively non toxic, widely available, and leaves no chemical residue.

Dry Heat Sterilization

- Kitchen Oven

    Dry heat sterilization is less effective in killing microorganisms than wet heat sterilization, however it can be used to sterilize towels and equipment that would be difficult to sterilize in a pressure cooker or by boiling. All items to be baked should first be washed with detergent, rinsed, and dried. To keep each item sterile until use, wrap each item with aluminum foil or paper tied with cotton twine. Items should be placed in the oven carefully, so they do not touch the oven elements. A shallow pan of water may be placed on the lower rack to prevent scorching. Nitrile gloves may be sterilized at 250°F (120°C), however nitrile deteriorates at higher temperatures.

    Baking Temperature/Time Duration
    338°F (170°C) /60 minutes
    320°F (160°C)/ 120 minutes
    302°F (150°C)/ 150 minutes
    284°F (140°C)/ 6 hours
    250°F (120°C)/12 hours (overnight)

Appendix G: Herbal Preparation Methods and Dosages

If gathering herbs, always check to see if the plant is endangered and always use an accurate field guide. Many poisonous species exist that look similar, so one must always be certain of identification. Do not gather near roads or areas which may have toxic residues in the soil. When purchasing, one must search for the purest, best quality organic herbs. Then, test dried herbs by placing a small amount in the palm of the hand and rubbing with a finger. The odor of fresh herb is aromatic and resinous. The odor of old herb may be stale or moldy. Return herbs that are old or stale, as the medicinal qualities will be lost. Use pure water and glass or enamel containers for preparing and holding medicinal preparations. As with all medicines, keep herbal medicines in a safe place that children cannot access.

Infusions

Infusions are used to extract the medicinal components of delicate plant parts, such as flowers and leaves. To make an infusion: heat water to boiling, add to herb, cover, and steep. Make fresh infusions every time, do not store for later use.

Decoctions

Decoctions are used to extract the medicinal components of tougher plant parts, such as roots and branches. To make a decoction: Heat the water in the pan to the point that steam begins to rise off the surface. Add the ground herb, cover, and turn heat down to simmer without boiling. Decoctions stored in the refrigerator will keep 1-2 days. A quarter cup of brandy, gin, or vodka can be added to one pint of decoction to prolong shelf life.

Tinctures

Tinctures are used to extract the alcohol soluble components of herbs. Tinctures have a long shelf life; they are easy to carry around; and due to their concentrated potency, a smaller quantity is necessary in any dosage. Fresh botanicals are usually used for tinctures. A 190 proof grain alcohol is used for fresh botanical tinctures, otherwise the botanicals will rot. The ratio of weight of herb to ounces of alcohol is given first in the recipe. Place the sealed tincture out of direct sunlight for at least two weeks. Add distilled water to dilute to the correct percentage of alcohol in the final tincture, if required. Tinctures kept in a cool dry place are good for several years.

Herb-Based Vaginal Pessaries

Wool is the preferred absorbent. Wool absorbs fluids, yet remains warm and releases the absorbed fluid readily to the surrounding tissue. For comparison, cotton is cooling and does not readily release fluids it has absorbed.

Use a piece of tooth floss to tie a knot around the piece of clean wool. The piece of wool should be approximately a fingers width when compressed. A plastic tampon applicator may be used for insertion: Wad the wool into the end of the tampon case with the string hanging down (through the case) like a tampon. Insert the wool pessary high in the vagina. Then, the barrel and plunger of a syringe, an infant medicine dropper, or a kitchen baster may be used to apply herbal liquid infusions or decoctions into the vagina onto the absorbent wool to saturate the wool pessary. Pessaries may be worn for up to 6 hours before replacing. Pessaries should be removed if irritation develops.

Vaginal Fumigation

Vaginal fumigation is an ancient process where the fume from steaming or burning herbal medicines is introduced into the vagina.[539] "Fumigation was used to fill the uterus with vapor, open its orifice, and sometimes even rectify its position."[540] Hippocrates wrote about steam fumigation of garlic to treat cancer of the uterus. Fumigation with sulfur was prescribed by Dioscorides to expel the fetus. In Ethiopian medicine, sulfur was used to facilitate the contraction of the uterus (as an oxytocic agent) during childbirth by direct fumigation of the female organ with sulfur vapor. In ancient India, the smoke from burning neem wood (neem is a known contraceptive) was introduced into the vagina via fumigation for contraceptive purposes.

To steam fumigate: Drill a hole through the center of the seat of a stool or chair. Affix a small plastic funnel or tube on the hole on top 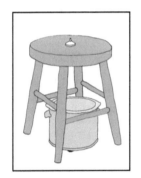 of the chair. Prepare a decoction. Place the decoction, ideally in an electric crock pot under the chair on the floor. Test the temperature of the steam first, and then using a blanket as a tent, carefully sit on the chair, so that the steam will enter the vagina via the funnel. Check the cervix occasionally and note its changes in softness and amount of relaxation. A cervix in its normal state feels like a nose while a cervix beginning to dilate has softness comparable to lips. (Note: Once the temperature has come down to a comfortable level, the herbal decoction may be used following the fumigation as a douche, sitz bath, and pessary.)

Essential Oils

Essential oils are highly concentrated and are not to be used internally. Essential oils if used externally should be used with extreme caution. Essential oils do not need to touch the skin to enter the body. Essential oils inhaled or in contact with mucosa can be rapidly absorbed into the body. The entry of the essential oil via the blood/brain barrier is very rapid, with plasma concentrations reaching their peak 18 minutes after exposure.[541] Essential oils can increase, decrease, or even stop uterine contractions.[542]

Dosages

Methods and herbal dosages listed in this book are for educational purposes only. Using these dosages without consulting a physician or qualified health professional would be practicing self medication. Practicing self medication is dangerous and is not recommended. Please consult your health professional.

Each individual has unique characteristics and sensitivities that make it impossible to have a one-size-fits-all dosage. Some of the dosage adjustments a qualified herbalist might suggest follow.

The dosages in this book have been averaged from several sources and are calculated for an adult person who weighs 150 lbs. (68 kg); a person who weighs less or more would need to have the dosage adjusted to their body size. An adult who is sensitive to medications, would in addition need the starting dosage reduced by 50%.

Vegetarians and vegans are often more sensitive to herbs, especially estrogenic herbs. (Non-vegetarian consumption increases the amount of daily estrogens via animal products. Non-vegetarians

375

become accustomed to higher estrogen levels.) A vegan or vegetarian would need to have the starting dosage reduced by at least 30%.

Younger people have organs that metabolize, utilize and eliminate herbs differently than adults. Generally, younger people are more sensitive to herbal medicines. For young women between the ages of 14 - 18, the starting dosage would need to be reduced by 30%. For young women under age 14, the starting dosage would need to be reduced by 50%.

A qualified herbalist would also adjust dosage to individual plant characteristics: Different batches of herbs will have differing amounts of medicinal components. The potency of an herb will vary depending on the growing conditions, genetic variability, gathering, storage, and preparation methods. A trained herbalist would, throughout treatment, monitor a patient's individual responses to herbs and adjust dosage, as necessary.

Appendix H: Weights and Measures

Weights and Measures

1 ounce = 28.35 grams

1 fluid ounce = 29.56 ml

1 tsp. = 4.9 ml = 60 drops

1 Tbs. = 3 tsp. = ½ fl. oz. = 14.8 ml = 180 drops

½ pint = 1 cup = 16 tsp. = 48 tsp. = 8 fl. oz. = 236.6 ml

½ quart = 1 pint = 2 cups = 32 Tbs. = 106 tsp. = 16 fl. oz. = 473.2 ml

1 quart = 2 pints = 4 cups = 64 Tbs. = 212 tsp. = 32 fl. oz. = 946.4ml

Ounces of Herbs to Kitchen Measures (approximate):

l oz. powder = 3 Tbs.

 l oz. roots (cut and sifted) = ¼ cup

1 oz. leaf (cut and sifted) = 1 cup

Drams, Drachmas, Grains, and Minims

1tsp = 1 dram = 60 grains = 60 minima

1 grain = 65 mg

1 Tbs. = 3 tsp. = 3 drams = 180 grains = 180 minima

1 dram = 1 drachma

Appendix I: Antibiotics [543]

Infection of the uterus is extremely serious and life threatening but fortunately very rare (approximately 1 in 100,000 in clinical abortion). There is no recommended FDA approved dosage of antibiotics used preventatively for abortion. Using antibiotics without reason can stimulate the growth of bacteria that are resistant to antibiotics. Antibiotics can be secured before a self-induced abortion attempt or emergency medical services can be sought if a woman shows signs of infection after an abortion (See Post-Abortion Care and Resources).

Words to the Wise: Antibiotics should be used with physician oversight. Antibiotics can save lives, but can also cause negative side-effects. Some antibiotics can interfere with other prescription medications. Some antibiotics can interfere with the effectiveness of oral contraceptive pills, so other contraceptive measures should be used during and for seven days after antibiotic use. Milk, zinc, iron, or calcium taken at the same time as antibiotics can interfere with antibiotic absorption. Antibiotics can affect drugs with a narrow therapeutic index (like warfarin, digoxin, theophylline, phenytoin, etc.). Alcohol must not be consumed during treatment with metronidazole and for 48 hours after, as this may lead to an allergic reaction in some individuals. Grapefruit juice should not be consumed while taking erythromycin, as this can cause dangerous heart arythmias. Allergic reactions to antibiotics can cause anaphylactic shock and death.

Antibiotic Regimes

Antibiotics can interfere with the natural flora of the intestinal tract and disrupt body balance. Antibiotic use and disruption in beneficial intestinal flora, in scientific studies on mice, has been linked to the development of asthma and allergies.[544] To help prevent candida and other possible health problems when using antibiotics, eat foods with beneficial bacteria (like yogurt and miso) every day during the treatment and for one week following the treatment. Eating raw fruits and vegetables also helps to establish beneficial intestinal flora.

There are two antibiotic regimes for abortion. One regime is preventative, taken immediately after an abortion to help prevent an infection. The other regime is for when signs of infection are present. Different antibiotic regimes are recommended for breastfeeding and non-breastfeeding women, as certain antibiotics have been found to be detrimental to a breastfeeding infant when passed through a woman's milk.

Always carefully monitor temperature after an abortion and during antibiotic treatment.

❖ Preventative Antibiotic Regime:
  ➢ Non-Breastfeeding Woman Preventive Regime
     (take with lots of water):
     ▪ Take 100 mg doxycycline, two times a day on the day of the abortion.
  ➢ Breastfeeding Woman Preventive Regime
     (take with lots of water):
     ▪ Take 500 mg erthromycin, four times a day, for seven days.

❖ Antibiotic Regime for Symptoms of Fever and Infection:

Because the type of bacteria that is causing the infection is not known, a broad spectrum antibiotic regime is used. Continue to give the antibiotics for fever and infection until there has been no sign of fever for 48 hours. If fever is still present after 48 hours of starting antibiotics, seek immediate medical attention.

➢ Non-breastfeeding woman with signs of fever/infection:
  ▪ Take all three medicines (with lots of water):
    • 3.5 g ampicillin, all at once, one time only.
    • 100 mg doxycycline, two times a day.
    • 400 – 500 mg metronidazole, three times a day.

➢ Breastfeeding Woman with signs of fever/infection:

All of the following antibiotics are generally believed to be safe for the breastfeeding infant; however it is better to take the doses immediately after a feeding.

  ▪ Take these three medicines (with lots of water):
    • 2 g ampicillin, initial dose, then 1 g ampicillin, four times a day.
    • 80 mg gentamicin, three times a day.
    • 500 mg metronidazole, three times a day.

  ▪ OR Take these three medicines (with lots of water):
    • 500 mg ciprofloxacin, two times a day.
    • 100 mg doxycycline, two times a day.
    • 500 mg metronidazole, two times a day.

Appendix J: Contraception

A woman should research contraceptive options and use a method of choice. A woman's reproductive years on average span thirty years of her life. Each woman needs to stay informed of available contraceptive options. Some women will use every available contraceptive method.

There are many contraceptive options available to women and men. This section will not go into detail on the more common methods, as many written resources are already available on the more widely available contraceptive options: condoms, birth control pills, spermicides, etc. Instead, we will focus on the latest pharmaceutical and the alternative methods of contraception.

Emergency Contraception Pills

Emergency Contraception Pills (ECP), also known as morning after pills, are synthetic hormones or steroids taken orally in the few days after sex when a woman believes she may become pregnant. The hormones or steroids in emergency contraception disrupt the body's hormone levels and makes pregnancy less likely. Depending on where a woman is during her cycle, ECP can prevent ovulation, fertilization, or sperm transport. Around the world, ECP pills (under various brand names) are available either over-the-counter or from a pharmacist in 50 countries.

(92% effective) Mifepristone, a single dose of 100 mg, can be taken as an emergency contraception option.[545] Mifepristone is contraindicated in women who have an IUD, an ectopic pregnancy, adrenal failure, bleeding disorders, inherited porphyria, or anticoagulant or corticosteroid therapy.

(85-89% effective)[546] Levonorgestrel, also known as Plan-B, is a progestogen- only ECP. Plan-B is the only dedicated FDA approved Levonorgestrel ECP specifically marketed for emergency contraception in the United States. ECPs are available either over-the-counter or from a pharmacist without having to see a clinician in 43 countries, where more than 50 emergency contraceptive products are specifically packaged, labeled, and marketed. Progestogen-only ECPs work best the sooner they are taken after unprotected sex, but can be used up to 72 hours after unprotected intercourse.

(56% effective) Contraceptive pills may be used as ECP. With more than 60 million women worldwide on contraceptive pills, this option of emergency contraception may be more available than progestogen-only ECPs. However, the drawback to using contraceptive pills as for emergency contraception is that they are less effective than other ECP options. Birth control pills as emergency contraception can be used within 120 hours of unprotected intercourse, however the sooner the pills are taken the more effective they are. The use of contraceptive pills as ECP, can make a woman's menstruation come a few days later than usual. Women who have had a past heart attack or stroke, blood clots in the legs or lungs, or cancer of the breast, reproductive organs, or liver are not advised to use contraceptive pills as ECP. Various brands of contraceptive pills contain varying amounts of hormones.

382

To use contraceptive pills as ECP, one must take 100 mcg ethinyloestradiol and 0.5 mg levonorgestrel, to be repeated 12 hours later. It is essential to follow the latest guidelines exactly for the particular brand of pill; to find the latest guidelines, go to the online ECP web database of Princeton University, www.not-2-late.com.

Words to the Wise: Schedule your dosages of EPCs so that the second dose is taken before bed. Take anti-nausea medicine dimenhydrinate (like Dramamine™) one hour prior to the dose, if you are sensitive to nausea. If vomiting occurs within three hours of a dose, that dose should be repeated to make sure that enough hormones have entered the system to provide contraception.

Women who take ECP should watch for severe abdominal pains, chest pain or shortness of breath, severe headaches, vision problems, or severe pain or numbness in the extremities. Seek immediate medical attention if any of these problems occur.

Both men and women above the age of 18 can purchase FDA approved ECP without a prescription. If a person is under the age of 18, she or he may require a doctor or pharmacist's prescription to obtain ECP in the United States. Not all pharmacies stock ECP, so call ahead.

Alternative Contraception Options

Natural Spermicides

The following recipes are considered tried and true among midwives and natural health practitioners. They are best used in combination with a barrier method, such as a cervical cap or diaphragm. However, they can be used alone, but they will not be as effective when used alone.

Recipe 1
1 Tbs. (15 ml) 100% Aloe Vera Juice
4 drops fresh lemon juice

Recipe 2
1 tsp. Vitamin C Powder
2 Tbs. Personal Lubricant

To make a contraceptive sponge, cover a sea sponge with silk and tie with a ribbon. Mix the chosen recipe well. Dip your sponge in your spermicide or apply to a diaphragm or cervical cap and insert at least 10 minutes prior to intercourse. A small syringe, like an infant medicine syringe available at most pharmacies, can also be used to apply spermicides. Wait 8 hours after the last sexual act to remove the sponge or diaphragm, as removing earlier will remove the spermicide and not kill all the sperm. Do not leave the diaphragm or sponge in place for longer than 24 hours.

Phytoestrogen Contraception

In ancient times women are documented as using estrogenic herbs in the week following their period as a contraceptive measure. The week following the menstrual period is when a woman's natural estrogen levels are at their lowest. For women seeking naturally derived means of birth control, a possibility exists that utilizing estrogenic herbs (like pomegranate seeds) at this time of their cycle could interfere with ovulation and prevent pregnancy. No studies have been done on this contraceptive method.

To determine the correct dosage of estrogen, a woman can monitor estrogen levels while taking herbs with a body-fluid based observation lens (see Resources). The lens is a small microscope which allows a woman to see the characteristic crystallization of estrogen in a woman's saliva or vaginal fluids during ovulation. Altering the hormonal balance in the body by increasing estrogen immediately after menstruation (when estrogen is normally is at its lowest) would likely interfere in the ability of the body to ovulate normally that month.

1. First, for a month or two, a woman should observe her normal estrogen levels with the lens while utilizing non hormonal contraception like condoms.

2. When a woman can recognize the changes that occur in her saliva during her normal ovulation, she may begin taking estrogenic herbs in the week following her next period. A woman should continue using condoms or her chosen nonhormonal contraceptive

while testing and observing estrogen levels with the following method.

3. Increase the oral consumption of the estrogenic herbal substance (pomegranate seed) until the characteristic ferning indicative of estrogen is observed with the observation lens.

4. Monitor estrogen levels with the lens and adjust dosages to keep the body at observable estrogen for the six days after menstruation.

5. Continue monitoring estrogen levels throughout the entire month. If the characteristic ferning pattern reappears, ovulation would be indicated and further methods to prevent implantation would be needed if unprotected intercourse occurs around ovulation

Online Resources

❖ Abortion Support and Counseling

➢ www.YourBackline.org
Backline offers a confidential space for women and their loved ones to talk openly about pregnancy, parenting, abortion, and adoption. The Talk Line is available toll free, seven days a week. Backline takes calls from women and their loved ones all over the United States who are in the process of making decisions, or have already made decisions, about pregnancy. Backline understands that these decisions can be complex, and they support you no matter what you choose to do.
Backline Talk Line
Phone: 1.888.493.0092
Hours:
Monday - Thursday
5:00 p.m. - 10:00 p.m., Pacific Standard Time
Friday - Sunday
10:00 a.m. - 3:00 p.m., Pacific Standard Time

➢ www.AbortionConversation.com
Articles on tips for teens and parents for talking about abortion, emotional and spiritual health after abortion, and the pro-choice movement.

➢ www.Scarleteen.com
Sex Ed for the Real World
Scarleteen is the highest rated online sex education site for teens and young adults. Run by and maintained by young adult volunteers around the world, Scarleteen is built around what users ask for and takes an informal approach which teens and young adults can relate to.

➢ www.4Exhale.org
Exhale offers a free and confidential, After-Abortion Talkline that provides emotional support, resources and information. The talkline is available to women and girls who have had abortions and to their partners, friends, allies and family members. All calls are completely confidential and counselors are non-judgmental. Website has free supportive ecards to send in support of women

who have had an abortion. Spanish-speaking counselors are available every Wednesday on request. Cantonese-, Mandarin-, Vietnamese- and Tagalog-speaking counselors are available on request.

Toll-free talkline (available in the U.S.): 1.866.4 EXHALE
Toll calls outside of the U.S.: 1.510.446.7977
Monday – Friday:
5 p.m. – 10 p.m. PST
Saturday – Sunday:
12 p.m. – 10 p.m. PST

➤ www.TheAbortionProject.org
Project Voices is an online space to share your experience of abortion and read other women's stories.

❖ Adoption
   ➤ www.Adoption.com
   ➤ www.OpenAdoption.org

❖ Abortion Assistance – United States

   ➤ Overground Railroad
The Overground Railroad helps to support, transport, accommodate, and provide escorts for women to other states if they must travel between states to obtain safe and legal abortions. For information, contact National Organization for Women and Unitarian Church Ministers.
      ■ www.NOW.org - National Organization for Women
      Chapters exist across country in every state, usually in large cities.
      ■ www.UUA.org - Unitarian Universalist Association of Congregations.

   ➤ www.ProChoice.org
National Abortion Federation Hotline
Phone: 1.800.772.9100 (Mon – Sat: 9:30 am - 5:30 pm)

   ➤ www.ProChoiceResources.org
Hershey Abortion Assistance Fund – loans to women and teens.
Phone: 1.888.439.0124 (Wednesdays 5:00pm-7:00pm CST)

➢ www.WRAAP.org

Women's Reproductive Rights Assistance Project provides money to low-income women for emergency contraception and abortion. WRAAP services are provided free of charge in clinics all over the United States.
Phone: 1.323.223.7727

➢ www.CAIRProject.org

Community Abortion Information and Resources - call this 800 number to find a clinic or find money to help pay for an abortion.
Phone: 1.888.644.CAIR (1.800.644.2247)
Email: cairwa@nnaf.org

➢ www.NNAF.org

The National Network of Abortion Funds is a United States based network of local groups who help women pay for and travel to abortion services.
Phone: 1.617.524.6040
Fax: 1.617.524.6042
Email: INFO@NNAF.org

❖ Abortion Clinics

➢ AbortionClinicDirectory.com

The Abortion Clinic Directory is a directory of United States abortion clinics and information on surgical and medical abortion.

➢ GYNPages.com/ACOL/International.html
Listing of Abortion Clinics around the World

➢ ProChoice.org

The National Abortion Federation's website helps individuals find the clinics in the USA and Canada that abide by standards governing quality of care.
National Abortion Federation operates a toll free hotline at:
1.800.772.9100 in the US
1.800.424.2280 in Canada.

> MarieStopes.org.uk

Marie Stopes International is the United Kingdom's leading provider of sexual and reproductive health services. Marie Stopes also has projects around the world in over 40 countries providing safe abortion and women's health services.
Abortion Information and Appointments:
Phone (UK): 0845.300.80.90

❖ Medical Abortion –Misoprostol and mifepristone are approved for use with a prescription in the United States. Importing drugs without a prescription is illegal in the United States, however federal authorities have generally allowed the practice.[547] U.S. Customs stopped seizing mailed prescriptions from Canada in October 2006.[548] Misoprostol (Cytotec™) is reputed to be less difficult to obtain than mifepristone and is still 85-90% effective when used alone (see Medical Abortion). Arthrotec™ is a pharmaceutical that contains misoprostol and a painreliever and is sold as a treatment for arthritis and is often available without a prescription.

Medical abortion prescriptions can sometimes be obtained from a sympathetic doctor or pharmacist. Sometimes pills are available over-the-counter in ethnic markets in the United States and Mexico, and they are often advertised for sale online.

Warning! - Online sources of medical abortion pharmaceuticals are suspect. WomenonWeb.org analyzed pills obtained from Abortion-Pill-Online.com and found pills advertised as mifepristone did not contain mifepristone.[549] Some sites, like drugdelivery.ca are reported to have taken women's money, but the pills never arrived.
Suspected scam websites are listed:
www.womenonwaves.org/article-445-en.html

If you order pharmaceuticals from an online pharmacy make sure the online pharmacy has at least a contact phone number and a contact address (not just an outsourced call center), the website has a reputable domain name (not an ISP address), the shipment is trackable by a recognizable service (UPS, DHL, USPS, etc.), and SSL encryption is used.

(Medical Abortion cont.)

Also, check to see how long the website has been around:

Go to www.Google.com and type:

1. cache: www.website.com
2. site: www.website.com
3. link: www.website.com

The cache, site, and link information will indicate when the site was last seen on the search engine, how many pages of the website are in the search engine, and how many other websites are linked to the suspected website.

❖ Menstrual Extraction

➢ Manual Vacuum Aspiration Procedure Education:
- www.Hesperian.org
- www.WHO.int

➢ Networking:
- www.SisterZeus.com will help you connect to women interested in forming self-help groups in your area.
- National Women's Health Network
  514 10th Street NW, Suite 400
  Washington, DC 20004
  Email: nwhn@nwhn.org

- The Women's Health Voice
  Email: healthquestions@nwhn.org
  1.202.628.7814
  Monday – Friday 9AM-5PM (EST)
- Network for Reproductive Options (Oregon)
  Online: NROptions.org
  1.541.345.5702
  "Self-help Slide Show" Presentation
  Email: NRO@efn.org

➢ Supplies:
- Antibiotics (may be regulated by U.S. Customs)
  • Pet stores – Fish diseases are treated using human antibiotics.

- Ethnic markets – Latin, Russian, and Chinese small markets may have antibiotics available for sale.
- In Mexico – Antibiotics are sold over the counter.
- Internet – Some websites facilitate physician referral/prescriptions or no-prescription-needed sale of antibiotics.
  - www.AllPharmacyMedicines.com
- Speculums
  - www.FWHC.org offers a Self Exam Kit - Includes: Speculum, hand held mirror, small flashlight, and informational brochure.
- Karman Cannula (may be regulated by U.S. Customs) Obtained from sympathetic doctor or manufacturer:
  - www.Narang.com
  - www.MediPlusIndia.com
  - www.Suru.com
- Ring Forceps
  - www.WidgetSupply.com
- Mityvac™ Hand Held Vacuum/ Brake Bleeding Pump Kit
  - www.IdealTrueValue.com
  - www.ToolSource.com

- ❖ Herbal Abortion
  - ➤ Aloe Vera
    - Fresh aloe leaves
      - www.SunFood.com
    - Fresh aloe plants:
      - www.TheGrowers-Exchange.com
      - Available fresh in floral and horticultural shops.
  - ➤ Angelica
    - www.FrontierCoop.com
    - www.Herb-Pharm.com
    - www.MountainRoseHerbs.com
    - www.TaylorGarden.com
  - ➤ Arbor Vitae
    - www.MountainRoseHerbs.com
    - www.Herb-Pharm.com

- ➢ Great Arum
  - ▪ www.HortusB.com
- ➢ Avocado
  - ▪ Fruit/Seeds available fresh in grocery stores.
- ➢ Birthwort
  - ▪ Known as Bu Fei E Jiao San at www.MaxNature.com
- ➢ Barrenwort
  - ▪ www.Starwest-Botanicals.com
  - ▪ www.WildRoots.com
- ➢ Black Cohosh
  - ▪ www.FrontierCoop.com
  - ▪ www.MountainRoseHerbs.com
  - ▪ www.Herb-Pharm.com
- ➢ Blue Cohosh
  - ▪ www.FrontierCoop.com
  - ▪ www.MountainRoseHerbs.com
  - ▪ www.Herb-Pharm.com
- ➢ Castor Oil
  - ▪ www.MountainRoseHerbs.com
  - ▪ www.FrontierCoop.com
- ➢ Castor Beans
  - ▪ www.Ebay.com
- ➢ Chamomile
  - ▪ www.FrontierCoop.com
  - ▪ www.Herb-Pharm.com
- ➢ Chaste Tree
  - ▪ www.FrontierCoop.com
  - ▪ www.Herb-Pharm.com
- ➢ Cotton Fresh Root Bark Tincture
  - ▪ www.Herb-Pharm.com
- ➢ Daphne
  - ▪ www.Chinese-Herbs-Medicine.net
- ➢ Dittany
  - ▪ Available dried in international grocery stores.
  - ▪ www.Store.sheepish.us
    Sheepish
    326 Main Street
    Racine, WI, USA 53403
    Phone: 1.262.635.3244

393

- ➢ Garlic
  - ▪ Available fresh in grocery stores.
- ➢ Ginger
  - ▪ Available fresh in grocery stores.
- ➢ Hellebore, Black
  - ▪ www.WitchnKnight.com
- ➢ Hibiscus
  - ▪ Petal powder known as Jaswand:
    - • www.NatureWithLove.com
    - • www.AyurvedaGarden.com
- ➢ Horseradish
  - ▪ Available fresh in groceries during month of April
  - ▪ www.Herb-Pharm.com
- ➢ Juniper
  - ▪ www.FrontierCoop.com
  - ▪ www.Herb-Pharm.com
  - ▪ www.MountainRoseHerbs.com
  - ▪ www.TaylorGarden.com
- ➢ Lupine
  - ▪ Must be wild harvested or grown from seed.
- ➢ Male Fern
  - ▪ www.BlessedHerbs.com
- ➢ Mistletoe
  - ▪ www.FrontierCoop.com
  - ▪ www.MountainRoseHerbs.com
  - ▪ www.Herb-Pharm.com
- ➢ Mugwort
  - ▪ www.MountainRoseHerbs.com
  - ▪ www.FrontierCoop.com
- ➢ Nutmeg
  - ▪ www.MountainRoseHerbs.com
  - ▪ www.FrontierCoop.com
- ➢ Onion
  - ▪ Available fresh in grocery stores.
- ➢ Papaya
  - ▪ Available fresh in grocery stores.
- ➢ Parsley
  - ▪ Available fresh in grocery stores.
  - ▪ www.FrontierCoop.com

- ➢ Pennyroyal
  - ▪ www.MountainRoseHerbs.com
  - ▪ www.FrontierCoop.com
- ➢ Pineapple
  - ▪ Available green in tropical areas and some grocery stores in temperate climates.
- ➢ Pomegranate
  - ▪ Available October – January fresh in groceries
  - ▪ www.DiamondOrganics.com
- ➢ Queen Anne's Lace
  - ▪ Information: www.RobinRoseBennett.com)
  - ▪ www.SunStoneHerbs.com
  - ▪ www.HealingSpiritsHerbFarm.com
  - ▪ www.CedarSpringHerbFarm.com
- ➢ Rosemary
  - ▪ www.FrontierCoop.com
  - ▪ www.MountainRoseHerbs.com
  - ▪ www.Herb-Pharm.com
- ➢ Rue
  - ▪ www.SomaLuna.com
  - ▪ www.MountainRoseHerbs.com
  - ▪ www.Herb-Pharm.com
- ➢ Saffron
  - ▪ www.MountainRoseHerbs.com
  - ▪ www.FrontierCoop.com
- ➢ Stoneseed
  - ▪ Milestone Nursery
    PO Box 907
    Lyle, WA 98635
    Phone: 1.509.365.3642
- ➢ Tansy
  - ▪ www.Starwest-Botanicals.com
  - ▪ www.HerbalRemedies.com
  - ▪ www.WildRoots.com
- ➢ Wild Ginger
  - ▪ www.TaylorGarden.com

- ❖ Homeopathic Abortion
  - ➤ Abroma radix and Carica Papaya
    - ▪ SBL PVT. LTD.
      SBL House, 2
      Commercial complex
      Shrestha Vihar
      Delhi-110092, INDIA
      Phone: 91.11.22162353
      Email: sbl@vsnl.com
      Online: www.sblglobal.com
  - ➤ Gossypium Herbaceum
    - ▪ www.ABCHomeopathy.com
    - ▪ www.RemedySource.com
  - ➤ Humphrey's 11™
    - ▪ www.MediChest.com
    - ▪ www.TheHerbalMan.com
    - ▪ www.AmericaRX.com
  - ➤ Macrotinum
    - ▪ www.ABCHomeopathy.com
    - ▪ www.RemedySource.com
  - ➤ Pulsatilla
    - ▪ www.ABCHomeopathy.com
    - ▪ www.RemedySource.com

- ❖ Acupuncture Abortion
  - ➤ Acupuncturist Referral
    - ▪ www.Gancao.net
  - ➤ Acupuncture Supplies
    - ▪ www.LhasaOMS.com
    - ▪ www.A1hpi.com

- ❖ Yoga
  - ➤ To find a Teacher:
    - ▪ Online: www.IAYT.org
    - ▪ www.AmericanYogaAssociation.org

❖ Psychic Abortion
  ➢ Linda Baker
    1202 35th Street
    Renton, Washington, USA 98056-1964
    Phone: 1.425.271.1251
    Website: www. LindaBak.com
    Email: lindabak@hotmail.com

    Offers Audio Recording:
    Abortion – A Spiritual Approach
    Side A: Abortion: A Spiritual Approach
    Side B: Healing from Past Miscarriage or Abortion

    Linda Baker says, "Some people had successful miscarriages by putting the tape on at night and just letting it run all night, playing both sides continuously…When possible it is good for both parties to listen to the tape and to be in full agreement in desire for the miscarriage, as with reaching any goal, the clearer the energy is, the more likely the goal will be achieved."[550]

  ➢ Teresa Robertson, RN, CNM, MSN Intuitive Counselor
    Newland Healing Arts Mansion
    3011 N. Broadway, Suite 23
    Boulder, CO 80302
    Phone: 1.303.258.3904
    Website: www.LivingIntuitive.com
    Email: Teresa@BirthIntuitive.com

  ➢ Palden Jenkins
    16 Chilkwell Street
    Glastonbury
    Somerset BA6 8JG
    United Kingdom
    Phone: 01458.835079
    Website: www.Palden.co.uk
    Email: Palden.Jenkins@btopenworld.com
    Article 'Psychic Abortions,' 1999:
    www.palden.co.uk/palden/p4-childbirth.html

- ❖ Fetal Homicide State Laws in United States:
  - ➢ National Conference of State Legislatures
    www.ncsl.org/programs/health/fethom.htm

- ❖ Contraception
  - ➢ Emergency Contraceptive Pill Information
    - ▪ www.Not-2-Late.com
  - ➢ Body-fluid observation lens:
    - ▪ Fertility Scope™
      - • Info: www.FertilityScope.com
      - ♦ www.Early-Pregnancy-Tests.com
    - ▪ Maybemom™ Mini Ovulation Microscope
      - • Info and Ordering: www.MaybeMom.com
    - ▪ Fertile Focus™
      - • Info: Fertile-Focus.com
      - ♦ www.Drugstore.com
      - ♦ www.Early-Pregnancy-Tests.com
      - ♦ www.CVS.com

    - ▪ Fertility Tracker® Saliva Fertility Monitor
      - • Info: www.FertilityTracker.com
      - ♦ www.Amazon.com
      - ♦ www.Early-Pregnancy-Tests.com
      - ♦ www.BabyHopes.com

- ❖ Museums
  - ➢ Museum of Menstruation and Women's Health
    www.MUM.org

  - ➢ The Rags: paraphernalia of menstruation
    www.PowerHouseMuseum.com/rags/

  - ➢ Case Western Reserve University
    Allen Memorial Medical Library, 3rd Floor
    11000 Euclid Avenue (at Adelbert Road)
    Cleveland, Ohio 44106-1714
    Monday- Friday: 10:00 - 5:00 PM (Free)
    www.case.edu/affil/skuyhistcontraception/index.html

> ➤ Abortion and Contraception Museum
> Dr. Christina Fiala
> Chairman of the International Association of Abortion and
> Contraceptive Specialists
> Vienna, Austria
> At the Mariahilfer Gurtel 37
> 1st Floor
> (1150 Vienna)
> Wednesday-Sunday: 2:00 - 8:00 PM
> Museum of Contraception and Abortion (online)
> www.Contraceptive-Museum.org

❖ Cultural Works
> ➤ Poetry:
>> ▪ Judith Arcana, poet *What if your Mother.*
> ➤ Performance Art:
>> ▪ Cindy Cooper, *Words of Choice,* a play made up of works by
>> several writers.
>> ▪ Lisa Link, ongoing Instillation art *Warnings.*
>> ▪ Ju-Yeon Ryu, dancer and choreographer *Beyond Good and
>> Evil – Coin Locker Babies,* a dance portraying the life stories
>> of three Asian women.
>> ▪ Alicia Shvarts, performance artist, senior art project
>> censored by Yale University, April 2008.
> ➤ Ongoing online oral history projects:
>> ▪ Project Voice - TheAbortionProject.org
>> ▪ I'm not sorry - ImNotSorry.net
> ➤ Print and online magazine:
>> ▪ Our Truths/Neustras Verdades - OurTruths.org
> ➤ Online Exhibition:
>> ▪ I had an Abortion – WomenOnWeb.org
>> ▪ Midwest Teen Sex Show - Online video episodes
>> exploring teen sexuality.
>> www.MidwestTeenSexShow.com

➢ Film:

- Arnold Schulman, *Love with a Proper Stranger* (1963) U.S. romantic comedy.
- Dorthy Fadiman, *When Abortion was Illegal: Untold Stories* (1992) U.S. documentary.
- Gary Bennett, *Rain Without Thunder* (1993) Futuristic U.S. documentary.
- Tran Anh Hung, *Scent of Green Papaya* (1993) Vietnamese drama.
- Andrea Dorfman, *Parsley Days* (2000) Canadian comedy-drama.
- Edet Belzberg, *Children Underground* (2001) Documentary about abandoned Romanian children during the rule of Nicholae Ceauşescu.
- Timur Bekmambetov, *Night Watch [Nochnoi Dozor]* (2004) Russian fantasy thriller with a psychic abortion.
- Imelda Stauton, *Vera Drake* (2004) British drama.
- Jennifer Baumgardner and Gillian Aldrich, *Speak Out: I had an Abortion* (2005) at SpeakOutFilms.com.
- Christian Mungiu, *4 months, 3 weeks and 2 days* (2007) Romanian drama.

All illustrations are copyright © Sage-femme Collective.

Cover - 'Papaya Fibonacci Spiral.'
Leonardo of Pisa, known as Fibonacci, in his *Liber Abaci* AD 1202, conceptualized the population potential of a pair of rabbits into a visual mathematical representation and created the golden spiral. Colors were selected from a ripe papaya.

Herbal - Herb illustrations are derivative works based upon the following domain-free botanical illustrations:

Aloe - *Aloe succotrina* - Elizabeth Blackwell. *A Curious Herbal.* 1739.

Angelica - *Angelica archangelica* – William Woodville. *Medical Botany.* 1790.

Arum - *Arum drancululus* – Basilius Besler. *Hortus Eystettensis. 3rd ed..* 1713.

Avocado - *Persea americana* – *Yearbook of the United States Department of Agriculture.* 1911.

Arbor vitae - *Arbor vitae* – Elizabeth Blackwell. *Herbarium.* 1750.

Barrenwort - Epimedium grandiflorum - Otto Wilhelm Thomé. *Flora von Deutschland. Österreich und der Schweiz.* 1885.

Birthwort - *Aristolochia clematitis* –James Philips. *A Supplement to Medical Botany.* 1794.

Black Cohosh – *Cimicifuga racemosa* – Robert Bentley and Hanry Trimen. *Medicinal Plants.* 1880.

Black Hellebore – *Helleborus niger* - William Woodville. *Medical Botany.* 1790.

Blue Cohosh- *Chaulopyllum thalictroides* - *Drugs and Medicines of North America.* 1884-1887

Castor – *Ricinus communis* – Franz Eugen Köhler. *Köhler's Medizinal-Pflanzen.* 1883-1914.

Chamomile – *Anthemis nobilis* – Franz Eugen Köhler. *Köhler's Medizinal-Pflanzen.* 1883-1914.

Chaste tree - *Agnus castus* – Pierre Joseph Redouté. *Traité des arbres et arbustes que l'on cultive en France en pleine terre* by Duhamel du Monceau. 1801-1819.

401

Cotton – *Gossypium barbadense* – John Abbot. *The natural history of the rarer lepidopterous insects of Georgia.* 1797.

Daphne - *Daphne mezereum* - Otto Wilhelm Thomé. *Flora von Deutschland. Österreich und der Schweiz.* 1885.

Dittany – *Origanum dictamnus* – Elizabeth Blackwell. *A Curious Herbal.* 1739.

Garlic – *Allium sativum* – Woodville. *Medical Botany.* 1790

Ginger – *Zingiber officinalis* – Franz Eugen Köhler. *Koehler's Medicinal Plants* . 1887.

Hibiscus – *Hibiscus rosa-sinensis* – Jean Henri Jaume Saint-Hilaire. *Traite des arbrisseaux et des cultives en France et en pleine,* 1825.

Horseradish – *Cochlearia armoracia* – Woodville. *Medical Botany.* 1790.

Juniper – *Juniperus communis* –Otto Carl Berg & Carl Friedrich Schmidt. *Darstellung und Beschreibung sämtlicher in der Pharmacopoea Borusica aufgeführten offizinellen Gewächse* 1858-1863.

Lupine – *Lupinus angustifolius* – Basilius Besler. *Hortus Eystettensis.* 1713.

Male Fern – *Polypodium filix-mas* -William Woodville. *Medical Botany.* 1790.

Mistletoe – Viscum album – Otto Wilhelm Thomé. *Flora von Deutschland. Österreich und der Schweiz.* 1885.

Mugwort – *Artemisia vulgaris* – Otto Carl Berg & Carl Friedrich Schmidt. *Darstellung und Beschreibung sämtlicher in der Pharmacopoea Borusica aufgeführten offizinellen Gewächse.* 1858-1863.

Nutmeg – *Myristica moschata* - William Woodville. *Medical Botany.* 1790.

Onion – *Allium cepa* – *Vervolg op de Afbeeldingen der artseny-gewassen met derzelver Nederduitsche en Latynsche beschryvingen.* 1813.

Papaya – *Carica papaya* – Franz Eugen Köhler. *Köhler's Medizinal-Pflanzen.* 1883-1914.

Parsley – *Petroselinum neapoltanum* - Franz Eugen Köhler. *Köhler's Medizinal-Pflanzen.* 1883-1914.

Pennyroyal – *Hedeoma pulegoides* – Basilius Besler. *Hortus Eystettensis.* 3rd Ed. 1713.

Pineapple – *Ananas comosus* – Franz Eugen Köhler. *Neueste und wichtigste Medizinalpflanzen in naturgetreuen.* 1898.

Pomegranate – *Punica granatum* – Franz Eugen Köhler. Köhler's Medizinal-Pflanzen 1887.

Queen Anne's Lace – *Daucus carota* – Otto Wilhelm Thomé *Flora von Deutschland, Österreich und der Schweiz.* 1885.

Rosemary – *Rosmarinus officinalis* – Franz Eugen Köhler. Köhler's Medizinal-Pflanzen 1887.

Rue – *Ruta graveolens* – Otto Carl Berg & Carl Friedrich Schmidt. *Darstellung und Beschreibung sämtlicher in der Pharmacopoea Borusica aufgeführten offizinellen Gewächse,* 1858-1863.

Saffron – Crocus sativus – Otto Wilhelm Thomé *Flora von Deutschland, Österreich und der Schweiz.* 1885.

Squirting Cucumber – *Momordica elaterium* - William Woodville. *Medical Botany.*

Stoneseed – *Lithospermum officinale* – William Woodville. *A Supplement to Medical Botany.* 1794.

Tansy – *Tanacetum vulgare* – Otto Carl Berg & Carl Friedrich Schmidt. *Darstellung und Beschreibung sämtlicher in der Pharmacopoea Borusica aufgeführten offizinellen Gewächse* 1858-1863.

Wild Ginger – *Asarum canadense* - Otto Wilhelm Thomé. *Flora von Deutschland. Österreich und der Schweiz.* 1885.

Homeopathy - Homeopathy illustrations are derivative works based upon the following domain-free botanical illustrations:

Abroma radix - *Abroma augusta* - Francisco Manuel Blanco,*Flora de Filipinas.* 1880-1883.

Carica papaya – Franz Eugen Köhler. *Köhler's Medizinal-Pflanzen.*1883-1914.

Gossypium forte – *Gossypium barbadense* - John Abbot. *The natural history of the rarer lepidopterous insects of Georgia.* 1797.

Macrotinum - *Cimicifuga racemosa* - Robert Bentley and Henry Trimen. *Medicinal Plants, being descriptions with original figures of the Principal Plants employed in medicine.* 1880.

Pulsatilla pratensis - *Kräuterbuch.* 1914.

Sepia officinalis - Brehms Tierleben. *Allgemeine Kunde des Tierreiches.* 1893.

Endnotes

[1] Alfred Swaine Taylor, *The Principles and Practice of Medical Jurisprudence* (London: J. & A. Churchill, 1873), 179-91.

[2] Jodi L. Jacobson, "The Global Politics of Abortion," *Worldwatch Paper* 97 (July 1990), 56.

[3] World Health Organization, *Unsafe Abortion: Global and Regional Estimates of the Incidence of Unsafe Abortion.* (Geneva, World Health Organization, 2004).

[4] Christopher Tietze and Sarah Lewit, "Abortion," *Scientific American* 220 (1969), 21.

[5] F. Glenc, "Induced Abortion – a Historical Outline," *Polski Tygodnik Lekarski* 29, no. 45 (1974), 1957-8.

[6] Malcolm Potts and Martha Campbell, "History of Contraception," *Gynecology and Obstetrics* 6, chap. 8 (2002). http://big.berkeley.edu/ifplp.history.pdf (accessed August 14, 2008).

[7] Aristotle, *"History of Animals,"* book 7, chap. 3, 583b.

[8] Soranus, *Gynecology.* trans. Owsei Temkin (Baltimore: The John Hopkins University Press, 1991), 67.

[9] Susan A. Cohen, "New Data on Abortion Incidence, Safety Illuminate Key Aspects of Worldwide Abortion Debate," *Guttmacher Policy Review* 10, no.4 (Fall 2007). http://www.guttmacher.org/pubs/gpr/10/4/gpr100402.html (accessed June 28, 2008).

[10] Laura Gil, "Assessing Maternal Mortality due to Induced Abortion: A Systematic Review of the Literature," *Geneva Foundation for Medical Education and Research.* http://www.gfmer.ch/Medical_education_En/PGC_RH_2004/Gil_r eview.htm (accessed July 15, 2008).

[11] M. Sood, Y. Juneja, and U. Goyal, "Maternal Mortality and Morbidity Associated with Clandestine Abortions," *Journal of the Indian Medical Association* 93, no. 2 (Feb 1995), 77-9.

[12] M.E. Chowdhury, R. Botlero, M. Koblinsky, S.K. Saha, G. Dieltiens, and C. Ronsmans, "Determinants of Reduction in Maternal Mortality in Matlab, Bangladesh: a 30-year cohort study," *Lancet* 370, no. 9595 (2007), 1320.

[13] Robert E. Meyer and Paul A. Buescher, "Maternal Mortality Related to Induced Abortion in North Carolina: A Historical Study," *Family Planning Perspectives* (July 1994),

http://findarticles.com/p/articles/mi_qa3634/is_199407/ai_n871115
9 (accessed July 15, 2008).

[14] Susan A. Cohen, "New Data on Abortion Incidence, Safety Illuminate Key Aspects of Worldwide Abortion Debate," *Guttmacher Policy Review* 10, no. 4. (Fall 2007).

[15] John M. Paxman, Alberto Rizo, Laura Brown and Janie Benson, "The Clandestine Epidemic: The Practice of Unsafe Abortion in Latin America," *Studies in Family Planning*, . 24, no. 4 (Jul. - Aug., 1993), 205-26.

[16] D.S. Vladutiu, C. Spanu, I.M. Patiu, C. Neamtu, M. Gherman, and M. Manasia, "Abortion Prohibition and Acute Renal Failure: the Tragic Romanian Experience," *Renal Failure* 17, no. 5 (September 1995), 605-609.

[17] Cristian Pop-Eleches, "The Impact of an Abortion Ban on Socioeconomic Outcomes of Children: Evidence from Romania," *Journal of Political Economy* 114, no. 4 (2006).

[18] University of Maryland, "Orphaned Children Show Higher Intelligence and Fare Better in Foster Care than in Institutions." *Science Daily* (December 28, 2007). http://www.sciencedaily.com/releases/2007/12/071221130041.htm (accessed July 6, 2008).

[19] UNICEF, "Africa's Orphaned and Vulnerable Generations: Children Affected by AIDS," *Unicef, UNAids, and Pepfar.* (2006).

[20] J.N. Ferguson, L.J. Young, E.F. Hearn, M.M. Matzuk, T.R. Insel, and J.T. Winslow, "Social Amnesia in Mice Lacking the Oxytocin Gene," *Nature Genetics* 25 (2000), 284–98.

[21] D. Maestripieri, "The Biology of Human Parenting: Insights From Nonhuman Primates."*Neuroscience & Biobehavioral Reviews* 23 (1999), 411-22.

[22] C.S. Carter, L. Ahnert, K.E. Grossman, S.B. Hrdy, M.E. Lamb, et al. , *Attachment and Bonding: A New Synthesis.* (Cambridge: MIT Press, 2006).

[23] Michael Kosfeld, Markus Heinrichs, Paul J. Zak, Urs Fischbacher, and Ernst Fehr, "Oxytocin Increases Trust in Humans," *Nature* 435 (June 2, 2005), 673-76.

[24] Paroma Basu, "Psychologists Glimpse Biological Imprint of Childhood Neglect," *University of Wisconsin – Madison News.* November 21, 2005.

[25] Paul J. Zak, Robert Kurzban, and William T. Matzner, "The Neurobiology of Trust," *Annals of the New York Academy of Sciences* Annals of the New York Academy of Sciences 1032 (2004), 224-27.

[26] Lester R. Brown and Hal Kane, *Full House: Reassessing the Earth's Population Carrying Capacity* (Washington D.C: WorldWatch Institute, 1994).

[27] Thoraya Ahmed Obaid, Executive Director UNFPA in a speech "Saving Women's Lives," Smith College, March 26, 2003 http://www.unfpa.org/news/news.cfm?ID=271 (accessed August 30,2008).

[28] Julian Borger, "Feed the World? We are fighting a losing battle, UN admits," *Guardian* (February 26, 2008). http://www.guardian.co.uk/environment/2008/feb/26/food.unitedn ations (accessed July 18, 2008).

[29] N. Zill and K. O'Donnell, *Child Poverty Rates by Maternal Risk Factors: An Update.* (Rockville, MD: WESTAT, 2004).

[30] James Demeo, *Saharasia: The 4000 BCE Origins of Child Abuse, Sex-Repression, Warfare, and Social Violence in the Deserts of the Old World. Evidence for a World-wide, Climate-Linked Geographical Pattern in Human Behavior.* (Ashland, Oregon: Natural Energy Works, 2006).

[31] Steven D. Levitt and Stephen J. Dubner, *Freakonomics* (New York: HarperTorch, 2005), 117-144.

[32] Daniela Draghici, "A Personal View of Women's Sexual and Reproductive Lives in Romania," http://www.prochoiceforum.org.uk/psy_ocr9.asp (accessed April 25, 2008).

[33] Dan-Stefan Vladutiu, Costel Spanu, Ioan-Mihai Patiu, Cristina Neamtu, Mirela Gherman, and Mahai Manasia, "Abortion Prohibition and Acute Renal Failure: The Tragic Romanian Experience," *Renal Failure* 17, no. 5, (September 1995), 605-9.

[34] Cristian Pop-Eleches, "The Impact of an Abortion Ban on Socioeconomic Outcomes of Children: Evidence from Romania, " *Journal of Political Economy* 114, no. 4, (2006).

[35] Steven D. Levitt and Stephen J. Dubner, *Freakonomics.* (New York: HarperTorch, 2005), 117-44.

[36] Ibid., 135-44.

[37] Thomas Merrick, "Population and Poverty: New Views on an Old Controversy." *International Family Planning Perspectives* 28 (2002).

[38] NARAL Pro-Choice America, "State and Federal Legislation" (June, 2003), http://www.naral.org/choice-action-center/in_your_state/bill-tracker/ (accessed August 13, 2008).

[39] L. Finer and S. Henshaw, "Abortion Incidence and Services in the United States in 2000," *Perspectives on Sexual* and Reproductive *Health* 35, no. 1 (Jan-Feb 2003), 6-15.

[40] Guttmacher Institute, *U.S. Teenage Pregnancy Statistics: National and State Trends and Trends by Race and Ethnicity,* http://www.guttmacher.org/pubs/2006/09/11/USTPstats.pdf, (accessed Sept. 12, 2006).

[41] S. Henshaw and L. Finer, "The Accessibility of Abortion Services in the United States, 2001," *Perspectives on Sexual and Reproductive Health* 35, no. 1 (Jan-Feb 2003), 16-24.

[42] R. Almeling, L. Tews, and S. Dudley, "Abortion training in U.S. obstetrics and gynecology residency programs," *Family Planning Perspectives* 32, no. 6 (Nov-Dec 2000), 268-71, 320.

[43] Alfred J. Butler, *Arab Conquest of Egypt* (Oxford: Clarendon Press, 1902).

[44] Brian Levack, *The Witch Hunt in Early Modern Europe* (New York: Longman, 1995).

[45] Gunnar Heinsohn and Otto Steiger, "The Elimination of Medieval Birth Control and the Witch Trials of Modern Times," *International Journal of Women's Studies* (May 3, 1982), 193-214.

[46] Gunnar Heinsohn and Otto Steiger, "Birth Control: the Political-Economic Rationale Behind Jean Bodin's 'Démonomanie'," *History of Political Economy* 31, no. 3 (Fall 1999), 423-448.

[47] Stéphane Barry and Norbert Gualde, "La plus grande épidémie de l'histoire" *L'Histoire N° 310* (June 2006), 45-6.

[48] Jo Murphy-Lawless, "Fertility, Bodies and Politics: The Irish Case," *Reproductive Health Matters* 2 (1993), 56. Chrystel Hug, *The Politics of Sexual Morality in Ireland* (London: Macmillan, 1999), 164.

[49] Ursula Barry, "Movement, Change, and Reaction: The Struggle Over Reproductive Rights in Ireland," *The Abortion Papers: Ireland* ed. Ailbhe Smyth (Dublin: Attic Press, 1992), 116. Pauline Conroy-Jackson, "Outside the Jurisdiction: Irish Women Seeking Abortion," *The Abortion Papers: Ireland* ed. Aibhe Smyth (Dublin: Attic Press, 1992), 133-4.

[50] Roe v. Wade, 410 U.S. 113 (1973).

[51] S. Holland, *Bioethics: A Philosophical Introduction* (New York: Blackwell Publishing, 2003).

[52] Adam Aiger-Treworgy, "Huck, the Constitution and 'God's Standards'," *MSNBC News* (January 15, 2008). http://firstread.msnbc.msn.com/archive/2008/01/15/579265.aspx (accessed July 15, 2008).

[53] Interview of John McCain by Dan Gilgoff, http://www.beliefnet.com/story/220/story_22001_1.html (accessed July 15, 2008).

[54] Official Website for John McCain, "Human dignity and the sancity of Life: Overturning Roe v. Wade," http://www.johnmccain.com/Informing/Issues/95b18512-d5b6-456e-90a2-12028d71df58.htm (accessed July 16, 2008).

[55] U.S. Department of Health and Human Services, "Fetal Homicide," *National Conference of State Legislatures.* (April 2008), http://www.ncsl.org/programs/health/fethom.htm (accessed July 4, 2008).

[56] Sacred Congregation for the Doctrine of the Faith, "Declaration on Procured Abortion," http://www.vatican.va/roman_curia/congregations/cfaith/documents/rc_con_cfaith_doc_19741118_declaration-abortion_en.html (accessed July 16, 2008).

[57] John M. Riddle, *Contraception and Abortion* (Cambridge, Massachusetts: Harvard University Press, 1994), 138.

[58] Sahih Muslim, *The Book of Destiny (Kitab-ul-Qadr)*, http://www.searchtruth.com/book_display.php?book=33&translator=2 (accessed July 2, 2008).

[59] Elaine Martin, "Rethinking the Practice of Mizuko Kuyo in Contemporary Japan: Interviews with Practioners at a Buddhist Temple in Kyoto," http://bama.ua.edu/~emartin/publications/mkarticl.htm (accessed July 2, 2008).

[60] Haraprasad Shastri, ed., *Hajar Bachharer Purana Bangala Bhasay Bauddhagan O Doha*, (Bangiya Sahitya Parisat, 1916).

[61] Claufdia Dreifus, "The Dalai Lama," *The New York Times*, (November 28, 1993).

[62] S. Cromwell Crawford, *Dilemmas of Life and Death: Hindu Ethics in a North American Context* (Albany: State Univ. New York Press, 1995).

[63] Atharva Veda Samhita, VI-138.

[64] Pablo A. Nepomnaschy, "Cortisol Levels and Very Early Pregnancy Loss in Humans," *Proceedings of the National Academy of Sciences of the United States of America*, Published online before print Feb. 22, 2006. http://www.pnas.org/

[65] David E. Samuel, "A Review of the Effects of Plant Estrogenic Substances on Animal Reproduction," *The Ohio Journal of Science* 67, no.5 (September 1967), 308.

[66] T.S. Rumsey, T.H. Elsasser, and S. Kahl, "Roasted Soybeans and an Estrogenic Growth Promoter Affect Growth Hormone Status and Performance of Beef Steers," *Journal of Nutrition* 126, no. 11 (Nov 1996), 2880-7. S. Hewitt, J. R. Hillman and B. A. Knights, "Steroidal Oestrogens and Plant Growth and Development," *New Phytologist* 85, no. 3 (July 1980), 329-50.

[66] John A. McLachlan, "Environmental Signaling: What Embryos and Evolution Teach Us about Endocrine Eisrupting Channels." *Endocrine Reviews* 22, no. 3 (2001), 319-41.

[67] Ibid.

[68] Women on Waves Foundation, Amsterdam, Netherlands. http://www.womenonwaves.org/index.php (accessed July 18, 2008).

[69] United Nations, "Thailand Population Policy Data Bank," Population Division of the Department of Economic and Social Affairs of the United Nations Secretariat. http://www.un.org/esa/population/publications/abortion/doc/thailand.doc (accessed July 21, 2008).

[70] Soranus, *Gynecology*, trans. by Owsei Temkin (Baltimore: John Hopkins University Press, 1991), 65.

[71] Li Feng-cai *et al.*, "Clinical Observations on the Preventive Treatment of Artificial Abortion with *Song Tu Fang* (Relax Earth Formula), & the Occurence of Disease." *Xin Zhong Yi (New Chinese Medicine)*, #8, (2007), 37-38. Bob Flaws, trans. "Chinese Medical Preventative Treatment before Artificial Abortion," as published oneline: http://www.bluepoppy.com/cfwebstorefb/index.cfm?fuseaction=feature.display&feature_id=1411 (Accessed August 29, 2008).

[72] Victoria Blinder, Batya Elul, and Beverly Winikoff, "Mifepristone-misoprostol Medical Abortion: Who will Use it and Why?" *American Journal of Obstetrics & Gynecology* 179, no. 5 (November 1998), 1376. Irving Spitz, Lauri Benton, Wayne Bardin, and Ann Robbins, "The

Safety and Efficacy of Early Pregnancy Termination with Mifepristone and Misoprostol: Results from the First Multicenter U.S. Trial." *New England Journal of Medicine* 338 (1998), 1241-7.

[73] Batya Elul, et al., "Can Women in Less-Developed Countries Use a Simplified Medical Abortion Regimen?" *Lancet* 357, no. 9266 (2001), 1402-5. Beverly Winikoff, Charlotte Ellertson, Batya Elul, and Irving Sivin, "Acceptability and Feasibility of Early Pregnancy Termination by Mifepristone-Misoprostol," *Archives of Family Medicine* 7 (1998), 360-6.

[74] K. Coyaji, B. Elul, U. Krishna, S. Otiv, S. Ambardekar, A. Bopardikar, V. Raote, C. Elleartson, and B. Winikoff, "Mifepristone Abortion Outside the Urban Research Hospital Setting in India." *Lancet* 357, no. 9250 (2001), 120-2.

[75] C. Ellertson, B. Elul, S. Ambardekar, L. Wood, J. Carroll, K. Coyaji, "Accuracy of Assessment of Pregnancy Duration by Women Seeking Early Abortions." *Lancet* 355, no. 9207 (2000), 877-81.

[76] Women on Web official website, www.womenonweb.com

[77] S.K. Henshaw and L.B. Finer, "The Accessibility of Abortion Services in the United States, 2001," *Perspectives on Sexual and Reproductive Health* 35, no. 1(2003), 16–24.

[78] Ranjun Basu, Tina Gunlach, and Margaret Tasker, "Mifepristone and Misoprostol for Medical Termination of Pregnancy: The Effectiveness of a Flexible Regime." *Journal of Family Planning and Reproductive Health Care* 29, no. 3 (2003), 139 - 41.

[79] A. Jost, "New Data on the Hormonal Requirement of the Pregnant Rabbit; Partial Pregnancies and Fetal Anomalies Resulting from Treatment with a Hormonal Antagonist, Given at a Sub-Abortive Dosage," *Comptes Rendus de l'Academie des Sciences Serie 3 Sciences de la Vie* 303 (1986), 281–4. R.P Hardy, "Effects of the Anti-Progestin RU 38486 on Rat Embryos Growing in Culture," *Food and Chemical Toxicology* 29 (1991), 361–2. O.M. Avrech, A. Golan, Z. Weinraub, I. Bukovsky, and E. Caspi, "New Tools for the Trade," *Fertility and Sterility* 57 (1992), 1139–40. J.P Wolf, C.F. Chillik, C. Dubois, A. Ulmann, E.E. Baulieu, and G.D. Hodgen, "Tolerance of Perinidatory Primate Embryos to RU486 Exposure in Vitro and in Vivo." *Contraception* 41 (1990), 85–92.

[80] R. Henrion, "RU 486 abortions." *Nature* 338 (1989),110. J.C. Pons, M.C. Imbert, E. Elefant, C. Roux, P. Herschkorn, and E. Papiernik. "Development after Exposure to Mifepristone in Early Pregnancy."

410

Lancet 338 (1991),763. A. Ulmann, I. Rubin, and J. Barnard, "Development after In-Utero Exposure to Mifepristone." *Lancet* 338 (1991), 1270. J.C. Pons and E. Papiernik, "Mifepristone Teratogenicity." *Lancet* 338 (1991), 1332–3. B.H. Lim, D.A.R Lees, S. Bjornsson, C.B. Lunan, M.R. Cohn, P. Stewart and A. Davey, "Normal Development after Exposure to Mifepristone in Early Pregnancy." *Lancet* 336 (1990), 257–8.

[81] M. Philip, Caitlin Shannon, and Beverly Winikoff, eds., "Misoprostol and Teratogenicity: Reviewing the Evidence," *Report of a Meeting at the Population Council*, Critical Issues in Reproductive Health, Population Council and Gynuity Health Projects, New York, NY. (May 22, 2002).

[82] M. Wheeler, P. O'Meara, and M. Stanford, "Fetal Methotrexate and Misoprostol Exposure: The Past Revisited," *Teratology* 66, no. 2 (Aug 2002),73-6.

[83] E.J. Lazda and V.R. Sams, "The Effects of Gemeprost on the Second Trimester Fetus," *British Journal of Obstetrics and Gynaecology*. 102, no. 9, (1995), 731-4.

[84] "Instructions for Use: Abortion Induction with Misoprostol in Pregnancies up to 9 weeks LMP," Gynuity Health Projects (2003). K. Blanchard, B. Winikoff, and C. Ellertson, "Misoprostol used alone for the termination of early pregnancy: A review of the evidence," *Contraception*. 59 (1999) 209-17.

[85] R. Peyron, E. Aubény, V. Targosz, et al., "Early Termination of Pregnancy with Mifepristone (RU 486), and the Orally Active Prostaglandin Misoprostol." *New England Journal of Medicine* 328 (1993), 1509-13.

[86] H. el-Refaey, D. Rajasekar, M. Abdalla, L. Calder, and A. Templeton, "Induction of Abortion with Mifepristone (RU 486), and Oral or Vaginal Misoprostol," *New England Journal of Medicine* 332, no. 15 (April 13, 1995), 983-7.

[87] J. L. Carbonell Esteve, L. Varela, A. Velazco, R. Tanda, and C. Sánchez,"Oral Methotrexate Followed by Vaginal Misoprostol 7 Days after for Early Abortion A Randomized Trial," *Gynecologic and Obstetric Investigation* 47 (1999), 182-7.

[88] Mitchell D. Creinin, Courtney A. Schreiber, Paula Bednarek, Hanna Lintu, Marie-Soleil Wagner, and Leslie A. Meyn, "Mifepristone and Misoprostol Administered Simultaneously Versus 24 Hours Apart for Abortion: A Randomized Controlled Trial," *Obstetrics & Gynecology* 109 (2007), 885-94 .

[89] J. L. Carbonell Esteve, L. Varela, A. Velazco, R. Tanda, E. Cabezas, and C. Sánchez, "Early Abortion with 800 µg of Misoprostol by the Vaginal Route." *Contraception* 59 (1999), 219-25.

[90] Oi Shan Tang, B.Y. Miao, Sharon W.H. Lee, and Pak Chung Ho, "Pilot Study on the Use of Repeated Doses of Sublingual Misoprostol in Termination of Pregnancy up to 12 weeks Gestation: Efficacy and Acceptability," *Human Reproduction* 17, no. 3 (March 2002), 654-8.

[91] C. Bique, M. Usta, B. Debora, E. Chong, E. Westheimer, and B. Winikoff, "Comparison of misoprostol and manual vacuum aspiration for the treatment of incomplete abortion," *International Journal of Gynaaecology & Obstetrics*. Vol 98 (2007), 222-6. B. Dao, J. Blum, B. Thieba, et al. "Is misoprostol a Safe, Effective, and Acceptable Alternative to Manual Vacuum Aspiration for post abortion care? Results from a randomized trial in Burkina Faso, West Africa," *BJOG: An International Journal of Obstetrics & Gynaecology*. Vol 114 (2007) 1368-75.

[92] J.Y. Simpson, *Clinical Lectures on Diseases of Women*. (Philadelphia: Balchard & Lea, 1863).

[93] Rebecca Chalker, "The Whats, Whys, and Hows of Menstrual Extraction," *On the Issues* XXVI (1993), 42-56.

[94] Catherine S. Todd, "Manual Vacuum Aspiration for Second Trimester Pregnancy Termination," *International Journal of Gynecology & Obstetrics*. Vol 83, Issue 1 (2003), 5-9.

[95] Catherine S. Todd, "Buccal Misoprostol as Cervical Preparation for Second Trimester Pregnancy Termination," *Contraception* vol 65, Issue 6 (2002), 415-418.

[96] Marreen Paul and Kristin Nobel, "Papaya: A Simulation Model for Training in Uterine Aspiration," *Family Medicine* 37, no. 4 (2005), 242-4.

[97] There was one known miss-construction of the Del-EM™, where the check valve was put on the wrong way. Instead of establishing a vacuum, air was accidentally pushed into the uterine cavity causing an air embolism; the woman recovered completely.

[98] Benson, J. et al. "Meeting Women's Needs for Post-Abortion Family Planning: Framing the Questions," *Issues in Abortion Care* 2(1992). (Adapted from *Complications of Abortion: Technical and Managerial Guidelines for Prevention and Treatment*), 3.6.1. http://www2.alliance-hpsr.org/reproductive-health/publications/clinical_mngt_abortion_complications/chap3.html (accessed August 30, 2008).

[99] R.C. Bretherton, "Vacuum Aspiration of the Uterus." (Letter), *Medical Journal of Australia,* August 12, 1978; 2(4), 164. http://www.popline.org/docs/0300/783347.html (accessed August 30, 2008).

[100] John M. Riddle, *Eve's Herbs,* (Cambridge: Harvard University Press, 1997), 58.

[101] San'at Art Magazine, "From a History of Headwear in Uzbekistan," http://sanat.orexca.com/eng/3-4-05/from-history.shtml (accessed August 20, 2008).

[102] Rustam Mirzaev website, "The Blue Ceramics of Uzbekistan," http://www.travelcentre.com.au/travel/Central_Asia/blue_ceramics_of_uzbekistan.htm(accessed August 20, 2008).

[103] Advantour website, "Tajikistan – Traditional Crafts," http://www.advantour.com/tajikistan/crafts.htm(accessed August 20, 2008).

[104] Aristophanes, Frag. 309; Pollux, v. 101, vii.

[105] Larche Museum Collection. Lima, Peru.

[106] Jacobsthal, "On the Evolution of Forms of Ornament," *Nature.* 30, no. 768 (1884), 272-4.

[107] Uni Tiamat, *Herbal Abortion: The Fruit of the Tree of Knowledge.* (Peoria, IL: Sage-femme, 1994), 25.

[108] Lewis R. Goldfrank, *Goldfrank's Toxicologic Emergencies.* (Prentice Hall, 1998), 447.

[109] Ilene B. Anderson, Walter H. Mullen, James E. Meeker, Siamak C. Khojasteh-Bakht, Shimako Oishi, Sidney D. Nelson, and Paul D. Blanc, "Pennyroyal Toxicity: Measurement of Toxic Metabolite levels in Two Cases and Review of Literature," *Annals of Internal Medicine* 124, no. 8 (April 15, 1996), 726-34.

[110] Linda McNatt, "Woman Charged with Shooting Self to Cause an Abortion," *The Virginia-Pilot* (March 1, 2006). http://hamptonroads.com/node/71871 (accessed July 5, 2008).

[111] Uni Tiamat, *Herbal Abortion: The Fruit of the Tree of Knowledge.* (Peoria, IL: Sage-femme, 1994).

[112] Jeannine Parvati, *Hygieia: A Woman's Herbal.* (Berkeley, CA: Freestone Collective, Bookpeople, 1978), 23.

[113] M. Maud Grieve, *A Modern Herbal.* (New York: Dover, 1971.), 28.

[114] Ibid, 29.

[115] Christian Ratsch, *The Dictionary of Sacred and Medicinal Plants.* (Santa Barbara, CA: ABC_CLIO, 1992), 36.

[116] J.D. Keys, *Chinese Herbs, Botany, Chemistry, and Pharmacodynamics,* (Rutland, VT, USA: Charles E. Tuttle Co., 1976).

[117] E. Quisumbing, "Medicinal Plants of the Phillipines. Technical Bull. 16," (Manila: Dept. of Natural Resources, 1951), 1.

[118] C.R. McCuddin, "Samoan Medicinal Plants and their usage." *Office of Comprehensive Health Planning.* Dept. of Medical Services. Government of American Samoa, (1974).

[119] M.P. Singh, S.B. Malla, S.B. Rajbhandari, and A. Manandhar. "Medicinal plants of Nepal: Retrospects and Prospects," *Economic Botany* 33, no. 2 (1979), 185-98.

[120] W.S. Woo, E.B. Lee. K.H. Shin, S.S. Kang, and H.J. Chi, "A review of research on plants for fertility reduction in Korea," *Korean Journal of Pharmacognosy* 12, no. 3 (1981), 153-70.

[121] W. Wong, "Some Folk Medicinal Plants from Trinidad," *Economic Botany* 30 (1976),103-42.

[122] E.S. Ayensu, "Medicinal Plants of the West Indies," unpublished manuscript 1978, 110p. as cited in Ivan A. Ross, *Medicinal Plants of the World: Chemical Constituents, Traditional and Modern Medicinal Uses,* vol 2 (Totowa, NJ: Humana Press, 1999), 52.

[123] John M. Riddle, *Contraception and Abortion from the Ancient World to the Renaissance,* (Cambridge: Harvard University Press, 1992), 45.

[124] H.M.A. Razzack,"The Concept of Birth Control in Unani Medical Literature," unpublished manuscript (1980), 64. as cited in Ivan A. Ross, *Medicinal Plants of the World: Chemical Constituents, Traditional and Modern Medicinal Uses,* vol 2 (Totowa, NJ: Humana Press, 1999), 373.

[125] Daniel E. Moerman, *Medicinal Plants of Native America,* vols. 1-2 (Ann Arbor: University of Michigan, 1986), 37.

[126] Susan S.Weed, *Wise Woman Herbal for the Childbearing Year.* (Woodstock: Ash Tree Publishing, 1986), 70.

[127] Malcolm Stuart, *Herbs and Herbalism* (New York: Nostrand Reinhold, 1979), 25.

[128] Joseph Campbell, *The Masks of God: Creative Mythology* (New York: Viking, 1970),163.

[129] Kee Chang Huang, *The Pharmcology of Chinese Herbs* (Boca Roton: CRC Press, 1993), 247-8.

[130] M.L. Yeh, C.F. Liu, C.L. Huang, and T.C. Huang, "Hepatoprotective Effect of *Angelica archangelica* in Chronically Ethanol-Treated Mice," *Pharmacology.* 68, no. 2 (2003), 70-3.

131 D.P. Zhu."Dong Quai," *American Journal of Chinese Medicine* 15 ¾ (1987),117-125. C.F. Schmidt, B.E. Read, and K.K. Chen. "Chinese Drugs," *Chinese Medical Journal* 38 (1924),362.

132 B.E. Read. "Some of the Old Chinese Drugs used in Obstetrical Practice." *Journal of Obstetrics and Gynecology of the British Empire* 34 (1927), 498-508.

133 Y.M. Chen, "Observation of 737 Cases of Impotence treated by 'Kang Wei Ling,'" *Chung I Tsa Chih - Journal of Traditional Chinese Medicine* 22, no. 4 (1981), 36-7. Y.F. Fu, Y. Xia, Y.P. Shi, and N.Q. Sun. "Treatment of 34 Cases of Infertility Due to Tubal Occlusion with Compound Dang Quai Injection by Irrigation," *Jiangsu Journal of Traditional Chinese Medicine* 9, no. 1 (1988), 15-16.

134 S. Sigurdsson, H.M. Ogmundsdottir, J. Hallgrimsson, and S. Gudbjarnason, "Antitumour Activity of *Angelica archangelica* Leaf Extract," *In Vivo* 19 (2005), 191-4.

135 Daniel E. Moerman, *Medicinal Plants of Native America*, vols 1-2 (Ann Arbor: University of Michigan, 1986), 482.

136 Christian Ratsch, *The Dictionary of Sacred and Medicinal Plants* (Santa Barbara: ABC-CLIO, 1992), 40.

137 Ruth Trickey, *Women, Hormones, and the Menstrual Cycle.* (Allen and Unwin, 2003), 498.

138 M. Maud Grieve, *A Modern Herbal* (New York: Dover, 1971), 176-7.

139 Charles Montgomery Skinner, *Myths and Legends of Flowers, Trees, Fruits and Plants* (Philadelphia: J.B.Lippincott Co., 1911), 53.

140 X Xu, SI Cho, M Sammel, L You, S Cui, Y Huang, G Ma, C Padungtod, L Pothier, T Niu, D Christiani, T Smith, L Ryan and L Wang, "Association of Petrochemical Exposure with Spontaneous Abortion," *Occupational and Environmental Medicine* 55 (Boston: Department of Environmental Health, Harvard School of Public Health, 1998), 31-6.

141 London, Kathleen, "The History of Birth Control." *The Changing American Family: Historical and Comparative Perspectives.* (1982). http://www.yale.edu/ynhti/curriculum/units/1982/6/82.06.03.x.html (accessed March 16, 2008).

142 John M. Riddle, *Contraception and Abortion from the Ancient World to the Renaissance*, (Cambridge: Harvard University Press, 1992), 45.

143 T. J. Knab, "Metaphors, Concepts, and Coherence in Aztec" in. *Symbol and Meaning beyond the Closed Community: Essays in Mesoamerican.*

Gary H. Gossen (New York: State University of New York Institute for Mesoamerican Studies, 1986), 50.

[144] Charles Montgomery Skinner, *Myths and Legends of Flowers, Trees, Fruits, and Plants in all Ages*, (Philadelphia: J.B. Lippincott Co., 1911), 56-7.

[145] Julia F. Morton, "Some Folk Medicine Plants of Central American Markets," *Quarterly Journal of Crude Drug Research* 15 (1977), 165. Julia F. Morton, "Avocado," *Fruits of Warm Climates*. (Miami: Florida Flair Books, 1987), 91–102.

[146] J.T. Roig and Y. Mesa, *Plantas Medicinaes, Aromaticas O Venenosas De Cuba*, (Havana, Cuba: Misterio de Agricultura, 1945), 872.

[147] G.Tessman, "Die Indianer Nordost-Perus," *Grundlegende Forchunger Fur Eine Systematischen*, (Hamburg, Germany: 1930).

[148] Lisa Allen-Agostini, "Abortion a Public Health Issue," *The Trinadad Guardian*. (June 15, 2004). http://www.guardian.co.tt/archives/2004-06-15/features1.html (accessed July 20, 2008).

[149] Alan Guttmacher Institute, *Survey of Opinions on Abortion Practice in Brazil, Colombia, Chile, Mexico, Peru, and the Dominican Republic*, (1992).

[150] Feng, P.C., L. J. Haynes, K.E. Magnus, J.R. Plimmer, and H.S.A. Sherrat. "Pharmacological Screening of Some West Indian Medicinal Plants." *Journal of Pharmacy and Pharmacology* 14 (1962), 556-61.

[151] Veronica Rey-Ares, Nickolai Lazarov, Dieter Berg, Ulrike Berg, Lars Kunz, and Artur Mayerhofer. "Dopamine Receptor Repertoire of Human Granulosa Cells," *Reproductive Biology and Endocrinology* 2007, **5**:40.

[152] Edith Bevin, "Avocados Help Fight Cancer," *The Daily Telegraph*, (June 7, 2007).

[153] D. A. Levy, N. Mounedji, C. Noirot, and F. Leynadier, "Allergic Sensitization and Clinical Reactions to Latex, Food and Pollen in Adult Patients," *Clinical and Expermiental Allergy* 30 (2000),270-5. G. Crisi and D.V. Belsito, "Contact Urticaria from Latex in a Patient with Immediate Hypersensitivity to Banana, Avocado, and Peach," *Contact Dermatitis* 28 (1993), 247-8.

[154] T. C. Fuller and E. McClintock, *Poisonous plants of California*. (Berkley: University of California Press, 1986), 432. L. M. Hurt, "Avocado Poisoning." *LA. County Livestock Department Annual Report*, (1943), 43-4.

[155] J. A. Duke and E.S. Ayensu, *Medicinal Plants of China* (Algonac, Michigan: Reference Publications, Inc., 1999).

[156] Dioscoridies, *Materia Medica*, 4.19, (1.9).

[157] I. Berendes, Die Arzheimittellchredes Dioskurides (Stuttgart, Enke 2, 1902), 4, 376.

[158] Veronica Rey-Ares, Nickolai Lazarov, Dieter Berg, Ulrike Berg, Lars Kunz, and Artur Mayerhofer, "Dopamine receptor repertoire of human granulosa cells," *Reproductive Biology and Endocrinology* 2007, **5**:40.

[159] John M. Riddle, *Eve's Herbs*, (Cambridge: Harvard University Press, 1997), 58.

[160] Diorscorides, *De Materia medica* 3.7 (2.7).

[161] Avicenna, *Canon*, bk 2, tract. 2, chaps. 5, 6, 50 (Gerard of Cremora trans., 1557 ed., 2, fols. 99V, 102v-103; 1507 ed., fols. 89, 92v).

[162] Abu i-Fadl Dawad ibn Abi i-Bayan al-Isra'ili, *Al-Dustur al-bimaristani fi l-adwiya al-murakkada*, 8.124 (trans. Josè Luis Valverde Carmen Peña Muñoz, in *El formulario de los hospitales de ibn Abi l-Baya* (Granada, 1981), 87.

[163] F. von Defele, Antikonzeptionelle Arzneistoffe 2, 39 (1898).

[164] J. C. Saha, E.C. Savini, and S. Kasinathan, "Ecbolic Properties of Indian Medicinal Plants," *Indian Journal of Medical Research* 49(1961), 130-51.

[165] M.D. Rosenthal, "Effects of Aristolochic Acid on Phospholipase A Activity" *Biochimica et Biophysica Acta* (1989), 1001.

[166] Min Cui, Zhi-Hong Liu, Qi Qiu, Heng Li and Lei-Shi Li, 'Tumour Induction in Rats Following Exposure to Short-Term High Dose Aristolochic Acid I," (Nanjing: Research Institute of Nephrology, Jinling Hospital, Nanjing University School of Medicine, 2002).

[167] Cheung Siu-cheong and Li Ning-hon eds., *Chinese Medicinal Herbs of Hong Kong*, (Hong Kong: Commercial Press, 1978).

[168] G.A. Cooper-Driver, "Chemical substances in plants toxic to animals," *CRC Handbook of Naturally Occurring Food Toxicants*, (CRC Press, Boca Raton, 1983), 213-47.

[169] D. E. Moerman, *Medicinal Plants of Native America* vols. 1-2 (Ann Arbor: University of Michigan, 1986), 121.

[170] B.L. McFarlin, M.H. Gibson, J. O'Rear, and P. Harman, "A National Survey of Herbal Preparation Use by Nurse Midwives for Labor Stimulation. Review of the Literature and Recommendations for Practice." *Journal of Nurse Midwifery* 44 (1999), 205-16.

417

[171] N. Einer-Jensen, J. Zhao, K. P. Andersen, K. Kristoffersen, "Cimicifuga and Melbrosia Lack Oestrogenic Effects in Mice and Rats." *Maturitas* 25 (1996), 149-53.

[172] E. Liske, "Therapeutic Efficacy and Safety of *Cimicifuga racemosa* for Gynecologic Disorders," *Advances in Therapy* 15 (1998), 45-53.

[173] D. Dixon-Shanies, and N. Shaikh, "Growth Inhibition of Human Breast Cancer Cells by Herbs and Phytoestrogens," *Oncology Report* 6 (1999), 1383-7.

[174] H. Jarry, G. Harnischfeger, and E. Duker, "The Endocrine Effects of Constituents of *Cimicifuga racemosa* 2. In Vitro Binding of Constituents to Estrogen Receptors," *Planta Medica* (1985), 316-9.

[175] H. Jarry and G. Harnischfeger, "Endocrine Effects of Constituents of *Cimicifuga racemosa*. 1. The Effect on Serum Levels of Pituitary Hormones in Ovariectomized Rats." *Planta Medica* (1985), 46-9.

[176] D. Joy, J. Joy, and P. Duane, "Black Cohosh: A Cause of Abnormal Postmenopausal Liver Function Tests," *Climacteric* 11, no. 1 (2008), 84-8.

[177] Charles Montgomery Skinner, *Myths and Legends of Flowers, Trees, Fruits, and Plants* (Philedelphia: J.B. Lippincott, 1911), 136.

[178] R. B. Rao and R. S. Hoffman, "Nicotinic Toxicity from Tincture of Blue Cohosh (*Caulophyllum thalcitroides*), Used as an Abortifacient," *Veterinary and Human Toxicology* 44, no. 4 (2002), 221-2.

[179] A. Searpa .and Guerci, "Various Uses of the Castor oil Plant *Ricinus communis L.* A Review." *Journal of Ethnopharmacoly* 5, no. 2, (1982), 117-37.

[180] V.J. Brondegaard, "Contraceptive Plant Drugs." *Planta Medica* 23 (1973), 167-72.

[181] A.A. G. El-Dean Mahmoud, "Study of Indigenous (Folk Ways), Birth Control Methods in Alexandria." (master's thesis-University of Alexandria – Higher Institute of Nursing, 1972).

[182] D. Vitalyos, "Phytotherapy in Domestic Traditional Medicine in Matouba-Papaye (Guadaloupe)." Ph.D. Diss. – University of Paris (1979), 110.

[183] G.W. Harley, *Native African Medicine* (London: Frank Cars & Co. Ltd., 1970).

[184] W.S. Woo, E.B. Lee, K.H. Shin, S.S. Kang and H.S. Chi, "A Review of Research on Plants for Fertility Regulation in Korea." *Korean Journal of Pharmacognosy* 12, no. 3 (1981), 153-70.

[185] J. C. Saha, E.J. Savini and S. Kasinathan, "Ecbolic Properties of Indian Medicinal Plants. Part 1." *Indian Journal of Medicinal Research* 49 (1961), 130-51.

[186] G. Venkataraghavan, M. M. Naidu and M. Mahender, "Haematological Studies: An Experimental Feeding of Castor Bean Meal *(Ricinus communis)*, in Sheep." *Indian Veterinary Journal* 62, no. 5 (1985), 379-82.

[187] Pankaj Oudhia, "Research Note," (2003), http://www.botanical.com/site/column_poudhia/77_gyn.html (accessed April 14, 2008).

[188] S.K. Vedavathy, N. Rao, M. Rajaiah and N. Nagarju, "Folklore Information from Rayalaseema Region, Andhra Pradesh for Family Planning and Birth Control." *International Journal of Pharmacognosy* 29, no. 2 (1991), 113-6.

[189] A. Mathieu, "Observations on the Use of Castor Oil, Quinine, and Pituitary Extract in the Induction of Labor. An Analysis Based on the Study of 320 Consecutive Cases from Private Practice," *Surgery, Gynecology, and Obstetrics* 53 (1931), 676.

[190] M.B. Sahasrabudme, "Estrogen Potency of the Defatted Castor Seed." *Current Science* 14 (1945), 69.

[191] P.C. Feng, L.J. Haynes, K. E. Magnus and J. R. Plimmer, "Further Pharmacological Screening of Some West Indian Medicinal Plants." *Journal of Pharmacy and Pharmacology* 16 (1964), 115.

[192] S.A. Odunfa, "Microbiological and Toxicological Aspects of Fermentation of Castor Oil Seeds for Ogriri Production." *Journal of Food Science* 50, no. 6 (1985), 1758-9.

[193] F.K. Okwuasaba, S.C. Das, C.O. Isichei, M.M. Ekwenchi, and A.O. Olayinka, "Pharmacological Studies on the Antifertility Effects of RICOM-1013-J from Ricinus communis var minor and Preliminary Studies on Women Volunteers." *Phytotherapy Research* 11, no. 8 (1998), 547-51. S.C. Das., C.O. Isichei, F.K. Okuwuasaba, V.E. Uguru, O. Onoruvwe, "Chemical, Pathological, and Toxicological Studies of the Effects of RICOM-1013-J of Ricinus communis var minor on Women Volunteers and Rodents." *Phytotherapy Research* 14, no. 1 (2000), 15-19.

[194] Alexander Henry, *Posological and Therapeutic Tables* (Edinburgh: Maclachlan and Stewart, 1882), 63.

[195] David J. Spoerke Jr., *Herbal Medications* (Santa Barbara: Woodbridge Press, 1980), 168.

419

[196] H.M.A. Razzack, "The Concept of Birth Control in Unani Medicinal Literature," unpublished manuscript (1980), 64. as cited in Ivan A. Ross, *Medicinal Plants of the World: Chemical Constituents, Traditional and Modern Medicinal Uses, vol 2* (Totowa, NJ: Humana Press, 1999), 373.

[197] M. Magid and Wenzkowsky, "Illegal Methods of Abortion," *Dtsch Z Ges Gerichtl* 19 (1932), 501.

[198] Dioscorides, *Materia Medica* I.I03 (2.I-2).

[199] P.G. Merz, C. Gorkow, A. Schrodter, S. Rietbrock, C. Sieder, D. Loew, J.S. Dericks-Tan, and T.D. Taubert, "The Effects of a Special Agnus castus Extract (BP1095E1), on Prolactin Secretion in Healthy Male Subjects," *Experimental and Clinical Endocrinology and Diabetes* 104, no. 6 (1996), 447-53. H. Jarry, S. Leonhardt, C. Gorkow, and W. Wuttke, "In Vitro Prolactin but not LH and FSH Release is Inhibited by Compounds in Extracts of Agnus castus: Direct Evidence for a Dopaminergic Principle by the Dopamine Receptor Assay." *Experimental and Clinical Endocrinology* 102, no. 6 (1994), 448-54.

[200] E. Loch, et al, "Diagnosis and Treatment of Dyshormonal Menstrual Periods in the General Practice," *Gynakol Praxis* 14, no. 3 (1990), 489-95. D. Roeder, "Therapy of Cyclical Disorders with *Vitex agnus castus*," *Zeiterschrift fur Phytotherapie* 15, no. 3 (1994), 157-63

[201] N. Ando, I. Gorai, and T. Hirabuki. *et al.*, "Prolactin Disorders in Patients with Habitual Abortion," *Nippon Sanka Fujinka Gakkai Zasshi* 44 (1994), 650–56.

[202] Micheal A. Weiner, *Earth Medicine – Earth Food*, (NewYork: Maximillian, 1972), 11.

[203] Louis Bouton, *Plantes Médicinales de Maurice*, 13 (Port-Louis: Dupuy et Dubois, 1864).

[204] Charles R. Eckler, "A Contribution to the Pharmacology of Cotton Root Bark," *American Journal of Pharmacology* (May, 1920), 285.

[205] Mark D. Groover and Timothy E. Baumann, "They Worked Their Own Remedy: African-American Herbal Medicine and the Archeological Record," *South Carolina Antiquities 28* (1996), 24-25.

[206] James A. Duke, *Handbook of Medicinal Plants* (Boca Raton: CRC Press, 1985), 219.

[207] American Pharmaceutical Association, National Pharmaceutical Convention, American Pharmaceutical Association Meeting, 1866.

[208] Kee Chang Huang, *The Pharmacology of Chinese Herbs* (Boca Raton: CRC Press, 1993), 257.

209 S.K. Garg, S.K. Saksena, and R.R. Chaudhury, "Antifertility Screening of Plants. VI. Effect of Five Indigenous Plants on Early Pregnancy in Albino Rats," *Indian Journal of Medical Research* 58, no. 9 (1970), 1285-9.

210 G. A. Conway and J.C. Slocumb, "Plants used as Abortifacients and Emmenagogues by Spanish New Mexicans," *Journal of Ethnopharmacology* 1, no. 3 (1979), 241-61.

211 James A. Duke, *Handbook of Medicinal Plants* (Boca Raton: CRC Press, 1985), 219.

212 Carl Djerassi, *Politics of Contraception* (New York: W.H. Freeman & Co., Ltd., 1982), *302-4*.

213 Susan S. Weed, *Wise Woman Herbal for the Childbearing Year* (New York: Ash Tree Publishing, 1986), 11.

214 L. H. Peng, *Advances in Chinese Medicinals Materials Research* (Singapore/ Philadelphia: World Scientific Publishing Co., 1985), 639-45.

215 Judy Krizmanic, "How Green are your Garments?" *Vegetarian Times* (November 1992), 16.

216 Unesco, *Impact of Science on Society*, vol. 34-35 (1984-1985), 316.

217 Dioscorides, *Materia Medica*, 4.172 (3.4), cf. 4.170 (4.8-9).

218 C.R. Wang, H.Z. Huang, and R.S. Xu, "Studies on the Active Principals of the Root Yuanhua. Isolation and Structure of Yuanhua Fine," *Acta Chimica Sinica* 40 (1982), 835-9.

219 Y. Ma, H. Liu, S. Qu, X. Qiu, Y. Zhang, Y. Ding, and Y. Wei, "Effect of Yuanhua on Isolated Uterine Strips in Unpregnant Rats", *Zhongguo Zhong Yao Za Zhi* 23 (Lanzhou: Lanzhou Medical College 1998), 429-30.

220 C.R. Wang, Z.X. Chen, B.P. Ying. B.N. Zhou. J.S. Liu, and B.C. Pan, "Studies on the Active Principles of the Root of Yuan-Hua (*Daphne Genjwa*), Isolation and Structure of a New Antifertilite Diterpene Yuanhuadine," *Acta Chemica Sinica* 39, no. 5 (1981), 421-6.

221 Hubei College of Traditional Chinese Medicine, New Medical Communications (Hubei College of Traditional Chinese medicine), No. 1 (1974), 21.

222 89th Hospital of the Chinese PLA, "Summary of 100 cases of abortion induced by *Daphne genkwa.*" No. 1 (1974).

223 Zhu You-Ping Zhu, *Chinese Materia Medica: Chemistry, Pharmacology, and Applications* (Boca Raton, FL: CRC Press, 1998), 243. Hsun-Moo

Chang and Paul Pui-Hay But, *Pharmacology and Applications of Chinese Materia Medica* (World Scientific, 2001), 527.

[224] Y.G. Liang, "Morphological Observations of Placenta in 56 Cases of Mid-term Abortion Induced by Yuanhua Preparations," *Zhonghua Fu Chan Ke Za Zhi.* 14, no.4 (1979), 290-2. "Clinical Observations on 201 cases of Mid-term Abortion Induced by Yuanhuacine," *Zhonghua Fu Chan Ke Za Zhi.* 14, no. 4 (1979),287-9. (Chinese). X. M. Zhang, C.M. Wang, Y.H. Cen, H.S. Huo, J.Y. Ba, Z.T. Liu, and X.Q. Zhang, "Clinical Observation and Preliminary Study of Termination of Early Pregnancy by Administration of Yellow Daphne," *Shengzhi Yu Biyun* 4, no. 4,(Nov 1984), 42-6.

[225] Nancy J. Turner and Adam F. Szczawinski. *Common Poisonous Plants and Mushrooms of North America* (Portland, OR: Timber Press, 2003).

[226] I. H. Hall, R. Kasai, R. Y. Wu, K. Tagahara, K. H. Lee, "Antitumor Agents LV: Effects of Genkwadaphnin and Yuanhuacine on Nucleic Acid Synthesis of P-388 Lymphocytic Leukemia Cells," *Journal of Pharmaceutical Sciences* vol. 71, no. 11 (Sep 2006), 1263 – 7.

[227] Dioscorides, *Materia Medica,* 3.121 (2.5-6), 3-32 (1.7).

[228] E. F. Steinmetz. *Materia Medica Vegetabilis* 1 (Holland, 1954), 504.

[229] Eucharius Rösslin, *The Byrth of Mankynd, Otherwise Named the Womans Boke* (London: 1552), 137-41.

[230] International Plant Genetic Resources Institute (May 8-10 1996), CIHEAM, Vallezano-Bari, Italy.

[231] L.J. Harris, *The Book of Garlic* (New York: Holt, Rinehart, and Winston, 1975), 9.

[232] E. von Strubling, "Garlic in Ancient Times: A Contribution to the Dietetics and Nutrition of Man," *Ernahrunsforschang* 12 (1967), 591.

[233] L.J. Harris, *The Book of Garlic* (New York: Holt, Rinehart, and Winston, 1975), 21.

[234] Barbara G. Walker, *The Woman's Encyclopedia of Myths and Secrets* (SanFrancisco: Harper and Row, 1983), 158.

[235] J. Bachofen, *Myth, Religion, and Mother Right* (New Jersey: Princeton University Press, 1967), 192.

[236] L.J. Harris, *The Book of Garlic* (New York: Holt, Rinehart, and Winston, 1975), 85.

[237] Ibid., 10.

[238] S. Angus, *The Mystery-Religions,* (NewYork: Dover, 1975), 173.

[239] T.B. Criss and J.P. Markum, "A Lunar Effect on Fertility," *Social Biology* 28, nos. 1-2 (1981), 75-80.

[240] Sir E. A. Wallis Budge, *Gods of the Egyptians* (NewYork: Dover, 1969), 196.

[241] Harry E. Wedeck, *A Treasury of Witchcraft* (Secaucus, New Jersey: Citadel, 1975), 203.

[242] David Pickering, *Cassell's Dictionary of Superstitions* (New York: Sterling Publishing, 2003), 211.

[243] R. C. D. Casey, "Alleged Anti-fertility Plants of India," *Indian Journal of Medical Sciences* 14 (1960), 594. J. C. Saha, E. C. Savini, and S.Kasinthan, "Ecbolic Properties of Indian Medicinal Plants," *Indian Journal of Medical Research* 49 (1961), 131.

[244] H. Hikino, K. Aota, and T. Takemoto, "Structure and Absolute Configuration of Cyperotundone," *Chemical Pharmocology Bulletin* 14 (1966), 890.

[245] V. P. Kamboj, "A Review of Indian Medicinal Plants with Interceptive Activity," *Indian Journal of Medical Research* 4 (1988), 336-55.

[246] G. F. Asprey and P. Thorton, "Medicinal Plants of Jamaica, Part I, "*West Indian Medical Journal* 2, no.4 (1953), 233-52.

[247] C. H. Browner, "Plants used for Reproductive Health in Oaxaca, Mexico," *Economic Botany* 39, no.4 (1985), 482-504.

[248]A. Sharaf, "Food Plants as a Possible Factor in Fertility Control,"*Qualitas Plantarum et Materiae Vegetabiles* 17 (1969), 153.

[249] X. Xu, S.I. Cho, M. Sammel, L. You, S. Cui, Y. Huang, G. Ma, C. Padungtod, L. Pothier, T. Niu, D. Christiani, T. Smith, L. Ryan and L. Wang, "Association of Petrochemical Exposure with Spontaneous Abortion," *Occupational and Environmental Medicine* 55 (1998), 31-6.

[250] Y. X. Qian, "Spermicidal Effect in Vitro by the Active Principle of Garlic," *Contraception* 34 (1986), 295-302.

[251] Hippocrates, *Of Female Diseases. Hippocrates, The Writings of Hippocrates and Galen Book 1, LXXXV,* trans. John Redman Coxe (1846).

[252] James A. Duke, *The Green Pharmacy* (Emmaus, PA: Rodale, 1997), 329.

[253] J. M. Wilkinson, "Effect of Ginger Tea on the Fetal Development of Sprague-Dawley Rats," *Reproductive Toxicology* 14 (2000), 507–12.

[254] G. Dragendorff, *Die Heilpflanzen der Verschiedenen* (Enke, Stuttgart, Volker und Zeiten, 1898), 885.

[255] M.K. Alam,"Medicinal Ethnobotany of the Marma Tribe of Bangladesh." *Econonic Botany* 46, no.3 (1992), 330-5.

[256] V.R. Ramirez, L.J. Mostacero, A.E. Garcia, C.F. Mesia, P.F. Pelaez, C.D. Medina and C.H. Miranda, *Vegetales empleados en Medicina*

Tradicional Noreruana (Truillo, Peru: Banco Agrario del Peru & Nacl Univ Truillo, June 1988), 54.

257 I.H. Burkhill, *Dictionary of the Economic Products of the Malay Peninsula1* (Kuala Lumpur, Malaysia: Ministry of Agriculture and Cooperatives, 1966).

258 D.K. Holdsworth, "Medicinal Plants of Papua-New Guinea," *Technical Paper No. 175*, (Naumea, New Caledonia: South Pacifiic Commission, 1977).

259 S.K. Sharma and V.P. Singh, "The Antifungal Activity of some essential Oils." *Indian Drugs Pharm Ind* (1979), 14 (1), 3-6.

260 I.H. Burkhill, *Dictionary of the Economic Products of the Malay Penisula1* (Kuala Lumpur, Malaysia: Ministry of Agriculture and Cooperatives, 1966).

261 Pankaj Oudhia, "Traditional Medicinal Knowledge about Common Herbs Used for Abortion in Chhattisgarh, India," Research Note 10. http://www.botanical.com/site/column_poudhia/388_abortion.html (accessed November 16, 2007).

262 J.A. Murray, *The Plants and Drugs of Sind: Being a Systematic Account, with Descriptions, of the Indigenous Flora* (London: Richardson and Co. 1881).

263 Edward Bancroft, *An Essay on the Natural History of Guinan in South America* (London, 1769), 52.

264 Joseph E. Holloway, ed., *Africanisms in American Culture* (Indianapolis: Indiana University Press, 2005), 46.

265 M.P. Singh, H. Singh and K.N. Vovpa, "Antifertility Activity of Benzene Extract of *Hibiscus rosa-sinensis* Flowers in Female Albino Rats." *Planta Medica* 44 (1982), 171-4.

266 A.O. Prakash, "Glycogen Contents in the Rat Uterus: Response to Hibiscus rosa-sinensis Linn. Extracts." *Experientia 35, no. 8* (Aug 15, 1979), 1122-3.

267 S.D. Kholkute and K.N. Udupa, "Effects of *Hibiscus rosa- sinensis* on Pregnancy of Rats." *Planta Medica* 29(1976), 321-9. S.D. Kholkute, V. Mudgal, and P.J. Deshpande, "Screening of Indigenous Medicinal Plants for Antiferitlity Potentiality. *Planta Medica 29* (1976), 151-5. S.D. Kholkute, D. N. Srivastava, S. Chatterjee and K.N. Udupa, "Effects of Some Compounds Isolated from *Hibiscus rosa-sinensis* on Pregnancy in Rats. " *Journal of Research in Indian Medicine, Yoga, & Homeopathy* 11 (1976), 106-8.

424

[268] P.V. Tiwari, "Preliminary Clinical Trial on Flowers of *Hibiscus rosa-sinensis* as an Oral Contraceptive Agent," *Journal of Research in Indian Medicine, Yoga, & Homeopathy* 9, no.4 (1974), 96-8.

[269] V.R. Ramirez, L.J. Mostacero, A.E. Garcia, C.F. Mesia, P.F. Pelaez, C.D. Medina and C.H. Miranda, "Vegetales Empleados en Medicina Tradicional Noreruana Banco Agrario del Peru & Nacl Univ Trujillo," *Truillo* – Peru (June 1988), 54.

[270] Endang Purwaningsih, "The Effect of the Administration of *Hibiscus rosa-sinensis*, L Flower Extract on the Spermatogenetic Process in Strain AJ Male Mouse," *Jurnal Kedokteran Yarsi t 2*(2001), 21-9.

[271] S.D. Kholkute, S. Chatterjee, D.N. Srivastava and K.N. Udupa, "Effect of *Hibiscus rosa-sinensis* on the Reproductive Organs Of Male Rats." *Journal of Reproduction and Fertility* 38 (1974), 233-4.

[272] Pliny the Elder, *Natural History*, Book 20, xii

[273] Paul B. Hamel and Mary U. Chiltoskey, *Cherokee Plants and Their Uses - A 400 Year History* (Sylva, N.C.: Herald Publishing, 1975), 39.

[274] Jean Pulaiseul, *Grandmother's Secrets* (New York: G. P. Putnam's Sons, 1974), 147.

[275] Christian Ratsch, *The Dictionary of Sacred and Magical Plants* (Santa Barbara: ABC-CLIO, 1992), 102.

[276] Daniel E. Moerman, *Medicinal Plants of Native America*, Vols. 1-2 (Ann Arbor: University of Michigan, 1986), 248.

[277] Christian Ratsch, *The Dictionary of Sacred and Magical Plants*, (Santa Barbara: ABC-CLIO, 1992), 67.

[278] Joseph Kadans, *Encyclopedia of Medicinal Herbs* (New York: Arco Pub., 1972), 139.

[279] P. H. List and L. Horhammer, *Hager's Handbuch der Pharmazeutischen Praxis*, Vol 2-6 (Berlin: Springer, 1969-79), 256.

[280] John M. Riddle, *Contraception and Abortion from the Ancient World to the Renaissance*, (Cambridge: Harvard, 1992), 36.

[281] Anand O. Prakash, "Pontentialities of Some Indigenous Plants for Antifertility Activity," *International Journal of Crude Drug Research* 24 (1986), 22.

[282] "Final Report on the Safety Assessment of *Juniperus communis* Extract, *Juniperus oxycedrus* Extract, *Juniperus oxycedrus* Tar, *Juniperus phoenicea* Extract, and *Juniperus virginiana* Extract," *International Journal of Toxicology*, 20, Supplement 2 (2001), 41-56.

283 Dale R. Gardner, Kip E. Panter, and Lynn F. James, "Pine Needle Abortion in Cattle: Metabolism of Isocupressic Acid," *Journal of Agricultural and Food Chemistry* 47, no. 7 (1999), 2891 -7.

284 David G. Spoerke Jr., *Herbal Medications* (Santa Barbara: Woodbridge, 1980), 102.

285 Penelope Ody, *The Complete Medicinal Herbal* (New York: Dorling Kindersley, 1993), 72.

286 Jean Palaiseul, *Grandmother's Secrets* (New York: G.P. Putnam's Sons, 1974), 148.

287 Dioscorides, *De Materia Medica*, 2.109 (I.7-8).

288 Soranus, *Gynecology*, trans. Owsei Temkin (Baltimore: The John Hopkins University Press, 1991), 1.69 - 67.

289 Martin Levey and Noury al-Khaledy, *The Medical Formulary of al-Samarqandi, and the Relation of Early Arabic Simples to those found in the Indigenous Medicine of the Near East* (University of Pennsylvania Press, 1967) 66-67, 85-87.

290 A. Sharaf, "Food Plants as a Possible Factor in Fertility Control," *Plant Foods for Human Nutrition* 17, no.2 (1969), 153-60.

291 M. Mazur, P. Polakowski, and A. Szadowska, *Acta Physiologia Polonica* 17 (1996), 299-309.

292 R.F. Keeler, "Quinolizidine Alkaloids in Range and Grain Lupins." *Toxicants of Plant Origin* (Boca Raton, Fl: CRC Press, 1989).

293 A. M. Davis and D. M. Stout, " Anagyrine in Western American Lupines," *Journal of Range Management* 39 (1986), 29-30.

294 Australia New Zealand Food Authority, "Lupin Alkaloids in Food," Technical Report Series No.3. (2001).

295 G. Rotiroti, I. Skypala, G. Senna, and G. Passalacqua, "Anaphylaxis Due to Lupine Flour in a Celiac Patient," *Journal of Investigational Allergology & Clinical Immunology*, 17 (2007), 204-205.

296 Christina Hole, *Saints in Folklore* (New York: M. Barrows and Co. Inc., 1965), 137.

297 Charles Montgomery Skinner, *Myths and Legends of Flowers, Trees, Fruits, and Plants* (Philedelphia: J.B. Lippincott, 1911), 109.

298 Jean Pulaiseul, *Grandmother's Secrets*. (New York: G. P. Putnams's Sons, 1974), 176.

299 L. Lewin, *Die Fruchtabtreibung*, (1922), 216, 218.

300 David G. Spoerke Jr., *Herbal Medications* (Santa Barbara: Woodbridge, 1980), 113.

[301] Daniel E. Moerman, *Medicinal Plants of Native America*, vols. 1-2, (Ann Arbor: University of Michigan, 1986), 334.

[302] V. K. Chestnut, "Plants used by the Indians of Mendocino County, California," *The U.S. National Herbarium 7, no. 3* (1902), 344, 367.

[303] Christian Ratsch, *The Dictionary of Sacred and Magical Plants* (Santa Barbara: ABC-CLIO, 1992), 119.

[304] Robert W. Pelton, *The Complete Book of Voodoo* (New York: Putnam, 1972), 218, 221.

[305] K. Kelles, R. Hanser, and R.F. Chandler, eds., "Phoradendron Flavescens," *DeSmet PAGM : Adverse Effects of Herbal Drugs* 3, (1992-1997), 99-103.

[306] J. Bruneton, (C.K. Hatton, trans.), *Pharmacognosy, Phytochemistry, Medicinal Plants.* 2nd ed. (Andover, UK: Intercept Ltd; 1999).

[307] Christian Ratsch, *The Dictionary of Sacred and Magical Plants* (Santa Barbara: ABC-CLIO, 1992), 119.

[308] Emilè Male, *The Gothic Image*, (New York: Harper and Row, 1958), 153.

[309] Bertram S. Puckle, *Funeral Customs* (London: T. Werner Laurie Ltd., 1926), *116*.

[310] Micheal Castleman, *The Healing Herbs* (Emmaus: Rodale, 1991), 260.

[311] In March is a Celtic feast, called Ostara, celebrating the spring equinox. " Nettles in March" may have been considered a spring tonic. Around the first of May is the ancient Celtic holiday of Beltane, a sexual celebration where couples went to the newly plowed fields to lay down together and copulate in order to ensure the fertility of the coming years' crops. "Muggins in May" would have prevented pregnancy and reduced maternal mortality.

[312] Barbara G. Walker, *The Womans's Encyclopedia of Myths and Secrets* (San Francisco: Harper and Row, 1983), 58-60.

[313] Ibid., 233.

[314] Jean Pulaiseul, *Grandmother's Secrets* (New York: G. P. Putnam's Sons, 1974), 191.

[315] Penelope Ody, *The Complete Medicinal Herbal* (New York: Kindersley, 1993), 39.

[316] Barbara G.Walker, *The Womans's Encyclopedia of Myths and Secrets* (San Francisco: Harper and Row, 1983), 1091.

[317] Ibid., 281.

[318] Christian Ratsch, *The Dictionary of Sacred and Magical Plants* (Santa Barbara: ABC-CLIO, 1992), 56.

319 Ibid., 57.

320 Melvin R. Gilmore, "Some Native Nebraska Plants with Their Uses by the Dakota." *Collections of the Nebraska State Historical Society* 17(1913), 369.

321 James A. Duke, *Handbook of Medicinal Plants,* (Boca Raton: CRC Press, 1985), 69-70.

322Macolm Stuart, ed., *Herbs and Herbalism* (New York: Nostrand Reinhold, 1979), 31.

323 Elide A. Pastorello , Valerio Pravettoni, Laura Farioli, Frederica Rivolta, Amedeo Conti, Marco Ispano, Donatella Fortunato Donatella, Anders Bengtsson, and Matilde Bianchi, "Hypersensitivity to Mugwort (*Artemisia vulgaris*), in Patients with Peach Allergy is due to a Common Lipid Transfer Protein Allergen and is often without Clinical Expression," *Journal of Allergy and Clinical Immunology* 110, no.2 (2002), 310-7.

324 R.C. Green, "Nutmeg Poisoning" *Journal of the American Medical Association* 171, no. 10 (1959), 1342-4.

325 Walter Stanley Haines, *A Text-book of Legal Medicine and Toxicology* (W.B. Saunders, 1904), 93.

326 Kahun Papyrus, Section 3, paragraphs 26-32.

327Ebers Papyrus, [828].

328 Ibid.,[802].

329 W. Jochle, "Menses-inducing drugs: Their role in antique, medieval, and renaissance gynecology and birth control." *Contraception* 10 (1974), 425-39.

330 J. C. Saha and Kasinathan, "Ecbolic Properties of Indian Medicinal Plants - Part II." *Indian Journal of Medical Research* 49 (1961), 1094 - 8.

331 A. Petelot, "Les Plantes Medicinales du Chamboge du Laos et du Vietnam. Vols. 1-4." Archives des Recherches Agronomiques et Pastorales au Vietnam. No. 23 (1954).

332 R.N. Chopra, *Indigenous Drugs of India: Their Medicinal and Economic Aspects* (Calcutta, India: The Art Press, 1933), 550.

333M. Magid and M. Wenzkowsky, "Illegal Methods of Abortion." *Deutsche Zeitschrift fur die Gesamte Gerichtliche* 19(1932), 501+.

334A.A.G.el-Dean Mahmoud, "Study of Indigenous (Folk-ways), Birth Control Methods in Alexandria." Thesis-MS- Univ of Alexandria. Higher Inst of Nursing, 1972.

335H.M.A. Razzack, "The Concept of Birth Control in Unani Medical Literature," unpublished manuscript (1980), 64. as cited in Ivan A.

Ross, *Medicinal Plants of the World: Chemical Constituents, Traditional and Modern Medicinal Uses,* vol. 2 (Totowa, NJ: Humana Press, 1999), 64.

[336] Kathleen London, "The History of Birth Control." *The Changing American Family: Historical and Comparative Perspectives* (Yale University, 1982). http://www.yale.edu/ynhti/curriculum/units/1982/6/82.06.03.x.html (accessed March 16, 2008).

[337] S.A.Younis and E.G. Hagâp, "Preliminary Studies on the Red Onion Scaly Leaves: Abortive Action and Effects on Serum Enzymes in Mice," *Fitoterapia* 59, no.1 (1988), 21-4.

[338] K.C. Srivastava, "Aqueous Extracts of Onion, Garlic, and Ginger Inhibited Platelet Aggregation and Alter Arachidonic Acid Metabolism," *Biomedica Biochimica Acta* 43, no. 8-9(1984), 335-46.

[339] A. Sharaf, "Food Plants as a Possible Factor in Fertility Control," *Qualitas Plantarum Et Materiae Vegetabiles* 17(1969),153-. As cited in Ivan A. Ross, *Medicianl Plants of the World: Chemical Constituents, Traditional and Modern Medicinal Uses.* vol. 1 (Totowa, NJ: Humana Press, 1999), 78.

[340] H. Kreitmair, "Pharmacological Trials with Some Domestic Plants," *E Mereck's Jahresber* 50 (1936), 102-10.

[341] E.G. Ferro-Luzzi, "Food avoidance of pregnant women in Tamil Nadu. In Food, Ecology and Culture: Readings in the Anthropology of Dietary Practices," *Food, Ecology, and Culture* [John, RK Robson, editor] (New York, NY: Gordon and Breach Science Publishers, 1980), 101 - 8.

[342] R.C.F. Maughan, *Portugeuese East Africa: The History, Scenery, and Great Game of Maneca and Sofala* (London: Murray, 1906), 271.

[343] E. Quisumbing, "Medicinal Plants of the Phillipines," *Technical Bulletin* 16 (Manila: Dept. Natural Resources, 1951), 1.

[344] R. N. Chopra, R. L. Badhwar and S. Ghosh, "Poisonous Plants of India," *Manager of Publications.* 1 (Calcutta: Government of India Press, 1949).

[345] E. Quisumbing, "Medicinal Plants of the Phillipines," *Technical Bulletin* 16, (Manila: Dept. Natural Resources, 1951), 1.

[346] R.R. Rao and N.S. Jamir, "Ethnobotanical Studies in Nagaland, I . Medicinal Plants," *Economic Botany* (1982), 36:176-181.

[347] James Duke, *Amazonian Ethnobotanical Dictionary* (Boca Raton, FL: CRC Press, 1994), 42.

[348] T.S. Tang, "Macrocyclic Piperdine and Piperidine Alkaloids in *Carica papaya,"Tropical Foods Chemistry and Nutrition* 1 (1979), 55-68.

349 B. Vasileva, *Plantes Medicinales de Guinee* (Conarky, Republique, 1969).

350 G. Bourdy and A. Walter, "Maternity and Medicinal Plants in Vanuatu: The Cycle of Reproduction," *Journal of Ethnopharmacology* 37, no.3, (1992), 179-96.

351 V. P. Kamboj, "A Review of Indian Medicinal Plants with Interceptive Activity," *Indian Journal of Medical Research* 4 (1988), 336-55.

352 M. Gopalakrishnan and M. R. Rajekharasetty, "Effect of Papaya *(Carica Papaya)*, on Pregnancy and Estrous Cycle in Albino Rats of Wistar Strain," *Indian J Physical Pharmacol* 22 (1978), 66-70.

353 S. L. Bodhankar, S.K. Garg, and V.S. Mathur, "Antifertility Screening of Plants. Part IX. Effect of Five Indigenous Plants on Early Pregnancy in Female Albino Rats," *Indian Journal of Medical Research* 62 (1974), 831-7.

354 K.N. Sareen, N. Mistra, D.R. Varma, M.K.P. Amma, and M.L. Gujral, "Oral Contraceptives v. Anthelmintics as Antifertility Agents," *Indian Journal of Physiology and Pharmacology* 5 (1961), 125-35.

355 CFSAN/Office of Premarket Approval, FDA Biotechnology Consultation, BNF No. 000042, September 12, 1997. http://www.cfsan.fda.gov/~rdb/bnfm042.html(accessed November 23, 2007).

356 Thomas Cherian, "Effect of Papaya Latex on Gravid and Non-Gravid Rat Uterine Preparations in Vitro," *Journal of Ethnopharmacology* 70, no. 3 (July 15 2000), 205-12.

357 J. F. Morton. *Major Medicinal Plants* (Springfield, IL, USA: C.C. Thomas, 1977).

358 L.D. Kapoor, *Handbook of Ayurvedic Medicinal Plants* (Boca Raton, FL, USA:CRC Press, 2001), 100.

359 Kerharo and Bouquet, *Plantes Medicinales et Toxiques de la Cote-D'ivoire - Haute-Volta.* (Paris: Vigot Freres, 1950), 41–42. B. Oliver, "Medicinal plants in Nigeria." Nigerian College of Arts, Science and Technology 5, no. 52 (1960), 21.

360 Nakamura Y, Morimitsu Y, Uzu T, et al., "A Glutathione S-Transferase Inducer from Papaya: Rapid Screening, Identification, and Structure-Activity Relationship of Isothiocyanates." *Cancer Letters* 157(2000), 193-200.

361http://www.thaitable.com/Thai/recipes/Green_Papaya_Salad.htm (accessed November 23, 2007).

[362] Nina L. Etkin, *Plants in Indigenous Medicine and Diet: Biobehavioral Approaches* (Routledge 1986), 45.

[363] Paul of Aegina (Paulus Aegineta), *Libri medicorum* (Heiberg ed., I:276.), 3.61.5.26-28.

[364] Paul B. Hamel and Mary U. Chiltoskey, *Cherokee plants and their Uses: A 400 Year History* (Sylva, NY: Herald Publishing, 1975), 47.

[365] Joret and Homolle, *Jour. Pharm. Chim.*, (1855), 212.

[366] Edward Shorter, *Women's Bodies: A Social History of Women's Encounter with Health, III.* (New York: Basic Books, 1982), 220.

[367] Ibid., 219.

[368] Ibid.

[369] A. Austregesilo, "Acute Neuromyelitis," *The Journal of Nervous and Mental Disease*, 83, no. 3 (1936), 343.

[370] J. F. Morton, *Atlas of Medicinal Plants of Middle America.* (Springfield, IL: C.C. Thomas. 1981), 650.

[371] Tsonev, I., L. Rainova & M. Penova, "Concerning the Uterine Effect of Parsley, Petroselinum Sativum. II." *Farmatsiya* (Sofia, 1967), 17, 39.

[372] James A. Duke, *The Green Pharmacy* (Emmaus, PA, USA:Rodale, 1997), 362.

[373] E. S. Kryzhanovskaya, "Effect of Flavoring Substances on the Bodies of Pregnant and Nursing Women," *Voprosy Pitania* 6 (1970), 130.

[374] M. Blumenthal, ed., *The Complete German Commission E Monographs: Therapeutic Guide to Herbal Medicines* (Austin, TX, USA:. American Botanical Council, 1998).

[375] R. Ovcharov and S. Todorov, "[The Effect of Vitamin C on the Estrus Cycle and Embryogenesis of Rats]" (in Bulgarian). *Akusherstvo i ginekologiïa* 13, no. 3 (1974), 191-5. J.S. Vobecky, J. Vobecky, D. Shapcott, D. Cloutier, R. Lafond, and R. Blanchard, "Vitamins C and E in Spontaneous Abortion". *International Journal for Vitamin and Nutrition Research. Internationale Zeitschrift für Vitamin- und Ernährungsforschung. Journal international de vitaminologie et de nutrition* 46, no.3 (1976), 291-6.

[376] Nina Lilian Etkin, Carole H. Browner, Bernard R. Ortiz De Montellano, Memory Elvin-Lewis, James A. Duke, Robert T. Trotter, Michael H. Logan, Maurice M. Iwu, Anne Fleuret, Dale E.

Hammerschmidt, *Plants in Indigenous Medicine and Diet: Biobehavioral Approaches* (New York: Routledge, 1986), 40.

[377] David M. Friedman, *A Mind of Its Own: A Cultural History of the Penis* (New York: Penguin Books, 2001), 28.

[378] James A. Duke, *Handbook of Medicinal Plants* (Boca Raton: CRC Press, 1985), 307.

[379] Micheal A. Weiner, *Earth Medicine – Earth Food* (New York: Maxmillian, 1972), 13.

[380] Daniel E. Moerman, *Medicinal Plants of Native America,* vols. 1-2, (Ann Arbor: University of Michigan, 1986), 215.

[381] Malcolm Stuart ed., *Herbs and Herbalism* (New York: Nostrand Reinhold, 1979), 93.

[382] Susan S. Weed, *Wise Woman Herbal for the Childbearing Year* (Woodstock: Ash Tree Publishing, 1986), 8.

[383] J. A. Goyco, "A Study of the Relation between the Liver Protein Regeneration Capacity and the Hepatic Necrogenic Activity of Yeast Proteins," *Journal of Nutrition* 58, no. 3 (March 1956), 299-308.

[384] John M. Riddle, *Contraception and Abortion from the Ancient World to the Renaissance* (Cambridge: Harvard Press,1992), 54. Micheal Castleman, *The Healing Herbs* (Emmaus: Rodale, 1991), 289.

[385] D.W. Buechel, "Pennyroyal Oil Ingestion: Report of a Case," *Journal American Osteopath Association* 2 (1983), 793-4.

[386] J. C. Saha and S. Kasinathan, "Ecbolic Properties of Indian Medicinal Plants Part II," *Indian Journal of Medical Research* 49 (1961), 1094-8.

[387] Ibid.

[388] Y. N. Singh, "Traditional Medicine in Fiji: Some Herbal Folk Cures used by Fiji Indians," *Ethnopharmacology* 15, no.1 (1986), 57-8.

[389] E. S. Ayensu, *Medicinal Plants of the West Indies,* (unpublished manuscript 1978), 110. As cited in Ivan A. Ross, *Medicinal Plants of the World: Chemical Constituents, Traditional and Modern Medicinal Uses,* Vol . 2 ,(Totowa, NJ: Humana Press, 1999), 52.

[390] G. Dragendorff, *Die Heilpflanzen der Verschiedenen Volker und Zeiten,* (Stuttgart: F. Enke, 1898), 885.

[391] Ibid.

[392] G. E. Simpson, "Folk Medicine in Trinidad," *Journal of American Folklore* 75 (1962), 326-40.

[393] Mulyto, "Effects of *Ananas comosos* L. Fruits on Pregnant Mice," Thesis – MS-FAC Biol Univ Jenderal Soedirman Indonesia, 1986. As

cited in Ivan A. Ross, *Medicinal Plants of the World: Chemical Constituents, Traditional and Modern Medicinal Uses,* Vol . 2 (Totowa, NJ: Humana Press, 1999), 52.

[394] S. X. Garg, S. K. Soksena, and R. R. Chaudhury, "Antifertility Screening of Plants.Part VI. Effect of Five Indigenous Plants on Early Pregnancy in Albino Rats," *Indian Journal of Medical Research* 58 (1970), 1285-9.

[395] S. D. Feurt and L. E. Fox, "Report on Wax from Several Species of Tillandesia and from *Ananas comosus,*" *Science* (1955), 121.

[396] A. O. Prakash and R. Mathur, "Screening of Indian Plants for Antifertility Activity," *Indian Journal of Expimental Biology* 14 (1976), 623-6.

[397] J. Morton, *Fruits of Warm Climates.* (Creative Resource Systems, Inc., 1987), 18-28.

[398] Bible, 2 Kings 5:18.

[399] Barbara G. Walker, *Woman's Encyclopedia of Myths and Secrets* (San Francisco, CA, USA: Harper and Row, 1983), 646.

[400] R.M.A. Razzack, "The Concept of Birth Control in Unami Medical Literature," unpublished manuscript, (1980), 64. As cited in: Ivan A. Ross, *Medicinal Plants of the World: Chemical Constituents, Traditional and Modern Medicinal Uses,* vol . 2, (Totowa, NJ: Humana Press, 1999), 64.

[401] S. Venkataraghavan and T.P. Sundaresan, "A Short Note on Contraceptive in Ayurveda," *Journal of Scientific Research in Plants & Medicines* 2½ (1981), 39.

[402] J.M. Watt and M.G. Breyer-Brandwyk, *The Medicinal and Poisonous Plants of Southern and Eastern Africa, 2nd Ed,* (London: E.S. Livingstone, Ltd., 1962).

[403] Ibid.

[404] B.N. Dhawan and P.N. Saxena, "Evaluation of some Indigenous Drugs for Stimulant Effect on the Rat Uterus , A Preliminary Report," *Indian Journal Medical Research* 46, no. 6 (1958), 808-11.

[405] Danny A. van Elswijk, Uwe p. Schobel, Ephraim P. Lansky, Hubertus Irth, Jan van der Greef, "Rapid Dereplication of Estrogenic Compounds in Pomegranate (*Punica Granatum*), Using On-Line Biochemical Detection Coupled to Mass Spectrometry," *Phytochemistry* 65, no.2 (2004), 233-41.

[406] A. Sharaf and S.A.R. Nigm, "The Oestrogenic activity of Pomegranate Seed Oil," *Journal Endrocrinology* 29 (1964), 91.

407 A. Sharaf, "Food Plants as a Possible Factor in Fertility Control," *Plant Foods for Human Nutrition* 17, no. 2 (Netherlands, Springer, 1969), 153-60.

408 Y.S. Shubert, E.P. Lansky and I. Neeman, "Antioxidant and Eicosanoid Enzyme Inhibition Properties of Pomegranate Seed Oil and Fermented Juice Flavanoids," *Journal of Enthnopharmacology* 66, no. 1(1999), 11-7.

409 A. Sharaf, "Food Plants as a Possible Factor in Fertility Control," *Plant Foods for Human Nutrition* 17, no.2 (Netherlands, Springer, 1969), 153-60.

410 William Andrew Chatto, *Facts and Speculations on the Origin and History of Playing Cards* (London: John Russell Smith, 1848), 226.

411 Barbara G. Walker, *Woman's Dictionary of Symbols and Sacred Objects.* (HarperOne, 1988), 201-2.

412 Ibid., 218-220.

413 Ibid., 786.

414 Ibid., 366, 804.

415 Edith Hamilton, *Timeless Gods and Heroes* (Boston: Little Brown and Co., 1940), 236.

416 Alan E.Simmons, *Growing Unusual Fruit* (New York: Walker and Co., 1972), 284.

417 David G. Spoerke Jr., *Herbal Medications* (Santa Barbara, CA, USA: Woodbridge Press, 1980), 143.

418 A. Cornelius Celsus, trans. W.G. Spencer, *De Medicina* vol. 2 (Harvard University Press, 1961).

419 Jeannine Parvati, *Hygieia: A Woman's Herbal* (Berkeley, CA, USA: Freestone Collective, 1978), 77.

420 R. Chaudhury, "The Quest for a Herbal Contraceptive." *National Medical Journal of India* 6, no. 5 (Sep-Oct 1993), 199-201.

421 Kong Yun Cheung, Jing-Xi Xie, and Paul Pui-Hay But, "Fertility Regulating Agents From Traditional Chinese Medicines," *Journal of Ethnopharmacology.* 15(1986), 18-9. B.B.Kaliwal, R. Nazaar Ahamed, and M. Appaswomy Rao, "Abortifacient Effect of Carrotseed *(Daucus carota),* Extract and Its Reversal by Progesterone in Albino Rats," *Comparative Physiology and Ecology* 9 (1984), 74.

422 Kant, Ashwini, Dennis Jacob, and N.K. Lohia, "The Oestrogenic Efficacy of Carrot *(Daucus carota),* Seeds," *Journal* of *Advanced Zoology* 7 (1986), 36-41.

[423] Robin Bennett, "Wild Carrot Seeds for Herbal Contraception," *Northeast Herbal Association Newsletter* 6 (Marshfield, VT, USA : NEHA, 1994), 32-4.

[424] Christian Ratsch, *The Dictionary of Sacred and Magical Plants* (Santa Barbara, CA, USA: ABC_CLIO, 1992), 175.

[425] Jean Pulaiseul, *Grandmother's Secrets* (New York: G. P. Putnam's Sons, 1974), 242.

[426] Joseph E. Meyer, *The Herbalist* (Glenwood, IL, USA: Meyer, 1918), 230.

[427] Micheal Castleman, *The Healing Herbs* (Emmaus, PA, USA:Rodale, 1991), 311.

[428] L. Ruetter, *Traite de Matiere Medicinale et de Chimie Vegetale* (Paris: 1923), 232.

[429] Ales Hrdlicka, *Physiological and Medical Observations Among the Indians of Southwestern United States and Northern Mexico*, Bulletin 34, Bureau of American Ethnology, 1908 (Reprinted Kessinger 2005),165.

[430] James A. Duke, *Handbook of Medicinal Plants* (Boca Raton, FL, USA: CRC Press, 1985), 412.

[431] I. P. Lemonica, D.C. Damasceno, L.C. Di-Stasi, "Study of the embryotoxic effects of an extract of rosemary (*Rosemary officinalis L.*), *Brazil Journal Medical Research* 29, no. 2 (Feb 1996), 223-7.

[432] M.K. Nusier, H.N. Bataineh, and H.M. Daradkah, "Adverse Effects of Rosemary on Reproductive Function in Adult Male Rats." *Experimental Biology and Medicine* , 232, no. 6 (June 2007), 809-13.

[433] Joseph E. Meyer, *The Herbalist*, (Glenwood, IL, USA: Meyer, 1918), 175.

[434] Christian Ratsch, *The Dictionary of Sacred and Magical Plants* (Santa Barbara, CA, USA: ABC_CLIO, 1992), 143.

[435] Barbara G.Walker, *The Woman's Encyclopedia of Myths and Secrets* (San Francisco: Haper and Row, 1983), 233.

[436] Robert W. Pelton, *The Complete Book of Voodoo,* (New York: Putnam, 1972), 218, 221.

[437] Ibid.

[438] Ibid., 188.

[439] George A. Conway and John C. Slocumb, "Plants Used as Abortifacients and Emmenagogues by Spanish New Mexicans," *Journal of Ethnopharmacology* 1 (1979), 247-8.

[440] M. O. Guerra and A. T. L. Andrade, "Contraceptive Effects of Native Plants in Rats," *Contraception* 18 (1974), 191-9.

[441] Norman P. Farnsworth, et al., "Pontential Value of Plants as Sources of New Antifertility Agents, Part I" *Journal of Pharmaceutical Sciences* 64 (1975), 576.

[442] David G. Spoerke Jr., *Herbs and Herbalism* (New York: Van Nostrand Reinhold, 1979), 152.

[443] Yun Cheug Kong, Jing-Xi Xie, and Paul Pui-Hay But, "Fertility Regulating Agents from Traditional Chinese Medicines," *Journal of Ethnopharmacology* 15 (1986), 4.

[444] J.L. Gutiérrez-Pajares, L. Zúñiga, and J. Pino, "Ruta graveolens Aqueous Extract Retards Mouse Preimplantation Embryo Development," *Reproductive Toxicology* 17, no.6 (Nov.- Dec. 2003), 667-72.

[445] T.G. De Freitas, P.M. Augusto, and T. Montanari, "Effect of *Ruta graveolens* L.on Pregnant Mice," *Contraception* 71, no.1 (Jan 2005), 74-7.

[446] Claire Kowalchik and William H. Hylton, eds., *Rodale's Illustrated Encyclopedia of Herbs* (Emmaus, PA, Usa: Rodale, 1987), 435.

[447] Carmen Ciganda and Amalia Laborde, "Herbal Infusions Used for Induced Abortion," *Clinical Toxicology* 41, no.3 (2003), 235-9.

[448] David G. Spoerke Jr., *Herbal Medications*, (Santa Barbara: Woodbridge Press, 1980), 152.

[449] Christian Ratsch, *The Dictionary of Sacred and Magical Plants* (Santa Barbara, CA, USA: ABC-CLIO, 1992), 144.

[450] James A. Duke, *Handbook of Medicinal Plants* (Boca Raton, Fl, USA: CRC Press, 1985), 148.

[451] M. Agha-Hosseini, L.Kashani, A. Aleyaseen, A. Ghoreishi, H. Rahmanpour, A. R. Zarrinara, and S. Akhondzadeh, "Crocus sativus L. (saffron), in the Treatment Of Premenstrual Syndrome: A Double-Blind, Randomised and Placebo-Controlled Trial," *British Journal of Obstetrics and Gynecology* 115, no. 4 (March 2008), 515-9.

[452] Alfred Swaine Taylor and Robert Eglesfeld Griffith, *On Poisons, in Relation to Medical Jurisprudence and Medicine* (Philadelphia: Lea and Blanchard, 1848), 413.

[453] P. Vlachos, N.N. Kanitsakis, and N.N. Kokonas, "Fatal Cardiac and Renal Failure due to *Ecballium elaterium* (squirting cucumber)," *Journal of Toxicology Clinical Toxicology* 32 (1994), 737-8.

[454] Alex Johnston, *Plants and the Blackfoot.* (Lethbridge, Alberta: Lethbridge Historical Society, 1987), 51.

[455] Arthur Cronquist, *An Integrated System of Classification of Flowering Plants* (Irvington, NY: Columbia University Press, 1981), 920.

456 J.J. Craighead, F.C. Craighead and R.J. Davis, *A Field Guide to the Rocky Mountain Wildflowers* (Boston:Houghton Mifflin, 1963).

457 John C. Hellson, *Ethnobotany of the Blackfoot Indians.* (Ottawa: National Museums of Canada. Mercury Series, 1974), 114.

458 Alice B. Kehoe, "Women's Life Course in Northern Plains Indian Societies: Achieving the Honored Rank of Old Lady," Opinion Papers; Speeches/Meeting Papers 1982-12-05 as cited online: http://eric.ed.gov/ERICWebPortal/custom/portlets/recordDetails/d etailmini.jsp?_nfpb=true&_&ERICExtSearch_SearchValue_0=ED23 2794&ERICExtSearch_SearchType_0=no&accno=ED232794 (accessed April 23, 2008).

459 Nancy J. Turner, Laurence C. Thompson, and M. Terry Thompson et al., *Thompson Ethnobotany: Knowledge and Usage of Plants by the Thompson Indians of British Columbia.* Victoria. (Royal British Columbia Museum 1990), 192. Nancy J. Turner, R. Bouchard, and Dorothy I.D. Kennedy, *Ethnobotany of the Okanagan-Colville Indians of British Columbia and Washington.* (British Columbia Provincial Museum, 1980), 91.

460 M. L. Drasher and P.A. Zahl, "The Effect of Lithospermum on the mouse estrous cycle," *Proceedings of the Society for Experimental Biology and Medicine* (1946), 63, 66.

461 E.R. Plunkett and R.I. Noble, "Éffect of the Injection of *Lithospermum ruderale* on Endocrine Organs of Rats," *Endocrinology* (1951), 49.

462 John M. Riddle, *Contraception and Abortion from the Ancient World to the Renaissance,* (Cambridge: Harvard, 1992), 116-7.

463 Frances Densmore, "Uses of Plants by the Chippewa Indians." SI-BAE Annual Report 44 (1928), 358.

464 W.H. Mechling, "The Malecite Indians with Notes on the Micmacs." *Anthropologica* 8 (1959), 243. R. Frank Chandler, Lois Freeman, and Shirley N. Hooper, 1979 "Herbal Remedies of the Maritime Indians." *Journal of Ethnopharmacology* 1 (1979), 62.

465 Susan S. Weed, *Wise Woman Herbal for the Childbearing Year* (Woodstock, NY, USA: Ash Tree, 1986), 8.

466 Nancy J. Turner and Adam F. Szczawinski, *Common Poisonous Plants and Mushrooms of North America* (Portland, OR, USA: Timber Press, 1991), 140.

467 Alma R. Hutchens, *Indian Herbology of North America* (Ontario, Canada: Merco, 1969), 136.

[468] J. C. Saha, E.C. Savini, and S. Kasinathan, "Ecbolic Properties of Indian Medicinal Plants," *Indian Journal of Medical Research* 49 (1961), 130-51.

[469] M.D. Rosenthal, "Effects of Aristolochic Acid on Phospholipase A Activity," *Biochimica et Biophysica Acta* (1989),1001.

[470] Alfred Swaine Taylor, *The Principles and Practice of Medical Jurisprudence,* vol. 2 (Philadelphia: Henry C. Lea, 1873), 191.

[471] Min Cui, Zhi-Hong Liu, Qi Qiu, Heng Li and Lei-Shi Li, 'Tumour Induction in Rats Following Exposure to Short-Term High Dose Aristolochic Acid I ," (Nanjing: Research Institute of Nephrology, Jinling Hospital, Nanjing University School of Medicine, 2002).

[472] Etienne Van de Walle and Elisha P. Renne, *Regulating Menstruation: Beliefs, Practices, Interpretations* (Chicago: University of Chicago Press, 2001), 233.

[473] "Preparing for Labor and Birth with Homeopathy - Study on the Influence of a Homeopathic Treatment in Preparation for Labor and Birth." Dolisos Homeopathy Study. Pierre Dorfman, Marie Noel Lasserre, and Max Tetau, "Preparation a l'accounchement par homeopathie: Experimentation en double-insu versus placebo" (Preparation for Birth by Homeopathy; Experimentation by Double-Blind Versus Placebo), *Cahrs de Biotherapie.* 94 (April 1987), 77-81.

[474] Dr. R. Dubey, "Indian Drugs and Their Clinical Application," *The Homeopathic Prestige* (June 2001)published by Pratap Homoeo Pharmacy & Clinic, 944-A Nehru Road, Arjun Nagar, Kotla Mubarakpur,New Delhi-3.

[475] Becky A. Peckmann, *Christian Midwifery,* 3rd ed.,(Marble Hill, Missouri: Napsac, 1997), 280.

[476] William Boericke, *New Manual of Homeopathic Materia Medica and Repertory* (Jain Publishers. 2002), 301-302.

[477] Interviews with clinic doctors and counselors conducted by Robin Abrams and Talcott Camp, ACLU Reproductive Freedom Project, Metairie and New Orleans, Louisiana, August, 1990. http://www.skepticfiles.org/aclu/nowayout.htm (accessed November 3, 2007).

[478] K. Spindler, *The Man in the Ice* (Weidenfeld & Nicolson, London, 1994). Dorfer L, et al., "A Medical Report from the Stone Age?" *Lancet* 354 (Sep 18, 1999), 1023-5.

[479] Alternative Doctor Website, "Did Acupuncture Really Originate in Sri Lanka?" http://www.alternative-doctor.com/specials/SLacupuncture.htm (accessed September 10, 2008).

[480] John Amaro, "The 'Forbidden Points' of Acupuncture!'" *Dynamic Chiropractic* 18, no. 10 (May 1, 2000) http://www.chiroweb.com/archives/18/10/01.html (accessed May 16, 2008).

[481] M.T. Shih and F.M. Chen, "An Evaluation of Induction of Labor by Acupuncture." *Acupuncture Research Quarterly* (Taiwan) 1 (1977), 138.

[482] Anon, *Outline of Chinese Acupuncture* - English Version (Peking: Academy of Traditional Medicine, Foreign Languages Press, 1975), 305.

[483] J. Occonnar and D. Besky, *Acupuncture: A Comprehensive Text 6th ed.* (Seattle: Eastland Press, 1988), 678.

[484] Giovanni Maciocia, *Obstetrics and Gynecology in Chinese Medicine.* (Philadelphia: Elsevier Health Sciences, 1998), 485.

[485] Ibid. 151.

[486] Rina Nissim, *Natural Healing in Gynecology: A Manual for Women.* (Pandora Press, 1986).

[487] Andrew Orr, "Natural Induction Using Acupuncture-My research" Earth Mama's Web, http://www.earthmamasweb.com/articles/pregnancy/induct.html (accessed March 20, 2007).

[488] Jeanne Elizabeth Blum, *Woman Heal Thyself* (Boston: Tuttle Co. Inc., 1995), xv.

[489] T. Ots and C. Schulte-Uebbing, "Should Certain Acupuncture Points not be Punctured during Pregnancy?" *Deutsche Zeitschrift fur Akupunktur* 42 (1999), 18-24.

[490] R.A. Dale, "The Contraindicated (forbidden) Points of Acupuncture for Needling, Moxibustion and Pregnancy." *American Journal of Acupuncture* 25, no.1 (1997), 51-3.

[491] A.J. Norheim, "Adverse Effects of Acupuncture: A Study of the Literature for the Years 1981-1994." *Journal of Alternative and Complementary Medicine* 2, no. 2 (1999), 291-7.

[492] Stephen Birch, "The Problem of Acupoint Contraindications in Pregnancy," *Stichting (Foundation), for the Study of Traditional East Asian Medicine.* http://www.paradigm-pubs.com/Birch-Contra (accessed May 13, 2008).

439

493 Sally Griffyn and Michaela Clarke, *Ashtanga Yoga for Women* (Berkeley, CA:Ulysses Press, 2003), 109.

494 Ibid.

495 J.S. Sambhi, "Abortion by Massage," *IPPF Medical Bulletin* 11, no. 1 (Feb 1977), 3. F. Havranek, "Abortion Induced by Massage," *Cesk Cynekol.* 42, no. 7(Aug 1977), 532. "Health Consequences of Induced Abortion in Rural NE Thailand." *Studies in Family Planning* 12, no. 2 (Feb 1981), 58-65.

496 Murray A. Rubinstein, *Taiwan: A New History,* (Armonk, NY: M.E. Sharpe, 2007), 92.

497 Macolm Potts and Martha Campbell, "History of Contraception," *Gynecology and Obstetrics*, 6, chp. 8 (2002). http://big.berkeley.edu/ifplp.history.pdf (accessed Sept, 20, 2008).

498 Ales Hrdlicka, "Physiological and Medical Observations among Indians of the Southwestern United States and Northern Mexico," *Bureau of American Ethnology.* Bulletin 34 (1908), 164.

499 Ibid.

500 Ibid.

501 Ibid., 165.

502 T. Narkavonkit, "Massage Abortion in Thailand," *Nation Review* (Bangkok, Thailand: June 24, 1979), 8 – 9.

503 Malcolm Potts, Maura Graff, and Judy Taing, "Thousand Year Old Depiction of Massage Abortion," *Journal of Family Planning and Reproductive Health Care* (2007), 33-7.

504 Andrea Whittaker, *Intimate Knowledge: Women and Their Health in North-east Thailand* (Sydney: Allen & Unwin, 2000), 159.

505 M. Gallen, *Abortion Practices in the Philippines: An Exploratory Study Among Clients and Practitioners.*(Washington, DC: International Committee on Applied Research in Population, 1980).

506 Diane McDonald, "Touching the Core: The Heart and Intelligence of Mayan Abdominal Massage," *Massage and Bodywork* (August/September 2002).

507 Gunnar Landtman, *The Kiwai Papuans of British New Guinea* (London: Macmillan and Co, Ltd., 1927).

508 A. L. Kroeber, *Handbook of Indians of California. Bulletin 78 (Washington:* Bureau of Indian Ethnology, 1925).

509 Thurnwald Hilde, "Women's Status in Buin Society,' *Oceania.* 5 (1934), 142-70.

510 A. M. Vergiat, *Moeurs et Coutumes des Manja* (Paris: Payot, 1937).

[511]Soranus, *Gynecology*. trans. by Owsei Temkin (Baltimore: The John Hopkins University Press, 1991), 1.59-65.

[512] Walter S. Wells and William Braithwaite, *An Epitome of Braithwaite's Retrospect of Practical Medicine and Surgery v.1*(NewYork: Dick and Fitzgerald, 1860), 23.

[513] Gin contains juniper oils, which give the alcohol its distinctive flavor. (see Juniper).

[514] John M. Graham Jr., "Marshall J. Edwards: Discoverer of Maternal Hyperthermia as a Teratogen," *Birth Defects Research Part A: Clinical and Molecular Teratology* 73, no. 11(2005), 857-64.

[515] John M. Graham, Matthew J. Edwards, and Marshall J. Edwards, "Teratogen Update: Gestational Effects of Meternal Hyperthermia Due to Febrile Illness and Resultant Patterns of Defects in Humans," *Teratology* 58 (1998), 209-221.

[516] De-Kun Li, Teresa Janevic, Roxana Odouli, and Liyan Liu, "Hot Tub Use during Pregnancy and the Risk of Miscarriage," *American Journal of Epidemiology* 158 (2003), 938-41.

[517] M.A.S. Harvey, et al., "Suggested Limits to the Use of Hot Tub and Sauna by Pregnant Women," *Canadian Medical Association Journal* (1981), 125-30.

[518] M.J. Edwards, et al., "Hyperthermia and Birth Defects," *Reproductive Toxicology* 9, no. 5 (1995), 411.

[519] Earnest and Pearl Beaglehole, *Hopi of the Second Mesa*. (Menasha, WI, USA: American Anthropological Association, 1935).

[520] C.I. Shade, "Ethnological Notes on the Aleuts," manuscript submitted in accordance to degree requirements of AB with distinction, Harvard University Department of Anthropology, 1949, As cited in: George Devereux, *A Study of Abortion in Primitive Societies* (New York: International Universities Press, Inc., 1976), 177.

[521] George Devereux, "Mohave Indian Infanticide," *The Psychoanalytic Review* 35 (1948), 126-38.

[522] George Devereux, *A Study of Abortion in Primitive Societies*. (New York: International Universities Press, Inc., 1976), 361-71.

[523] Mush, "About a Window I Didn't Open," http://www.goblinbox.com/?cat=34 (accessed June 5, 2008).

[524] Teresa Robertson, "Midwife, Intuitive, and Healer: A conversation with Teresa Robertson," http://www.birthpsychology.com/lifebefore/concept12.html (accessed June 15, 2008).

525 Linda Baker, *Soul Contracts*. (New York: Writers Club Press, 2003), 126-127.

526 Ibid.

527 Teresa Robertson, "Midwife, Intuitive, and Healer: A conversation with Teresa Robertson,"
http://www.birthpsychology.com/lifebefore/concept12.html (accessed June 15, 2008).

528 Ibid.

529 Teresa Robertson, "Midwife, Intuitive, and Healer: A conversation with Teresa Robertson,"
http://www.birthpsychology.com/lifebefore/concept12.html (accessed June 15, 2008).

530 A.J. Wilcox, D.D. Baird, and C.R. Weinberg, "Time of Implantation of the Conceptus and Loss of Pregnancy." *New England Journal of Medicine* 340, no.23 (1999), 1796–9.

531 In the last twenty years, hundreds of women in the United States have been arrested for using drugs while pregnant. In 2004 in South Carolina, Gabriela Flores spent four months in jail awaiting trial for self-induced abortion with mifepristone. Also in South Carolina in 2001, Regina McKnight received a sentence of twelve years in prison for unintentionally aborting a late term infant from the use of cocaine; this sentence was overturned after McKnight served 8 years in jail. Theresa Lee Hernandez, a drug addict, had a late-term pregnancy loss. The miscarried fetus tested positive for methamphetamine, and Hernandez was charged with murder. Hernandez spent three years in jail awaiting trial on murder charges. For more information see: AdvocatesForPregnantWomen.org.

532 This measuring system is a very rough guide. A 6mm cannula will usually suffice for 6 – 8 weeks LMP. A 14mm cannula will usually suffice for the first half of the second trimester.

533 C. Todd, "Manual Vacuum Aspiration for Second Trimester Pregnancy Termination," *International Journal of Gynecology & Obstetrics*. Vol 83, Issue 1(2003), 5-9.

534 Catherine S. Todd, "Buccal Misoprostol as Cervical Preparation for Second Trimester Pregnancy Termination," *Contraception* vol 65, Issue 6 (2002), 415-418.

535 J . Carbonell , F . Gallego , M . Llorente , S . Bermudez , E . Sala, L . González , and C . Texido, "Vaginal vs. Sublingual Misoprostol With Mifepristone for Cervical Priming in Second-Trimester Abortion by

Dilation and Evacuation: A Randomized Clinical Trial," *Contraception* 75, no. 3 (2007), 230 – 7.

[536] Yu Lihua Zhang, "Observations on the Effect of Ear-AP for Dilation of Cervical Os on 56 Cases," Beijing: Second National Symposium on Acupuncture and Moxabustion and Acupuncture Anaesthesia, All China Society of Acupuncture and Moxabustion (1984), 87-8.

[537] H.Y. Zhang, L.H. Yu, and Q.Z. Ye, "Dilation of the Cervix Uteri by Ear-AP: Analysis of 120 Cases," *Journal of Acupuncture and Moxibustion* 8, no.2 (1988), 21-2.

[538] Claus C. Schnorrenberger, *Chen- Chiu – The Original Acupuncture: A New Healing Paradigm*, (Boston: Wisdom Publications, 2003), 189.

[539] Robert Jutte, *Contraception: A History* (Polity, 2008), 47.

[540] William John Stewart McKay, *The History of Ancient Gynæcology* (London: Baillière, Tindall and Cox, 1901), 41.

[541] Jaeger W et al.,"Pharmokinetic studies of the Fragrance Compound 1,8-cineole in Humans during Inhalation," *Chem. Senses* 21(1996), 477-80.

[542] M. Lis-Balchin and S. Hart, "A Preliminary Study of the Effect of Essential Oils on Skeletal and Smooth Muscle in Vitro," *Journal of Ethnopharmacology* 58 (1997), 183-7.

[543] Hesperian Organization, *Where There Is No Doctor (Berkeley, CA: Hesperian, 2007), 97, 256-257.*

[544] Mairi C. Noverr, Nicole R. Falkowski, Rod A. McDonald, Andrew N. McKenzie, and Gary B. Huffnagle. "Development of Allergic Airway Disease in Mice following Antibiotic Therapy and Fungal Microbiota Increase: Role of Host Genetics, Antigen, and Interleukin-13,"*Infection and Immunity* 73 (2005), 30-38.

[545] Premila W. Ashok, Catriona Stalder, Prabhath T. Wagaarachchi, Gillian M. Flett, Louise Melvin, and Allan Templeton, "A randomised study comparing a low dose of mifepristone and the Yuzpe regimen for emergency contraception," *British Journal of Obstetrics and Gynaecology* 109, no.5 (2002), 553–60.

[546] WHO Task Force on Postovulatory Methods of Fertility Regulation, "Randomised Controlled Trial of Levonorgestrel versus the Yuzpe Regimen of Combined Oral Contraceptives for Emergency Contraception," *Lancet* 352 (1998), 428-33. FDA (July 29, 1999), Plan B label information.

443

547 Kaiser Daily Health Policy Report July 12, 2006,
http://www.kaisernetwork.org/daily_reports/rep_index.cfm?hint=3&
DR_ID=38440 (accessed June 25, 2008).
548 John Carreyrou, "U.S. to Stop Seizing Canadian Medicine," *Wall Street Journal,* October 3, 2006.
549 Women on Waves, "Warning!! False medicines offered for sale on Abortion-pill-online.com," http://www.womenonwaves.org/article-445-en.html (accessed November 15, 2008).
550 Linda Baker, personal correspondence to Sage-femme Collective dated June 26, 2008.

Index

451

tachycardia, 37
Tai Chong, 314
Tai Xi, 313
Tanacetum vulgare. See tansy
tansy, 283–87
TCM. *See* Chinese, traditional
 medicine
teratogen, 27, 38, 44, 61
testosterone, 115, 116, 149
Thuja occidentalis. See arbor vitae
thujone, 100, 101, 103, 144, 145,
 146, 177, 190, 194, 212, 215,
 262, 264, 284, 286, 358
tinctures, 373
toxicity, 39
 defined, 358
Trillium Pend., 345
Umbelliferae, 81, 94, 97, 233, 235,
 257
unwanted child
 lack of nurturing, 5
vermifuge, 119, 133, 148, 196,
 203, 212, 227, 358
Viscum album. See mistletoe
Vitamin C, 36, 43, 100, 186, 222,
 236, 431
Vitamin P. *See* rutin

Vitex agnus castus. See chaste tree
Webster v. Reproductive Health
 1989, 10
weights and measures, 377
wild ginger, 288–91
women's rights
 economic prosperity, 10
 reproductive, 10
World Health Organization, 4, 65,
 366
Yin Bai, 314
Yin Ling Quan, 316
yoga, 31, 318–26
 garbhasana, 322
 marichiasana D, 320
 nidraasana, 319
 pasasana, 323
Yong Quan, 313
You Gui Wan, 347
Zhanohai, 313
Zhi Bian, 311
Zhi Yin, 311
Zigong, 369
Zingiber officinalis. See ginger
Zingiberaceae, 177
Zu Lin Qi, 312
Zu San Li, 316

Made in United States
Troutdale, OR
04/13/2024

19167765R10282